# Global Bioethics - Current Challenges, New Developments, and Future Directions

*Edited by Peter Clark*

Published in London, United Kingdom

Global Bioethics - Current Challenges, New Developments, and Future Directions
http://dx.doi.org/10.5772/intechopen.1005709
Edited by Peter Clark

Contributors
Chris Impey, Daniel DiSandro, David Fernando Espinosa Esqueda, Dorkina Myrick, Francesco Allegri, Francis Pamela Molina Sabogal, Franz Staudt, Fredy Abboud, Giovanny Armando Argoty Chamorro, Gunther Scherz, Jaison Lawrence Santhi, Joel Koshy, Josefina Lattus, Joseph Kelly, Kirk C. Allison, Laura Jiménez Trujano, María Del Pilar Sosa Rosas, Matthias Klüglich, Milena Mesropyan, Paola Gateño, Peter A. Clark, Rispah Torrorey-Sawe, Susan E. Zinner, Susanna Davtyan, Sylvia Ramirez, Una P. Canning, Wim Graafland



First published in London, United Kingdom, 2025 by IntechOpen
IntechOpen is the global imprint of INTECHOPEN LIMITED, registered in England and Wales, registration number: 11086078, 167-169 Great Portland Street, London, W1W 5PF, United Kingdom

For EU product safety concerns: IN TECH d.o.o., Prolaz Marije Krucifikse Kozulić 3, 51000 Rijeka, Croatia, info@intechopen.com or visit our website at intechopen.com.

British Library Cataloguing-in-Publication Data
A catalogue record for this book is available from the British Library

Global Bioethics - Current Challenges, New Developments, and Future Directions
Edited by Peter Clark
p. cm.
Print ISBN 978-1-83634-557-2
Online ISBN 978-1-83634-556-5
eBook (PDF) ISBN 978-1-83634-558-9

# Meet the editor

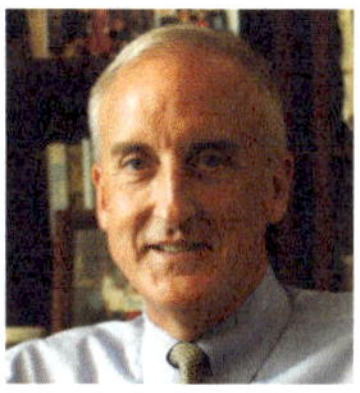

Peter A. Clark, S. J., Ph.D., is the John McShain Chair in Ethics and Director of the Institute of Clinical Bioethics at Saint Joseph's University in Philadelphia. He is also the bioethicist for the Jefferson Health System, St. Christopher's Hospital for Children, and Shriners Hospital for Children in Philadelphia, as well as Our Lady of Lourdes Hospital, Mercy Hospital in Baltimore, Catholic Charities of Maryland, Community Suburban Hospital, and Caritas Baby Hospital in Bethlehem, Palestine. As a bioethicist, Dr. Clark is responsible for the ethical training of medical fellows, residents, and interns in all acute care hospitals. He conducts weekly Ethics Teaching Rounds at the three acute care hospitals in the Jefferson Health System Northeast and Suburban Community Hospital, co-chairs the hospital ethics committees' Institutional Review Boards (IRBs) and the Corporate Ethics Committee, and is available for consultation 24/7 for all hospitals. Dr. Clark received his Ph.D. from Loyola University of Chicago in Medical Ethics and is the author of numerous articles in medical and bioethics journals on topics, which include medical futility, pain management, prejudice in the medical profession, the medical use of marijuana, safe injection sites, opioid prevention & education, tube feedings and PVS patients, male circumcision and HIV/AIDS, face transplantation, and the Ashley treatment, etc. He is also the author of *To Treat or Not to Treat: The Ethical Methodology of Richard A. McCormick as Applied to Treatment Decisions for Handicapped Newborns*, published by Creighton University Press, and *Death With Dignity: Ethical and Practical Considerations for Caregivers of the Terminally Ill*, published by University of Chicago Press. Dr. Clark is also editor of *Contemporary Issues in Bioethics and Bioethics: Medical, Ethical and Legal Perspectives*. Dr. Clark is also a reviewer for numerous bioethics journals and a member of various medical and ethical organizations, both nationally and internationally.

# Contents


**Preface** **IX**

**Section 1**
Inequalities in Health Care **1**

**Chapter 1** **3**
The 2024 H5N1 Virus Outbreak: Navigating the Tightrope between Containment and Caution
*by Jaison Lawrence Santhi, Daniel DiSandro, Joel Koshy, Fredy Abboud, Joseph Kelly and Peter A. Clark*

**Chapter 2** **25**
Global Bioethics: Addressing Current Challenges, Innovations, and the Needs of Underserved Populations
*by Rispah Torrorey-Sawe*

**Chapter 3** **41**
Responsibility, Trust, and Hope in Medical Ethics
*by Franz Staudt*

**Section 2**
Technological Advancements **65**

**Chapter 4** **67**
Human Enhancement and Our Future Off-Earth
*by Chris Impey*

**Chapter 5** **87**
The Ethical Issues of Neurotechnologies
*by Susanna Davtyan and Milena Mesropyan*

**Chapter 6** **99**
The Decline of *Ordre Public* and Morality in the Regulation of Patented Genetic Materials in the United States
*by Dorkina Myrick*

**Chapter 7** 121
A Narrative View on Drug Development and Its Ethical Aspects
*by Matthias Klüglich*

**Section 3**
Death and Dying 145

**Chapter 8** 147
Medical Homicide and Perverse Incentives in Global Perspective
*by Kirk C. Allison*

**Chapter 9** 179
Reflections on the Role of the Family in Euthanasia and Medical Decision-Making
*by Francis Pamela Molina Sabogal and Giovanny Armando Argoty Chamorro*

**Chapter 10** 191
Terminal Illness, Intolerable Suffering, a Bad Death, Loss of Autonomy: Where to Next for Assisted Dying's Burgeoning Inclusion Criteria – A Duty to Die?
*by Una P. Canning*

**Chapter 11** 209
The Future of Euthanasia in the Netherlands
*by Wim Graafland*

**Chapter 12** 225
Euthanasia: In Search of the Most Appropriate Approach
*by Francesco Allegri*

**Section 4**
Patient Critical Care 237

**Chapter 13** 239
Global Bioethics and Nursing
*by María Del Pilar Sosa Rosas, Laura Jiménez Trujano and David Fernando Espinosa Esqueda*

**Chapter 14** 255
Redefining Medical Ethics in Esthetic Practice: Balancing Patient Empowerment and Professional Responsibility
*by Sylvia Ramirez and Gunther Scherz*

**Chapter 15** 279
Expanding the Notion of 'Best Interests' in the UNCRC to Include Future Generations of Children
*by Susan E. Zinner*

**Chapter 16** 293
Rebuilding Lives: Areola and Nipple Complex Reconstruction
*by Paola Gateño and Josefina Lattus*

# Preface

Bioethics is a relatively new discipline of ethics that addresses ethical issues arising from medicine and medical research. Healthcare professionals are confronted daily with ethical dilemmas arising from their relationships with patients, clinical institutions, the pharmaceutical industry, biotech firms, and other entities. The ethical issues span the spectrum from the future of euthanasia, genetic engineering, ethical issues in neurotechnology, therapeutic versus enhancement procedures, nanotechnology, allocation of scarce resources, inequalities in healthcare, beginning-of-life issues to end-of-life issues. To analyze these issues, bioethicists employ various ethical theories to achieve clarity and consistency in their decision-making. These theories may differ in their approach, but they all utilize established ethical rules and principles to ensure prudent and coherent solutions in clinical situations where the interests or priorities of different individuals conflict. These ethical principles include autonomy, beneficence, non-maleficence, confidentiality, and justice, among others. These principles serve as the backbone for these ethical theories, helping us to apply a holistic approach and arrive at well-reasoned positions. The various articles in this book present ethical dilemmas that healthcare professionals face today and will continue to face in the future. The authors present various perspectives, which not only assist healthcare professionals and researchers today but also challenge them to explore and rethink some of the fundamental ideas in medicine and medical research, paving the way into new and uncharted territories. Technological and medical developments are happening at a rapid pace in the fields of medicine and bioethics, and we are being called to process our progress at a similarly fast pace. The speed of progress is sometimes outpacing our ability to discern the ethical rightness or wrongness of our actions. As a result, we are seeing the potential for depersonalization and dehumanization of people who are the most vulnerable in society. The central issue is that scientists will not stop the pace of progress. Therefore, bioethicists must answer the call to balance risks and benefits, considering the nature of the human person, and determine where to draw lines between therapeutic treatments and those that involve enhancement, as well as how to distribute our limited medical resources in a just manner globally. To accomplish this task, dialogue and transparency must continue to be enhanced and encouraged among bioethicists, researchers, scientists and clinicians. The issues confronting us now and in the future in medicine and research are only going to become more complex, comprehensive and challenging. It is the role of the bioethicist today to engage in a constructive dialogue with their colleagues in medicine, scientific research, law, and the biomedical-industrial complex so that new procedures and techniques are thoroughly vetted from all vantage points to preserve and defend the very dignity and respect of the human person. This job may appear daunting at first glance, but unless those trained in philosophical and theological ethics take the lead, the future of humanity will become compromised. This book aims to foster a dialogue with our colleagues across various disciplines, examining these critical bioethical issues from multiple perspectives to ensure the best interests of patients, families, and society as a whole are protected in the future.

**Peter A. Clark, Ph.D.**
John McShain Chair in Ethics,
Saint Joseph's University,
Philadelphia, Pennsylvania, USA

Section 1

# Inequalities in Health Care

Chapter 1

# The 2024 H5N1 Virus Outbreak: Navigating the Tightrope between Containment and Caution

*Jaison Lawrence Santhi, Daniel DiSandro, Joel Koshy, Fredy Abboud, Joseph Kelly and Peter A. Clark*


## Abstract

While avian influenza has a long history of reported outbreaks dating back to the nineteenth century, the 2024 outbreak presented a unique challenge: transmission among cattle. Officials grew concerned early because this was the first outbreak in history predominantly spreading among mammals, and because the outbreak has continued into 2025 with more mutations noted and more humans infected, the danger of pandemic-level evolution appears to be growing. This paper seeks to comprehensively analyze the current outbreak starting with the history and medical aspects of bird flu, including previous outbreaks, clinical features in humans, and methods of prevention. Next, we present the public health timeline of the current outbreak, highlighting critical milestones that suggest virus progression and exploring ways in which the US could have learned from the COVID-19 pandemic. The financial implications of this outbreak domestically and globally are then evaluated to fully display the virus's potential impact. Finally, we examine whether intervening on a virus that has infected less than 70 people and has killed only one is worth the potential harm using the principle of proportionate reason. This analysis informs our recommendations of increased communication, testing, transparent data sharing, vaccine research, and global surveillance to combat further damage.


**Keywords:** avian influenza, prevention, global health, proportionate reason, COVID-19

## 1. Introduction

The H5N1 virus, a member of the *Orthomyxoviridae* family of viruses and subtype of influenza A, first emerged in Southern China in 1996, initially causing poultry outbreaks in Hong Kong in 1997 and resulting in 18 human infections [1]. Although that initial outbreak was controlled, the virus itself was not eradicated and ended up resurfacing in 2003 to infect birds throughout Asia, Africa, Europe, and the Middle East [2]. Since the 2003 resurgence, the World Health Organization (WHO) has documented 890 human infections from over 23 countries [1].

In January 2022, the virus was first detected in the United States in the wild bird population and has since infected over 136 million commercial and wild birds [1]. Furthermore, the virus has spread to a variety of other mammals: from house cats to bears. Since 2023, H5N1 has been infecting dairy cattle, and data from 2024 show that the virus infected 67 Americans [3]. During the initial outbreak in US cattle, experts assured that H5N1 was not a threat to humans and that it should pass through as quickly as it infected the cattle. However, just 1 year later the virus has infected over 900 herds and dozens of people, killing one [3]. Although the Centers for Disease Control and Prevention (CDC) and its officials have labeled H5N1 as a low public health risk, recent developments have indicated that the possibility of a pandemic is not as far-fetched as it may seem [3]. While the number of human cases remains relatively low, experts are urging public health officials to address the lack of clear guidelines, insufficient testing protocols, and the delays in data collection and release to deal with this virus before it progresses. The current lack of focused effort is reminiscent of the protocols and procedures during the initial phase of the COVID-19 pandemic [3].

The goal of this paper is to analyze the H5N1 Avian Influenza virus from historical, medical, public health, financial, and ethical perspectives and to render a recommendation that combines these perspectives. The recommendation of the authors has the goal of using the public health failures of the COVID-19 pandemic to inform the development of policy and infrastructure to deal with H5N1 and similar viruses in the future.

## 2. Discovery and early global outbreaks

After spreading contagiously among poultry, avian influenza was first described and designated as "fowl plague" in Northern Italy in 1878. Until 1880, "fowl plague" was mistaken for fowl cholera, but subsequent research and comparison of the two disease-causing agents showed "fowl plague" to be different from fowl cholera [4]. In 1901, investigators discovered the viral nature of the "fowl plague"-causing agent. Fifty-four years later, research into the agent's structural properties landed it in the type A influenza virus family [5]. In 1981, "fowl plague" was renamed as "highly pathogenic avian influenza" (HPAI) at the First International Symposium on Avian Influenza [6].

Between 1901 and 1930, HPAI outbreaks were reported throughout the world [7]. Reports suggest an HPAI outbreak in Italy in 1894 and another in 1901, during which infected poultry helped transmit the disease into Germany and eastern Austria, and then into France and Belgium [8]. The HPAI endemic persisted in Central Europe until the 1930s [4]. Meanwhile, the United States witnessed its first HPAI outbreak in the fall of 1924. The first infections were reported in New York City. The disease was then propagated with variable intensities into the states of Pennsylvania, Connecticut, New Jersey, Illinois, Missouri, West Virginia, Indiana, and Michigan. The outbreak was controlled by April 1925 [4]. By the 1950s, HPAI infections had been identified in Europe, North America, South America, Africa, and Asia [4].

During the first half of the twentieth century, all isolated HPAI agents belonged to the H7 subtype, but the year 1959 marked the discovery of the first HPAI H5 subtype (H5N1), extracted from chicken in Scotland [9]. A second H5 strain of HPAI was isolated in South Africa in 1961 [10]. Since the 1950s, researchers have discovered 16 hemagglutinin subtypes (H1–H16) and 9 neuraminidase subtypes ("N") (N1–N9) in birds; hemagglutinin and neuraminidase are surface glycoproteins that characterize avian influenza viruses, as the latter have only one subtype of each on their surfaces [11]. Currently, H5N1 constitutes the primary health concern of health officials worldwide, as it has been the root cause of the most debilitating and deadly HPAI outbreaks in history.

### 2.1 Southern China (1996–1997)

In 1997, Hong Kong suffered an HPAI H5N1 outbreak, in which the H5N1 strain may have evolved from a progenitor common to the influenza A virus identified in commercial geese in China's Guangdong Province in 1996 [12, 13]. H5N1 infections first spread among poultry in March and April 1997, leading to the death of 4000 chickens. The first human infection was reported in a 3-year-old child in May 1997 [13, 14]. Rampant infections of poultry persisted throughout October, November, and December, with approximately 20% of local poultry being infected at the time. The second confirmed human infection occurred in November 1997, after which another 16 individuals tested positive, raising the total to 18 confirmed human infections, spread across different districts [13, 14]. Retrospective investigations and studies have suggested that human infections were caused by direct human-to-chicken and, possibly, human-to-human transmission of H5N1 through close physical contact [13]. It wasn't until December 1997 that the outbreak was curbed through large-scale culling of 1.5 million chickens in Hong Kong, temporary suspension of the import of live poultry from mainland China, and separation of waterfowls from chicken [13, 14].

However, Southern China's high population density, large dependence on agricultural activity, and attraction of migratory birds during winters render it a fitting environment for avian influenza outbreaks. HPAI H5N1 was later isolated from waterfowls in Hong Kong [15]. Multiple H5N1 strains, genetically and structurally similar to the viral agents isolated from Guangdong geese in 1997, reemerged in Southern China in 2001, marking one of many resurgences of poultry and human H5N1 infections in the subsequent years [10].

### 2.2 East and South China, Europe, Africa, and the Middle East (2003–2009)

In 2003, Hong Kong witnessed another HPAI H5N1 outbreak among poultry, as genetic reassortment in H5N1 resulted in genetically different strains, such that strains with phenotypic advantages outcompeted other strains. The strain with genotype (Z) was most prevalent during the outbreak, and two human infections were reported in November 2003 [16]. Subsequent H5N1 infections in Qinghai Lake in 2005 resulted in large-scale death of wild birds. Evidence points to migratory birds functioning as H5N1 vectors, carrying the virus into Qinghai Lake [10, 17]. By then, H5N1 had spread rapidly into Thailand, Indonesia, Japan, Cambodia, Vietnam, and Laos, showing the ease and subtlety with which H5N1 may be transmitted internationally [16].

Vietnam first encountered H5N1 following the transmission of the virus from Yunnan Province, China near the end of 2003 [17]. Rapid transmission among poultry was accompanied with 65 confirmed cases of human H5N1 infections between 2004 and 2005 [17]. Although nationwide interventions, such as vaccinating poultry and implementing poultry-focused surveillance programs, helped curtail the initial outbreak, H5N1 infections reemerged sporadically afterwards. By 2010, the total number of confirmed human cases in Vietnam reached 119, with a mortality rate of 49.6% [18].

In late 2003, HPAI H5N1 was identified as the cause of large-scale death of poultry in geographically distinct regions in Thailand [19]. The first confirmed case of human H5N1 infection was in January 2004; the disease-causing agent was identified as H5N1 (genotype Z)—related to the virus responsible for the concurrent outbreak in Vietnam [19]. Through enforcing strict poultry regulation and HPAI-infection prevention measures, Thailand minimized the severity of multiple outbreaks between 2003 and 2004 [17]. However, Thailand further experienced two other major H5N1 outbreaks in 2004–2005 and 2005–2006 [19]. By November 2005, there had been 20 confirmed cases of humans infected with H5N1, 13 of whom passed away [19]. Though the major outbreaks were put under control, the virus persisted in small indigenous environmental reservoirs, as 1141 H5N1 outbreaks had been reported in Thailand up until 2009 [17].

Similarly, Laos, Cambodia, Japan, Indonesia, Malaysia, and Myanmar encountered H5N1 through vectors migrating from surrounding H5N1-infected regions, some of which were deemed as infection epicenters [17]. Many affected countries resorted to large-scale culling of poultry, which in some countries (e.g., Malaysia) may have helped avert human H5N1 infections [17]. Meanwhile, H5N1 became endemic to many affected regions (e.g., Indonesia) [17, 20]. Common among affected regions was the resurgence of H5N1 infections, despite containment of previous outbreaks [17].

As increasing evidence pointed toward migratory birds transmitting H5N1, fears of an H5N1 pandemic were substantiated as H5N1-infected birds were found in Russia, Turkey, Croatia, and Romania in 2005 [10]. Germany, Sweden, Italy, France, Czech Republic, and other European countries followed, as each country's authorities issued reports of H5N1 infections of poultry in 2006 [21]. Between 2006 and 2007, HPAI H5N1 was propagated throughout Africa, the Middle East, and Northern and Western Europe [10].

### 2.3 Recent times (2020–2025)

More recently, a major H5N1 panzootic outbreak has begun. Two different lineages of H5N1 emerged in Europe in mid-2020. Migratory birds traveling through the East Atlantic Flyway transmitted one lineage across the northern coasts of Central Europe and then to North America [22]. The second lineage was introduced to Africa and was then propagated throughout the Middle East and Asia [22]. Genetic reassortment allowed for the emergence of H5N1 viruses adapted to more virulently infect wild birds [23].

The intra- and intercontinental transmission of H5N1 paved the way for a series of global H5N1 outbreaks between 2021 and 2022. Canadian and American authorities confirmed the detection of H5N1-infected wild birds in late 2021 [24]. The United States reported its first confirmed human H5N1 infection since 2016 in April 2022 [24]. Moreover, H5N1 reached South America through migratory birds traveling down the Pacific Migratory Flyway, as Columbia reported detecting HPAI H5N1 in birds in October 2022 [25]. Other South American countries, including Peru, Bolivia, Chile, Ecuador, Argentina, and Uruguay, later reported the first identifications of H5N1-infected animals [25]. Likewise, cases of H5N1-infected humans have been reported in different continents—Asia, Europe, North America, and South America—between 2020 and July 2023 [26]. Since 2020, the current panzootic has led to the death of over 100 million birds [27].

*DOI: http://dx.doi.org/10.5772/intechopen.1010912*

As the panzootic persists to this day, with the most recent outbreak in the United States in March 2024, there is growing concern of a possible pandemic looming in the horizon.

## 3. Medical analysis

### 3.1 Epidemiology

Given its long and widespread history, the reason the avian flu is considered as a public health emergency among many epidemiologists is its high case-to-death rate (52%). From January 2003 to March 2024, the WHO reported 463 deaths among a total of 888 reported cases [28].

Currently, the virus lacks sustained human-to-human transmission potential, indicating that the possibility of a pandemic caused by the virus is low. However, influenza viruses are known for their potential to undergo antigenic drift, which is a random change in the nucleotide sequence of a gene due to mutations during replication, and antigenic shift, or the reassortment of genes between two different viruses as they infect the same cell. When this happens in the hemagglutinin or neuraminidase genes of an influenza virus, the latter's ability to enter and infect cells can change. H5N1 is a specific subtype of influenza A that resulted from years of evolution, and epidemiologists worry that more random mutations may lead to increased entry and disease in human cells [29].

### 3.2 Pathogenesis in humans

The avian influenza virus is classified into 16 hemagglutinin (HA) and 9 neuraminidase (NA) subtypes based on surface glycoprotein variations. This allows 144 possible HA/NA combinations in birds. While most of these subtypes circulate among wild aquatic birds, some of them can occasionally spread to domestic poultry and mammals through saliva, nasal secretions, and feces. Only six subtypes—H3 (H3N8), H5 (H5N1, H5N6, H5N8), H6, H7, H9 (H9N2), and H10—have been reported to infect humans. Transmission is believed to occur primarily through direct contact with infected poultry or contaminated surfaces, although some theories suggest pigs may act as intermediates [30].

Once the virus attaches to the respiratory epithelium in humans, the HA glycoprotein facilitates entry into the cell, and the virus proceeds to replicate inside the cell's nucleus. The new virus particles travel to the cell membrane and the NA protein facilitates exit of the virus particles from the cell, which leads to the breakage of the cell membrane followed by the death of the cell, ultimately triggering an immune response [31].

### 3.3 Presentation and clinical features

From the limited data available on human infection of H5N1, patients mostly present with mild illness characterized most commonly by conjunctivitis, mild fever, and other symptoms of upper respiratory infection, like cough, sore throat, and rhinorrhea [32]. More severe disease is indicated by high fever (39 to 41°C) and shortness of breath. This can lead to complications of rapid-onset severe pneumonia, acute respiratory distress syndrome requiring mechanical ventilation, altered mental status, and seizures. There was a reported case of a patient presented with acute encephalitis caused by avian flu [33–35].

### 3.4 Treatment

Patients who have confirmed infections with bird flu should start antiviral therapy with oseltamivir (75 mg) twice daily orally for 5 days. According to the CDC, treatment should ideally begin within 48 hours of symptoms onset. Even if a patient has crossed the 48 hours threshold, it should be started as soon as possible. Alternate viral therapies like zanamivir and peramivir are also available in parenteral form for patients who cannot tolerate oral medications.

### 3.5 Prevention

Below are some of the recommended practices to prevent bird flu infections: [36].

1. Avoid coming in direct contact with sick or dead wild birds and poultry. If you must come in close contact with them, wear proper recommended personal protective equipment (PPEs).

2. To prevent nosocomial infections, infected patients should be placed in a negative pressure room with standard contact precautions (including gowns and gloves) and respiratory precautions (N95).

3. Poultry farmers and workers, bird flock owners should use PPEs.

4. There should be close surveillance, quarantine, and depopulation of infected flock in poultry farms.

5. Avoid consuming undercooked or uncooked bird meat or bird products like unpasteurized milk or raw eggs.

6. Appropriate post-exposure prophylaxis for individuals who came in direct contact with infected patients or sick/dead birds.

## 4. Public health response

With the history and medical features of the virus in mind, it is now critical to analyze the timeline of the current outbreak from a public health perspective and draw comparisons to the response to the early stages of the COVID-19 pandemic.

### 4.1 Timeline

Suspicion began in February 2024 when farmers in northern Texas noticed some of their cows had stopped making milk [37]. Veterinary researchers eventually discovered that H5N1 was the pathogen present in these cows, and the United States Department of Agriculture (USDA) announced dairy outbreaks in Texas as well as Kansas and Michigan on March 25, 2024 [38]. The proclamation of a dairy outbreak of bird flu was significant in its own right because cows represent a more biologically similar organism to humans than birds. However, with the official announcement came the first misstep, namely a transfer of control from local farmers and veterinarians to state and federal agencies [37]. The following months were defined by a lack of communication from the USDA to farmers, who had been requesting support for studies and research on their farms [37]. Additionally, now that the government was involved, farmers grew worried that their livestock and potentially their farms would be excluded from the dairy market upon a positive test result if they agreed to testing [37].

Evidence of this early disorganization manifested in the report of dairy herd infections in a total of nine states by April 25, 2024, at which time the USDA announced a mandate for testing of all cattle traveling across states [38, 39]. During this time, a dairy farm worker in Texas and two dairy farmers in Michigan had tested positive for H5N1, bringing the human case total to three by the end of May 2024 [38]. While these infections did not result in significant disease and were not thought to be transmitted human-to-human, the CDC and USDA began updating personal protective equipment guidelines for workers [38]. And by mid-July 2024, although the rate of newly infected dairy herds seemed to be slowing, the tally of human cases reached 13 after an outbreak on a poultry farm in Colorado [37]. This culminated in a July 30, 2024 announcement by the CDC to devote $10 million to stop bird flu infections among farm workers, including $5 million for vaccine development [40].

As the summer neared the end, the first outbreaks in California, the nation's largest milk producer, stoked worries of escalation. And in September, there was a confirmed case of H5N1 in a Missouri resident with no known direct exposure to animals followed by two close contacts of that individual developing symptoms [38]. It should be noted that these contacts were not tested for bird flu at the time of symptoms, and later studies revealed no evidence of past H5N1 infection [38]. However, a CDC study on blood samples from farm workers in Michigan and Colorado revealed that from June to August of 2024, there was serological evidence of prior H5N1 infection in 7% of dairy farm workers [41]. While this was useful data and informed the CDC's subsequent recommendation to actively monitor all exposed workers with regular testing for symptomatic individuals, it highlights the lack of surveillance and epidemiological data that defined much of the outbreak over the late Spring and Summer 2024 [37, 41]. And it is for this reason that leading international virologists and epidemiologists have been left surprised and disappointed by the US's handling of this situation [37].

As November and December 2024 progressed, the situation in California worsened, with human infections rising, bringing the US total case count to 67 by the end of 2024. Two supplies of raw milk out of California also tested positive for H5N1, sparking a December USDA federal order to test all raw milk nationwide [38].

Perhaps most significantly, the winter months of 2024 into 2025 also brought the first known severe human cases of H5N1 infection resulting in the prolonged critical care stay of a 13-year-old girl from British Columbia and the death of an elderly patient in Louisiana, who had many comorbidities, in January [38]. Around the same time, on January 3, 2025, the US Department of Health and Human Services (HHS) pledged $306 million to continue H5N1 response efforts, including more funding for hospital preparedness, testing, and surveillance [42]. HHS later awarded $590 million to Moderna to accelerate messenger RNA (mRNA) vaccine development against H5N1 [43]. As of January 16, 2025, the CDC has issued a recommendation for all clinicians in the country to test all hospitalized flu patients for subtyping to identify more potential bird flu cases [44].

In terms of where this situation could be headed, these most recent cases of severe illness not only represent the potential devastation of this virus in vulnerable individuals, but research on the latest strains of the virus suggest that a single mutation in the virus that is currently circulating could be enough to confer human specificity to the virus's receptors, allowing it to spread through human-to-human transmission [45]. Scientists have cited this as a reason why asymptomatic or mild spread through dairy farm workers is concerning, as any amount of time spent in the human body places selective pressure on those strains that may be more specific for human cell receptors [45]. Researchers also warn of coinfection with seasonal influenza, which through gene reassortment can cause a hybrid virus that is more suitable for human infection [45]. These concerns reemphasize a common feeling among virologists and epidemiologists that allowing the virus to circulate among cows and farm workers poses an exponential risk of progression to more efficient human transmission of the virus.

### 4.2 Comparison to COVID response

While we acknowledge that a congruent comparison of the public health response to the COVID-19 outbreak in 2020 is not possible given the difference in the virus transmission and its prevalence in humans, we regard comparison of some of the key timepoints as essential to evaluating if the response was adequate to protect US citizens and sufficiently mitigate risk of pandemic.

The main parallel and subject of criticism for this bird flu response has been nationwide testing capability. When analyzing the 2020 COVID outbreak, many experts concur that the CDC's hold on testing contributed significantly to the country's inability to respond adequately and suppress the rapid spread [46]. It wasn't until late February 2020 that the Food and Drug Administration (FDA) authorized private laboratories to begin making their own COVID tests, and it wasn't until mid-March 2020 that the first commercial test was approved [46]. Similarly, the CDC kept a hold on all bird flu testing until December 2024, although commercial and academic laboratories had been inquiring about it since April 2024 [37]. Experts, including the former top CDC official Ali Khan, agree that the CDC and FDA should have expanded to non-federal testing facilities months ago [37]. In drawing this comparison, we understand that the impetus during 2020 may have been greater since transmission through humans was so rapid relative to bird flu, but we maintain that the ability to expand testing should have been more efficient after the failures during the COVID outbreak.

While this is an unfortunate similarity that many agree have led to deficient surveillance in both public health events, we wanted to draw a key difference in the bird flu epidemic that is uniquely contributing to lackluster surveillance that may be out of the control of the government and their ability to respond to public health emergencies. Even when monitoring efforts were increased after initial outbreaks, farmers were reluctant to cooperate for a few reasons. First, they were worried that reporting test results or allowing their herds to be tested at all might make them subject to economic losses (although the government has reimbursed for lost livestock) [37]. Also, they do not want their workers tested, given the competitive and cutthroat nature of the dairy industry. Finally, it is in the general nature of rural communities to avoid government intervention and be skeptical of any government involvement in their businesses [37]. Jennifer Morse, Medical Director of the Mid-Michigan District Health Department, describes the rural communities she serves as "minimal-government-minded" [37]. She attributes the tough decisions that public health officials had to make during the COVID pandemic to growing antigovernment sentiment as well [37].

Overall, while not a perfect comparison, we argue that some of the milestones of this bird flu outbreak feel all too similar to the beginnings of the COVID-19 pandemic. It is with this timeline and comparison in mind that we offer the recommendations contained herein.

## 5. Financial considerations

The average retail price of a large dozen eggs in the US in December of 2023 was $2.51 [47]. In December of 2024, the same dozen of eggs would go on to be sold at an average price of $4.15, a staggering price hike of 65.38% in just 1 year [47]. With popular news headlines proclaiming predictions regarding the continued uptick of the price of eggs and other common household grocery staples, perhaps for the average American the financial consequences of the HPAI virus may be perceived to be limited to such a microcosmic level. However, the reality is that there are significant economic implications to the recent crisis surrounding HPAI—not just domestically, but globally as well.

Although the CDC reports that the current [January 2025] public risk is low, several experts in the field have expressed their concerns regarding the potential for pandemic levels of infectivity and transmission [37, 48, 49]. Despite a slow start, the response to HPAI detection in the United States has recently picked up steam—especially at the national level—highlighting some of the most financially taxing aspects of the response efforts. For instance, the USDA released a statement in March 2024 stating that it was going to provide $502 million to "prepare for potential additional detections of high pathogenic avian influenza," supplementary to the initially invested $793 million in emergency funding for the "implementation of quarantine restrictions, depopulating affected flocks, disposing of depopulated birds, cleaning and eliminating the virus from affected premises, and conducting surveillance in surrounding areas" [50]. Similarly, the US HHS has announced as recently as January 2025 that it will provide $306 million toward monitoring and preparedness initiatives, notably with the CDC distributing $111 million for monitoring and testing programs, as well as the National Institute of Health (NIH) distributing $11 million for research efforts into vaccines and other potential solutions [42].

Since March 2024, the CDC has monitored more than 12,700 people after reported exposure to infected animals, tested more than 580 people, and detected 67 confirmed cases [48]. Similarly, the USDA has monitored and confirmed over 929 cases in cattle, over 136 million cases among wild aquatic birds and across 1431 flocks of poultry, and approximately 500 cases in wild and captive wild mammals across the nation since the onset of the outbreaks [51]. Still, it appears that this is a race in which the response efforts are lagging behind the impact that the virus appears to be having, and the economy is suffering for it. Economists and financial experts have estimated that the outbreak in 2022 alone has resulted in losses ranging from $2.5 to $3 billion [52]. With the outbreak still ongoing in 2025, it is difficult to underscore the disastrous economic impact that the costs incurred up to this point and the potential costs for monitoring and containing this virus among animals and people alike in the future will eventually amount to.

From a global perspective, the response by the United States to this growing crisis demonstrates a crucial point. In the United States, federal agencies like the USDA have become involved in surveillance, testing, depopulating, and disposing of affected animals throughout the nation, and while testing and surveillance are necessary, it's no secret that this has raised manufacturing and distributive costs for goods created from those animals. Some of these added costs are passed onto the consumer as evidenced by price hikes discussed previously, but farmers, distributors, and others involved in the industry are undoubtedly financially impacted. This brings up an important question: in the event that HPAI is not well contained within the US and another pandemic arises, how will these same groups be affected in countries that do not have the infrastructure or the resources to implement proper animal testing and surveillance initiatives? This same question is certainly transposable to the consequences in the public health realm as well. If history is any indicator, the answers to these questions lie in the research that has shown that due to lack of proper testing and vaccination resources, the COVID-19 death toll was four times higher overall and 31% higher on a per capita basis in lower-income countries compared to their higher-income counterparts [53]. In addition, experts have estimated that due to the COVID-19 pandemic, 160 million people were pushed into poverty and 137 million people lost their jobs globally—the economic fallout from which entire nations are still on the road to recovery [53]. In the countries which the United Nations (UN) have deemed to be the least developed countries (LDCs), agricultural supply chain disruptions and labor shortages have forced drastic increases in the prices of staple foods and pushed millions into a state of food insecurity [54, 55].

Lukewarm efforts in engaging a crisis that has medical, public health, and financial implications have never boded well for the United States or the global society at large. For all the reasons mentioned above, it is imperative that appropriate caution is taken and an adequate response to the growing crisis of the HPAI virus is implemented sooner rather than later. If there was ever a time to act, it's now.

## 6. Ethical analysis

The Bird Flu pandemic is not inevitable but with the H5N1 virus circulating in poultry, cattle, and other domestic animals, mutations are happening and the situation is quickly changing. Many public health officials believe it is not if a pandemic will strike the United States but when. To date, the federal government has taken a very laissez-faire attitude toward this virus. There are ineffective guidelines, inadequate testing, and long delays in the release of data. One might think we would have learned some valuable lessons from the COVID-19 pandemic. It appears that we have not. Many in the area of infectious disease fear that the right combination of genetic mutations could create a new pandemic that we are unprepared to handle. The developments we are witnessing could be a precursor to what might be the next pandemic. "Human cases of H5N1 have been observed over the past year in the United States. Most cases had exposure to animals that were infected with H5N1, but cases without known animal exposure have been identified as well. Recently, a probable case in Delaware and a severe hospitalized case was identified in Louisiana. The patient in Louisiana has died" [56]. According to Rosemarie Tong, Director of the Center for Professional and Applied Ethics at the University of North Carolina, "during the first year of a pandemic fewer than 10% of us will have access to an effective vaccine. Federal stockpiles of experimental vaccines that may or may not work may be available for more of us, but it will take months for a truly effective vaccine to be developed, manufactured, and distributed" [57]. As a developed nation, we have an ethical responsibility to be better prepared so that fewer lives are lost if it does escalate into a pandemic. This means not only American lives but the lives of our fellow brothers and sisters around the world. Guidelines, recommendations, more surveillance, vaccine production and research, testing, and safeguards should be put in place immediately to prepare if the H5N1 does genetically mutate and we see human-to-human transmission. Ethically, to determine if a proper relationship exists between the specific value and the other elements of the act, the principle of proportionate reason could be applied to the situation.

Proportionate reason refers to a specific value and its relation to all elements in the action. It is a crucial element in an analysis of the morality of a human action. Proportionate reason is a moral principle that one may employ to determine objectively and concretely the rightness or wrongness of actions [58]. "The more adequate notion of 'proportion' refers to what truly gives an action its moral meaning: the relation of the means to the end. More broadly speaking, 'proportionate' refers to the relation between the specific value at stake and the premoral evils (the limitations, the harms, or the inconvenience) which may inevitably come about in trying to achieve the value" [59]. In general, proportionate reason refers to a specific value and its relation to all other elements of the act.

"One should not understand proportionate reason in purely mathematical terms, but rather as a balance between values and disvalues in determining whether the means (an act)is *proportionate* to the intended end or *reason*. The 'reason'd (*ratio*) here is not 'some serious reason' that an agent identifies to justify the evil effect of the act; alternatively, what many commentators 'mean by 'reason' [is] a concrete value which is at stake in the act of an agent.' The term 'proportionate' means a formal relation between the reason for the act and the premoral values and disvalues in the act. More specifically, the term signifies a proper structural relation (*debita proportio*) of the means to the end or of the end to further ends.' Thus, the proper understanding of proportionate reason contains these two dimensions: the reason (*ratio*) and the proper structural relation (*debita proportio*) of the premoral values and disvalues involved in the action. Proportionalism is the general analytic structure for determining the rightness or wrongness of actions within which one appeals to proportionate reason" [60].

In regard to the H5N1 flu, the specific value in this act is to immediately increase testing, surveillance, create adequate guidelines, gather data, and increase research into adequate vaccine development to combat H5N1 to preserve human life. In addition, we have the ethical responsibility to educate the public and encourage responsible behavior for all members of society. The harm, which may come about by trying to achieve this value, is the foreseen but unintended possibility that some may view this as overreacting causing fear in the public sector and engendering more distrust in the public health sector by Americans. The ethical question is whether the value of potentially saving lives outweighs the risks and harms of causing fear and increasing mistrust of Americans in regard to public health? To determine if a proper relationship exists between the specific value and the other elements of the act, ethicist Richard McCormick, S.J. proposes three criteria for the establishment of proportionate reason:

1. The means used will not cause more harm than necessary to achieve the value.

2. No less harmful way exists to protect the value.

3. The means used to achieve the value will not undermine it [61].

The application of McCormick's criteria to promoting immediate guidelines, testing, surveillance, collecting data, and starting to stockpile antiviral medications, such as oseltamivir, zanamivir, and peramivir, will focus on whether there are appropriate data and studies, accurate assessment tools, and uniform national guidelines that support the argument that there is a proportionate reason for taking these precautions. *First,* we know that with proper preparations, such as testing, surveillance, national guidelines for protection, and data collection, the United States will be prepared in the event that H5N1 does mutate and a pandemic does begin. Yes, one can argue that at the moment this is not a reality and that these precautions could cause fear among the public and increase the mistrust of the public health care system. To determine if there is a proportionate reason to allow for this, the specific value being sought must be at least equal to the value being sacrificed [62]. It can be argued that being prepared for a pending epidemic has the potential to save lives, especially among the most vulnerable members of our society. Therefore, the means used to achieve the value will not cause more harm than necessary. In fact, the means used has the potential of saving thousands of lives. Through education of the public about the importance of being prepared, it should help to eliminate the fear that could be caused and the mistrust that could result.

*Second*, at present, there does not seem to be a better alternative than to prepare for a possible epidemic. "This criterion demands that we choose the best means available to us at the time, even though this may have to change in the future" [62]. We have an ethical responsibility to educate the public about precautions against H5N1. "Health care experts emphasize that there are precautions Americans can take: Do not touch sick or dead bids, or other animals; get tested if you have flu-like symptoms; do not consume raw milk or meat or feed them to pets" [3]. Data collection about animal infections of H5N1 is essential. "Cats that became infected with bird flu might have spread the virus to humans in the same household and vice versa, according to data that briefly appeared online in the report from the CDC but then abruptly vanished. The data appears to have been mistakenly posted but includes crucial information about the risks of bird flu to people and pets" [63]. Experts believe that these data are important to insure public health but many wonder why these findings are not being released to the public. According to Jennifer Nuzzo, Director of the Pandemic Center at Brown University School of Public Health, "If there is new evidence about H5N1 that is been held up for political purposes, that is just completely at odds with what government's responsibility is, which is to protect the American people" [64]. Withholding these data from the public will cause more harm than good. Finally, in the last week there has been a controversy over the United States Agency for International Development (USAID) and its funding. As a result of the funding being paused, the USAID has stopped monitoring bird flu in 49 countries as it was doing 3 weeks ago [65]. Unless there is worldwide surveillance, this disease will spread and there is the real possibility of a worldwide pandemic. This could kill thousands of people worldwide. Unless the United States public health system takes on more testing, increased surveillance, and data collection on animal infections, establishes

*DOI: http://dx.doi.org/10.5772/intechopen.1010912*

guidelines for prevention, and increases outreach to farm workers in regard to protective gear, there is the inevitability of potential harm. Even though the H5N1 pandemic is not inevitable, it appears that developments in the cattle and poultry industry make the possibility of it impacting humans less remotely today. This virus is dangerous and the signals we are receiving clearly indicate that inevitable harm is very possible.

*Third*, it seems clear that establishing guidelines for protection, increasing testing, increasing worldwide surveillance, monitoring animal infections and human infections, and increasing the production of vaccines do not undermine the value of human life. One can argue that these interventions may cause fear in the public, when, at the present moment, there is no sign that an epidemic is imminent. It could also increase mistrust in our public health system when many are saying that a H5N1 vaccine could be dangerous. This mistrust could make Americans very skeptical of these precautions. However, if you examine the progression of the H5N1 virus in animals and now in humans, many infectious disease professionals and public health officials see these developments as classic steps toward a pandemic [3]. One can argue that there have been steps taken by the US government to prepare for this possible pandemic. But each step taken seems to be flawed. The USDA was slow to begin testing H5N1 vaccines for cows and released genetic information from the virus samples but failed to reveal where and when the samples were collected, which would help scientists. The USDA's program to test bulk milk began in December, a year after the outbreak, and still does not include the outbreak in Idaho. Ginkgo Bioworks already assesses half the nation's commercial milk supply for bacteria, antibiotics, and other substances. Why have we not added H5N1 to the list? [3]. Proactively increasing precautions, testing, guidelines, more surveillance and increasing the manufacture of vaccines may cause fear in the American public and could cause mistrust in the public health care system if the H5N1 pandemic does not materialize. However, if the pandemic does materialize, which many fear we are only a mutation away from happening, then many lives could be lost and much harm could come to the most vulnerable in society. The only way we can protect Americans and those in other countries is through education and prevention. The only way we can educate others is with the correct data, which will require more testing and surveillance and guidelines for precautions. The data obtained must be shared with other nations. Surveillance of the situation must occur worldwide. H5N1 is too precarious for us not to be proactive. The withdrawal of the US from the WHO and the stopping of monitoring of H5N1 by USAID this week will only cause more harm than good. Ethically, the greater good of humanity is at-risk and the common good of society can only be advanced by further testing, monitoring, data collection, and sharing of data and clinical research into potential new vaccines. In addition, with established medical guidelines and protocols in place, oversight committees can be established to protect individuals, families, and society as a whole from any misinformation and fears that may arise from this situation. Vaccine safety is a priority and safeguards can be put in place that protect all people. H5N1 has historically affected birds. However, we have seen a wide range of mammals being infected in the last 2 years. We know from experience, the more mammals infected by this type of virus, the more possibilities there are for this virus to mutate and infect humans. The principle of proportionate reason clearly justifies a proactive protocol to protect all humans. Failure to enact these safeguards will put lives in danger and may result in many deaths.

## 7. Recommendations

With all of these perspectives in mind, it is important to formally outline the recommendations we suggest moving forward to approach the H5N1 situation more appropriately. We will herein list four measures for improving the domestic situation as well as one recommendation to satisfy the US's global responsibility to its neighbors.

### 7.1 Communication

Arguably, the most primitive and important function of any public health institution when dealing with infectious disease is communication. At the federal level, this involves communication with not only citizens but also local officials and clinicians [66]. The recent layoff of thousands of federal public health officials imposed by the Trump administration poses a great danger to the CDC's ability to carry out this vital public health function [66]. For example, infections in a group of dairy farm workers in Colorado in July 2024 were defined by a lack of awareness of bird flu and hence lack of personal protective equipment when handling animals [67]. While national announcements for PPE for these workers had been made, this communication must still reach the workers themselves in order to be effective. Additionally, communication via the CDC can help inform clinicians' decision-making as clinicians must know whether or not to be considering bird flu in a patient with relevant presenting symptoms and what the epidemiology of bird flu is in their part of the country [66]. Thus, there are multiple levels of communication that must be clear.

### 7.2 Testing

On February 13, 2025, the CDC released results of a study that was conducted on 150 asymptomatic veterinarians from across the US, with the key finding that three were positive for antibodies against H5N1 virus [68]. Two of these veterinarians work in states, namely South Carolina and Georgia, with no reported outbreaks of H5N1 in dairy herds [68]. These data are merely the most recent representation of what a lack of surveillance testing can cause over time. Findings like these suggest that we truly are not aware of the full scope of the issue at the moment and that in order to be adequately aware of the situation, testing of asymptomatic dairy workers and veterinarians should be increased across the country [69].

### 7.3 Transparent and comprehensive data collection and sharing

As has been mentioned throughout this chapter, data collection and sharing has been deemed incomplete and lackluster by many who are evaluating this issue. The recent action by the CDC to add and subsequently remove data about cat infections from its website is the latest example and raises questions about data collection and sharing overall [63]. Of course, as mentioned in the Ethical Analysis, one of the harms of increasing preventive measures for a virus that has infected less than 100 humans and has caused only one death is increasing mistrust and doubt in public health, and we recognize that certain data without proper scientific backing may elicit unnecessary fear and cause unnecessary harm. However, in this circumstance, the now-deleted data seem to suggest a new mode of transmission or a new risk to humans, namely between cats and humans, and we regard sharing this type information to the public as more beneficial than harmful [63]. Transparency will result in a more educated public better prepared to handle any future changes to the virus.

### 7.4 Vaccine research and funding

It is clear from the COVID-19 pandemic and generally in past infectious disease outbreaks that vaccination is the most important piece of the puzzle. The Biden administration has awarded Moderna funding, both in July 2024 and January 2025, to begin and speed up mRNA vaccine development against H5N1, respectively [70]. While we regard this one of the positive aspects of the US response to H5N1 so far, the new presidential administration and public health appointments represent potential changes to the philosophy on vaccine development, especially for a virus with little human effects so far. We recommend a continuation of support for Moderna to develop this vaccine so that appropriate stockpiles are available should they be needed.

### 7.5 A note on the cattle industry

In an effort to create comprehensive recommendations, we ought to mention a recommendation for the cattle industry in preparation for future pathogenic threats. Rather than responding to one species at a given time after consequences arise, the goal should be to develop plans that can be modified or tailored to a range of pathogens. This necessarily entails improving surveillance and testing for any emerging disease and thus fits with our other recommendations as well, but we thought it imperative to specify this recommendation as well.

### 7.6 Global surveillance

The early days of the Trump administration in 2025 have brought large-scale trimming of the federal workforce. While the loss of workforce in the CDC is bound to affect public health in the US, perhaps the downsize most consequential to the bird flu situation is the layoff of nearly 95% of the USAID agency's workforce [66]. This sector of the federal government is responsible for international coordination and surveillance of infectious disease and global health [66]. Monitoring of bird flu in 49 countries has thus been halted due to this change, inevitably leaving cases undetected and coordination for research impossible [66]. As the COVID-19 pandemic showed us, leaving viruses to circulate undetected internationally, even if the situation in the US is manageable, leaves the door open for mutation and widespread devastation. Similarly, the executive order to withdraw from the WHO poses another risk to global vulnerability to infectious disease, as WHO membership provides a basis for global data sharing and evidence-based recommendation formation [71]. As an economic and political world leader, the US has an ethical responsibility to provide the means necessary to protect all from a bird flu outbreak and the damages that such an outbreak entails.

Additionally, from an economic perspective, the virus's effect on international trade and food supply has already manifested in price increases. And, the COVID-19 pandemic revealed the vicious cycle that is the relationship between disease and inequality. In 2020, individuals in communities experiencing poverty and discrimination, who were already lacking in many social determinants of health, were more likely to remain working through public health restrictions and thus more likely to contract and die from disease compared to their white counterparts [67]. This phenomenon drove individuals further into poverty, and the cycle continued. A similar trend could be seen domestically and internationally among vulnerable populations if H5N1 reaches a pandemic level. So, while not inevitable, if H5N1 progresses to a point where pandemic is within reach, the risks to the world are astronomical. The US has an ethical responsibility to mitigate them.

## 8. Conclusion

In summary, the H5N1 virus poses a unique and complex challenge to the US and the world. The history of influenza virus outbreaks and the trends of the current situation in the US warrant great attention and concern. And up to this point, many officials agree that the US response has been lacking in many facets, including testing, surveillance, research, and communication. An argument can be made that given the low impact on human lives thus far, increasing measures now creates more costs and harm than benefit. But we maintain that prevention requires proaction, and the risks of the progression of this virus are too great to be handling the situation with subpar effectiveness. The US has a responsibility not only to its own citizens but to the world to contain this outbreak and prevent devastation.


## Author details

Jaison Lawrence Santhi[1], Daniel DiSandro[2], Joel Koshy[3], Fredy Abboud[4], Joseph Kelly[5] and Peter A. Clark[4]*

1 Mercy Catholic Medical Center, Darby, PA, United States

2 Lewis Katz School of Medicine, Temple University, Philadelphia, PA, United States

3 Philadelphia College of Osteopathic Medicine, Philadelphia, PA, United States

4 Saint Joseph's University, Philadelphia, PA, United States

5 Sidney Kimmel Medical College, Thomas Jefferson University, Philadelphia, PA, United States

*Address all correspondence to: pclark@sju.edu

## References

[1] Centers for Disease Control and Prevention. Past Reported Global Human Cases with Highly Pathogenic Avian Influenza a(H5N1) (HPAI H5N1) by Country, 1997-2025. United States of America: Centers for Disease Control and Prevention; 2025. Available from: www.cdc.gov/bird-flu/php/avian-flu-summary/chart-epi-curve-ah5n1.html [Accessed: February 3, 2025]

[2] Peiris JS, de Jong MD, Guan Y. Avian influenza virus (H5N1): A threat to human health. Clinical Microbiology Reviews. 2007;**20**(2):243-267. DOI: 10.1128/CMR.00037-06

[3] Mandavilli A. A Dangerous Virus': Bird Flu Enters a New Phase. United States of America: The New York Times; 2025. Available from: www.nytimes.com/2025/01/27/health/bird-flu-h5n1.html?searchResultPosition=1

[4] Lupiani B, Reddy SM. The history of avian influenza. Comparative Immunology, Microbiology and Infectious Diseases. 2009;**32**(4):311-323. DOI: 10.1016/j.cimid.2008.01.004

[5] Schäfer W. Vergleichende Sero-Immunologische Untersuchungen Über Die Viren Der Influenza Und Klassischen Geflügelpest. Zeitschrift für Naturforschung B. 1955;**10**(2):81-91. DOI: 10.1515/znb-1955-0205

[6] Easterday BC. Historical perspective of the avian influenza symposium. Avian Diseases. 2003;**47**:3-5. Available from: http://www.jstor.org/stable/3298792

[7] Centers for Disease Control and Prevention. 1880-1959 Highlights in the History of Avian Influenza (Bird Flu) Timeline. United States of America: Centers for Disease Control and Prevention; 2024. Available from: https://www.cdc.gov/bird-flu/avian-timeline/1880-1959.html

[8] Wilksinson L, Waterson AP. The development of the virus concept as reflected in corpora of studies on individual pathogens. 2. The agent of fowl plague—A model virus. Medical History. 1975;**19**(1):52-72. DOI: 10.1017/S0025727300019931

[9] Pereira HG, Tumova B, Law VG. Avian Influenza A Viruses. Bulletin of the World Health Organization. 1965;**32**(6):855-860. Available from: https://pmc.ncbi.nlm.nih.gov/articles/PMC2555286/

[10] Lycett SJ, Duchatel F, Digard P. A brief history of bird flu. Philosophical Transactions of the Royal Society of London. Series B, Biological Sciences. 2019;**374**(1775):20180257. Available from: https://pmc.ncbi.nlm.nih.gov/articles/PMC6553608/

[11] Centers for Disease Control and Prevention. Types of Influenza Viruses. United States of America: Centers for Disease Control and Prevention; 2024. Available from: https://www.cdc.gov/flu/about/viruses-types.html#:~:text=Influenza%20A%20viruses%20are%20divided,N1%20through%20N11%2C%20respectively

[12] Duan L, Campitelli L, Fan XH, Leung YH, Vijaykrishna D, Zhang JX, et al. Characterization of low-pathogenic H5 subtype influenza viruses from Eurasia: Implications for the origin of highly pathogenic H5N1 viruses. Journal of Virology. 2007;**81**(14):7529-7539. DOI: 10.1128/jvi.00327-07

[13] Chan PK. Outbreak of avian influenza a(H5N1) virus

infection in Hong Kong in 1997. Clinical Infectious Diseases. 2002;**34**(Supplement_2):S58-S64. DOI: 10.1086/338820

[14] Tam JS. Influenza a (H5N1) in Hong Kong: An overview. Vaccine. 2002;**20**(Suppl. 2):S77-S81. DOI: 10.1016/s0264-410x(02)00137-8

[15] Webster RG, Guan Y, Peiris M, Walker D, Krauss S, Zhou NN, et al. Characterization of H5N1 influenza viruses that continue to circulate in geese in southeastern China. Journal of Virology. 2002;**76**(1):118-126. DOI: 10.1128/jvi.76.1.118-126.2002

[16] Kou Z, Lei FM, Yu J, Fan ZJ, Yin ZH, Jia CX, et al. New genotype of avian influenza H5N1 viruses isolated from tree sparrows in China. Journal of Virology. 2005;**79**(24):15460-15466. DOI: 10.1128/jvi.79.24.15460-15466.2005

[17] Gutiérrez R, Naughtin M, Horm S, San S, Buchy P. A(H5N1) virus evolution in South East Asia. Viruses. 2009;**1**(3):335-361. DOI: 10.3390/v1030335

[18] Creanga A, Le Hang N, Cuong VD, Nguyen HT, Phuong HV, Thanh LT, et al. Highly pathogenic avian influenza a(H5N1) viruses at the animal–human Interface in Vietnam, 2003-2010. The Journal of Infectious Diseases. 2017;**216**(suppl_4):S529-S538. DOI: 10.1093/infdis/jix003

[19] Auewarakul P. The past and present threat of avian influenza in Thailand. Emerging Infections in Asia. 2008;**1**(1):31-44. DOI: 10.1007/978-0-387-75722-3_2

[20] Rehman S, Effendi MH, Witaningruma AM, Nnabuikeb UE, Bilal M, Abbas A, et al. Avian influenza (H5N1) virus, epidemiology and its effects on backyard poultry in Indonesia: A review. F1000Research. 2023;**11**:1321. DOI: 10.12688/f1000research.125878.2

[21] Cattoli G, Fusaro A, Monne I, Capua I. H5N1 virus evolution in Europe—An updated overview. Viruses. 2009;**1**(3):1351-1363. DOI: 10.3390/v1031351

[22] Xie R, Edwards KM, Wille M, Wei X, Wong S-S, Zanin M, et al. The episodic resurgence of highly pathogenic avian influenza H5 virus. Nature. 2023;**622**(7984):810-817. DOI: 10.1038/s41586-023-06631-2

[23] Centers for Disease Control and Prevention. 2020-2024 Highlights in the History of Avian Influenza (Bird Flu) Timeline. United States of America: Centers for Disease Control and Prevention; 2024. Available from: https://www.cdc.gov/bird-flu/avian-timeline/2020s.html

[24] World Health Organization. Avian Influenza a(H5N1) – United States of America. United States of America: World Health Organization; 2024. Available from: https://www.who.int/emergencies/disease-outbreak-news/item/2024-DON512#:~:text=Public%20health%20response,HPAI%20A(H5N1)%20virus

[25] Ruiz-Saenz J, Martinez-Gutierrez M, Pujol FH. Multiple introductions of highly pathogenic avian influenza H5N1 clade 2.3.4.4B into South America. Travel Medicine and Infectious Disease. 2023;**53**:102591. DOI: 10.1016/j.tmaid.2023.102591

[26] Plaza PI, Gamarra-Toledo V, Euguí JR, Lambertucci SA. Recent changes in patterns of mammal infection with highly pathogenic avian influenza a(H5N1) virus worldwide. Emerging

Infectious Diseases. 2024;**30**(3):444-452. DOI: 10.3201/eid3003.231098

[27] American Academy of Ophthalmology. Novel H5N1 Bird Flu Outbreak. United States of America: American Academy of Ophthalmology; 2025. Available from: https://www.aao.org/education/bird-flu#:~:text=Highly%20pathogenic%20avian%20influenza%20(HPAI,(H5N1)%20viruses%20since%201997

[28] Dye C, Barclay WS. Should we worry about a growing threat from 'bird flu'? BMJ (Clinical research ed.). 2024;**385**:q1199. Available from: https://pubmed.ncbi.nlm.nih.gov/38834195/

[29] Macfarlane JT, Lim WS. Bird flu and pandemic flu. BMJ. 2005;**331**(7523):975-976. DOI: 10.1136/bmj.38649.389005.de

[30] AbuBakar U, Amrani L, Kamarulzaman FA, Karsani SA, Hassandarvish P, Khairat JE. Avian influenza virus tropism in humans. Viruses. 2023;**15**(4):833. DOI: 10.3390/v15040833

[31] Next.amboss.com. Available from: https://next.amboss.com/us/article/Bm0z3g?q=bird+flu [Accessed: February 24, 2025]

[32] Centers for Disease Control and Prevention. Signs and Symptoms of Bird Flu in People. United States of America: Centers for Disease Control and Prevention; 2024. Available from: https://www.cdc.gov/bird-flu/signs-symptoms/index.html

[33] Gao R, Cao B, Yunwen H, Feng Z, Wang D, Wanfu H, et al. Human infection with a novel avian-origin influenza a (H7n9) virus. New England Journal of Medicine. 2013;**368**(20):1888-1897. DOI: 10.1056/nejmoa1304459

[34] Lai C-C, Hsueh P-R. Human infection caused by avian influenza a (H10N5) virus. Journal of Microbiology, Immunology and Infection. 2024;**57**(3):343-345. DOI: 10.1016/j.jmii.2024.04.006

[35] Zhou M, Zhang X, Jieming Q. Coronavirus disease 2019 (COVID-19): A clinical update. Frontiers of Medicine. 2020;**14**(2):126-135. Available from: https://pmc.ncbi.nlm.nih.gov/articles/PMC7115348/

[36] Centers for Disease Control and Prevention. Prevention and Antiviral Treatment of Avian Influenza a Viruses in People. United States of America: Centers for Disease Control and Prevention; 2024. Available from: https://www.cdc.gov/bird-flu/prevention/index.html

[37] Maxmen A. How America Lost Control of the Bird Flu, Setting the Stage for another Pandemic. United States of America: KFF Health News; 2025. Available from: https://kffhealthnews.org/news/article/bird-flu-spread-cattle-poultry-pandemic-cdc/

[38] Scarpino SV, Krugman A. Timeline: H5N1 Bird Flu Outbreak in the U.S. United States of America: Think Global Health; 2025. Available from: https://www.thinkglobalhealth.org/article/timeline-h5n1-bird-flu-outbreak-us

[39] USDA. USDA Actions to Protect Livestock Health from Highly Pathogenic H5N1 Avian Influenza. United States of America: US Department of Agriculture; 2024. Available from: https://www.usda.gov/about-usda/news/press-releases/2024/04/24/usda-actions-protect-livestock-health-highly-pathogenic-h5n1-avian-influenza

[40] Douglas L, Steenhuysen J. US to Spend $10 Million to Curb Bird Flu in

Farm Workers, Including Vaccine Push. United States of America: Reuters; 2024. Available from: https://www.reuters.com/business/healthcare-pharmaceuticals/us-spend-10-million-curb-bird-flu-farm-workers-including-seasonal-flu-vaccine-2024-07-30/

[41] Mellis AM, Coyle J, Marshall KE, Frutos AM, Singleton J, Drehoff C, et al. Serologic evidence of recent infection with highly pathogenic avian influenza a(H5) virus among dairy workers — Michigan and Colorado, June–august 2024. MMWR. Morbidity and Mortality Weekly Report. 2024;**73**(44):1004-1009. DOI: 10.15585/mmwr.mm7344a3

[42] U.S. Department of Health and Human Services (HHS). HHS Awards $306 Million in Avian Flu Monitoring and Preparedness Funding. United States of America: U.S. Department of Health and Human Services (HHS); 2025. Available from: https://public3.pagefreezer.com/browse/HHS.gov/21-01-2025T07:38/https://www.hhs.gov/about/news/2025/01/03/hhs-awards-306-million-avian-flu-monitoring-and-preparedness-funding.html

[43] U.S. Department of Health and Human Services (HHS). HHS Provides $590 Million to Accelerate Pandemic Influenza mRNA-Based Vaccine Development, Enhance Platform Capability for Other Emerging Infectious Disease. United States of America: U.S. Department of Health and Human Services (HHS); 2025. Available from: https://public3.pagefreezer.com/browse/HHS.gov/21-01-2025T07:38/https://www.hhs.gov/about/news/2025/01/17/hhs-provides-590-million-accelerate-pandemic-influenza-mrna-based-vaccine-development-enhance-platform-capability-other-emerging-infectious-disease.html

[44] CDC Health Alert Network. Accelerated Subtyping of Influenza a in Hospitalized Patients. United States of America: CDC Health Alert Network; 2025. Available from: https://www.cdc.gov/han/2025/han00520.html

[45] Lin T-H, Zhu X, Wang S, Zhang D, McBride R, Wenli Y, et al. A single mutation in bovine influenza H5N1 hemagglutinin switches specificity to human receptors. Science. 2024;**386**(6726):1128-1134. DOI: 10.1126/science.adt0180

[46] Alexander M, Unruh L, Koval A, Belanger W. United States response to the COVID-19 pandemic, January-November 2020. Health Economics, Policy, and Law. 2021;**17**(1):62-75. Available from: https://pmc.ncbi.nlm.nih.gov/articles/PMC8060542/

[47] U.S. Bureau of Labor Statistics. Eggs, Grade a, Large, per Doz. in U.S. City Average, Average Price, Not Seasonally Adjusted. United States of America: U.S. Bureau of Labor Statistics; 2025. Available from: https://data.bls.gov/timeseries/APU0000708111

[48] Centers for Disease Control and Prevention. H5 Bird Flu: Current Situation. United States of America: Centers for Disease Control and Prevention; 2025. Available from: https://www.cdc.gov/bird-flu/situation-summary/index.html

[49] Buchler EG. How Serious Is Bird Flu? United States of America: The Hub; 2025. Available from: https://hub.jhu.edu/2025/01/13/bird-flu-meghan-davis-qa/

[50] Animal and Plant Health Inspection Service. USDA Provides Additional $502 Million for Highly Pathogenic Avian Influenza – Stands Ready to Combat Additional Detections. United States of America: Animal and Plant Health Inspection Service; 2024. Available

from: https://www.aphis.usda.gov/news/agency-announcements/usda-provides-additional-502-million-highly-pathogenic-avian-influenza

[51] Animal and Plant Health Inspection Service. Detections of Highly Pathogenic Avian Influenza. United States of America: Animal and Plant Health Inspection Service; 2024. Available from: https://www.aphis.usda.gov/livestock-poultry-disease/avian/avian-influenza/hpai-detections

[52] Farahat RA, Khan SH, Rabaan AA, Al-Tawfiq JA. The resurgence of avian influenza and human infection: A brief outlook. New Microbes and New Infections. 2023;**53**:101122. DOI: 10.1016/j.nmni.2023.101122

[53] Oxfam International. COVID-19 Death Toll Four Times Higher in Lower-Income Countries than Rich Ones. United States of America: Oxfam International; 2022. Available from: https://www.oxfam.org/en/press-releases/covid-19-death-toll-four-times-higher-lower-income-countries-rich-ones

[54] Food Security Information Network (FSIN). Global Report on Food Crises 2020. United States of America: Food Security Information Network (FSIN); 2020. Available from: https://www.fsinplatform.org/global-report-food-crises-2020

[55] UN Economic and Social Commission for Asia and the Pacific. Strengthening the Resilience of Least Developed Countries in the Wake of the Coronavirus Disease Pandemic. United States of America: UN Economic and Social Commission for Asia and the Pacific; 2021. Available from: https://www.unescap.org/kp/2021/CSNDR2021

[56] Philadelphia Department of Public Health, Division of Disease Control. Influenza H5N1 Update. United States of America: Philadelphia Department of Public Health, Division of Disease Control; 2024

[57] Tong R. Ethics and avian flu. North Carolina Medical Journal. 2007;**68**(1):69-70

[58] Walter JJ. The foundation and formulation of norms. In: Curran CE, editor. Moral Theology: Challenges for the Future, Essays in Honor of Richard a. McCormick, S.J. New York, NY: Paulist Press; 1990. p. 132

[59] Gula R. Reason Informed by Faith: Foundations of Catholic Morality. New York: Paulist Press; 1989. pp. 270-272

[60] Kockler N. The principle of double effect and proportionate reason. Virtual Mentor. 2007;**9**(5):369-374. DOI: 10.1001/virtualmentor.2007.9.5.pfor2-0705

[61] McCormick's criteria for proportionate reason first appeared inMcCormick R. Ambiguity In Moral Choice. Milwaukee, WI: Marquette University Press; 1973. He later reworked the criteria in response to criticism. His revised criteria can be found in Doing Evil To Achieve Good, eds. Richard McCormick and Paul Ramsey (Chicago, IL, United States of America: Loyola University Press, 1978)

[62] Gula R. Reason Informed by Faith: Foundations of Catholic Morality. New York: Paulist Press; 1989. pp. 274

[63] Mandavilli A, Anthes E. C.D.C. Posts, Then Deletes, Data on Bird Flu Spread between Cats and People. United States of America: The New York Times; 2025

[64] Mandavilli A, Anthes E. C.D.C. Posts, Then Deletes, Data on Bird Flu Spread between Cats and People. The New York Times; 2025

[65] Powers S. I Ran USAID: Killing it Is a Win for Autocrats Everywhere. United States of America: The New York Times; 2025

[66] Samantaroy S. US Response to Bird Flu Requires Global Collaboration - but CDC Updates Remain on Hold. United States of America: Health Policy Watch; 2025. Available from: https://healthpolicy-watch.news/response-to-bird-flu-requires-global-collaboration-open-communication/

[67] Maxmen A. Inequality's Deadly Toll. United States of America: Nature News; 2021. Available from: https://www.nature.com/immersive/d41586-021-00943-x/index.html

[68] Leonard J, Harker EJ, Szablewski CM, Margrey SF, Fred Gingrich K, Crossley K, et al. Notes from the field: Seroprevalence of highly pathogenic avian influenza a(H5) virus infections among bovine veterinary practitioners — United States, September 2024. MMWR. Morbidity and Mortality Weekly Report. 2025;**74**(4):50-52. DOI: 10.15585/mmwr.mm7404a2

[69] Anthes E. C.D.C. Study Finds Silent Bird Flu Infections in Dairy Veterinarians. United States of America: The New York Times; 2025. Available from: https://www.nytimes.com/2025/02/13/science/cdc-bird-flu-infections.html

[70] Kim J. U.S. Pays $590 Million to Moderna to Speed up Development of Bird Flu Vaccine. United States of America: NPR; 2025. Available from: https://www.npr.org/2025/01/18/nx-s1-5266868/bird-flu-vaccine-moderna

[71] Johns Hopkins Bloomberg School of Public Health. The U.S. and the WHO: An Imperfect but Essential Relationship. United States of America: Johns Hopkins Bloomberg School of Public Health; 2025. Available from: https://publichealth.jhu.edu/2025/the-consequences-of-the-us-withdrawal-from-the-who

Chapter 2

# Global Bioethics: Addressing Current Challenges, Innovations, and the Needs of Underserved Populations

*Rispah Torrorey-Sawe*


## Abstract

Bioethics in the twenty-first century is increasingly influenced by rapid technological advancements, medical innovations, and significant healthcare disparities. Emerging technologies, such as artificial intelligence, gene editing, and biotechnology present profound ethical challenges, particularly in ensuring equitable access to healthcare for all populations. This chapter explores how bioethics intersects with human rights, healthcare access, and social justice, emphasizing the ethical concerns of marginalized communities often excluded from global bioethical discourse. It critically examines the risks and benefits of AI in diagnostics, the moral complexities of genetic modifications, and the socioeconomic impacts of biotechnological advancements. The discussion also incorporates ethical frameworks that address inclusivity and equity in healthcare policy and practice. Cross-cultural perspectives are considered, advocating for ethical decision-making models that integrate diverse viewpoints while upholding fundamental human rights. Ethical considerations surrounding healthcare disparities are examined, particularly in the allocation of medical resources and the role of policy development in mitigating inequities. Additionally, the role of interdisciplinary collaboration in bioethics is highlighted, promoting responsible scientific progress. The chapter concludes by discussing the future directions of bioethics, emphasizing the need for robust policy development, ethical governance, and increased public engagement to navigate the evolving challenges in healthcare and medical technology. Strengthening global cooperation and fostering inclusive discussions will be essential in ensuring ethical medical innovations that benefit all populations, particularly those historically underserved.


**Keywords:** global bioethics, ethical challenges, medical innovations, healthcare disparities, underrepresented populations, human rights, sustainability, biotechnology, artificial intelligence, genetic editing, cross-cultural ethics, healthcare access, social justice

## 1. Introduction

Bioethics is an interdisciplinary field that examines the moral and ethical implications of advancements in biology, medicine, and technology. The term "bioethics" was first introduced in 1927 by German theologian Fritz Jahr, who proposed a "Bioethical Imperative" advocating for moral consideration toward all forms of life [1]. The modern evolution of bioethics gained momentum in the 1960s and 1970s, driven by rapid technological progress and complex medical practices. The advent of organ transplantation, for instance, raised profound ethical questions about donor consent, allocation of scarce resources, and the definition of death [2]. Simultaneously, with the expansion of clinical trials, it became increasingly clear that researchers needed to obtain informed consent from participants and take active steps to protect their well-being, which resulted in the creation of ethical guidelines and oversight bodies, like institutional review boards (IRBs) to ensure proper research conduct with human subjects [3]. During this period, the principle of patient autonomy became increasingly prominent, challenging paternalistic models of healthcare. Patients sought greater involvement in their medical decisions, prompting a reevaluation of clinician-patient relationships and the ethical obligations of healthcare providers [4].

In the twenty-first century, global bioethics stands at the intersection of rapid technological advancements and persistent healthcare disparities, especially affecting underserved populations. This chapter delves into the ethical challenges posed by emerging technologies—such as gene editing, artificial intelligence (AI), and biotechnology—while emphasizing the imperative to address the needs of marginalized communities often excluded from global bioethical discourse.

The advent of technologies like CRISPR-Cas9 has revolutionized possibilities in gene editing, offering potential cures for genetic diseases. Simultaneously, AI's integration into healthcare promises enhanced diagnostics and personalized treatments. However, these innovations raise profound ethical questions, particularly concerning equitable access and the potential exacerbation of existing health disparities. Marginalized communities frequently lack representation in research and access to cutting-edge treatments, underscoring the need for an inclusive bioethical framework.

## 2. Theoretical foundations of bioethics

Bioethics, as an interdisciplinary field, draws upon various ethical theories and moral principles to navigate complex issues in healthcare, medicine, and biotechnology. Understanding these foundational theories and principles is essential for analyzing and resolving bioethical dilemmas.

### 2.1 Overview of major ethical theories

1. *Utilitarianism*: This consequentialist theory posits that the morality of an action is determined by its overall benefit or harm. In bioethics, utilitarianism guides decisions by evaluating potential outcomes to maximize overall well-being.

2. *Deontology*: Rooted in the philosophy of Immanuel Kant, deontology emphasizes duties and adherence to moral rules. It asserts that certain actions are inherently

right or wrong, regardless of their consequences. In bioethical contexts, deontological approaches focus on respecting individuals' rights and fulfilling moral obligations.

3. *Virtue ethics*: Originating from Aristotelian philosophy, virtue ethics centers on the character and virtues of moral agents rather than specific actions. In bioethics, this perspective encourages healthcare professionals to cultivate virtues such as compassion, honesty, and courage, guiding ethical behavior in medical practice.

### 2.2 Application of ethical theories in bioethical contexts

These ethical theories provide distinct frameworks for addressing bioethical issues:

- *Utilitarianism*: Applied in public health policies, utilitarianism supports measures that promote the greatest good for the largest number, such as vaccination programs and resource allocation during pandemics.

- *Deontology*: Influences practices like obtaining informed consent, ensuring that patients' autonomy and rights are respected, regardless of the potential outcomes.

- *Virtue ethics*: Encourages medical practitioners to develop moral character, fostering trust and empathy in patient-caregiver relationships.

### 2.3 Discussion of core moral principles

In addition to these theories, bioethics often relies on four fundamental principles to guide ethical decision-making:

1. *Autonomy*: Respecting an individual's right to make informed decisions about their own healthcare. This principle underpins practices like informed consent and honors patients' personal values and choices.

2. *Beneficence*: The obligation to act in the best interest of the patient, promoting their well-being and taking positive steps to prevent harm.

3. *Non-maleficence*: A commitment to "do no harm," ensuring that medical interventions do not cause unnecessary injury or suffering to patients.

4. *Justice*: Ensuring fairness in the distribution of healthcare resources and treatments, and addressing disparities to provide equitable care for all individuals.

## 3. Methodologies in bioethics

Bioethics employs a range of methodologies to systematically analyze and address ethical dilemmas in healthcare, research, and policy. These methodologies provide structured approaches to navigate complex moral issues, ensuring that decisions are well-reasoned and ethically sound.

### 3.1 Approaches to ethical analysis and reasoning

1. *Principle-based methods*: These methods rely on foundational ethical principles to guide decision-making [5]:

    - *Consequentialist methods*: Focus on the outcomes of actions, aiming to maximize overall good or minimize harm.

    - *Deontological methods*: Emphasize duties and adherence to moral rules, assessing the inherent rightness or wrongness of actions.

    - *Principlism*: A pluralistic approach that balances multiple ethical principles, such as autonomy, beneficence, non-maleficence, and justice, to resolve moral dilemmas.

2. *Case-based methods (Casuistry)*: This approach analyzes specific cases by drawing parallels to precedent-setting cases, focusing on practical decision-making over theoretical constructs.

3. *Virtue ethics*: Centers on the moral character and virtues of individuals, promoting traits like compassion, honesty, and courage as guides for ethical behavior.

4. *Ethics of care*: Highlights the importance of interpersonal relationships and context-specific considerations, emphasizing empathy and care in moral reasoning.

5. *Communitarian perspectives*: Focus on communal values and social contexts, advocating for the common good and societal well-being in ethical deliberations.

### 3.2 Role of case studies and thought experiments

Case studies and thought experiments are vital tools in bioethics:

- *Case studies*: Provide real-world contexts to apply ethical theories, facilitating practical understanding and highlighting the nuances of moral dilemmas.

- *Thought experiments*: Utilize hypothetical scenarios to challenge existing beliefs, explore potential consequences, and refine ethical principles.

Engaging with these tools enhances critical thinking and aids in developing well-rounded ethical judgments.

### 3.3 Interdisciplinary collaboration in bioethical decision-making

Bioethical issues often intersect with various disciplines, necessitating collaborative approaches:

- *Integration of empirical research*: Incorporating data from social sciences, medicine, and public health to inform ethical analyses and ground normative conclusions in real-world contexts [6].

- *Cross-cultural engagement:* Recognizing diverse cultural perspectives enriches ethical deliberations, promoting inclusivity and global relevance in bioethical standards.

- *Policy development*: Collaborating with legal experts, policymakers, and community stakeholders ensures that ethical guidelines are practical, enforceable, and aligned with societal values.

## 4. Ethical challenges in emerging technologies

The rapid advancement of technologies such as artificial intelligence (AI), biotechnology, and nanotechnology has introduced profound ethical considerations that society must address. These emerging technologies, while offering significant benefits, also pose challenges related to privacy, bias, accountability, and the potential for misuse.

### 4.1 Artificial intelligence (AI)

- *Bias and discrimination*: AI systems can inadvertently perpetuate existing societal biases if trained on skewed datasets. For example, AI tools used in hiring processes have been found to favor certain demographics over others, leading to discriminatory practices. Ensuring fairness requires meticulous attention to the data used and the algorithms' design (https://www.reuters.com/sustainability/society-equity/comment-business-leaders-risk-sleepwalking-towards-ai-misuse-2024-11-19).

- *Transparency and accountability*: According to Ref. [7] in his article on transparency and accountability in AI systems: safeguarding well-being in the age of algorithmic decision-making indicated that the widespread adoption of artificial intelligence (AI) across various sectors has sparked concerns about its effects on individuals and society, particularly due to the opacity of its decision-making processes and the challenges in ensuring accountability. This review explored the primary legal and ethical issues related to fostering transparency and accountability in AI systems. It highlighted four key thematic areas: technical methodologies, legal and regulatory considerations, ethical and societal implications, and interdisciplinary, multi-stakeholder approaches. By synthesizing current research and offering strategic insights for policymakers, this confirms advanced discussions on responsible AI governance and sets the stage for future research. The ultimate objective is to safeguard societal and individual well-being by ensuring AI technologies are designed and implemented in a transparent, accountable, and ethical manner.

### 4.2 Biotechnology

Biotechnology and genetic engineering offer significant opportunities to enhance human health, improve agriculture, and promote environmental sustainability. A breakthrough in the 1970s was the development of biosynthetic human insulin (BHI) through recombinant DNA technology, revolutionizing diabetes treatment. However, alongside these technological advancements, there are considerable risks that must be carefully managed to prevent potential harm to both people and the environment.

Recognizing these challenges, international organizations such as the United Nations Educational, Scientific and Cultural Organization (UNESCO) and the Convention on Biological Diversity have established ethical frameworks to guide responsible decision-making in this field.

While advancements in genome editing present significant scientific potential for human benefit, UNESCO emphasizes the importance of adhering to the ethical principles outlined in the Universal Declaration on the Human Genome and Human Rights (1997). Caution is required when considering genetic modifications that can be inherited by future generations, such as germline therapy and human embryo interventions. In response to these concerns, UNESCO's International Bioethics Committee has recommended a temporary suspension of human germline genome engineering until the safety and efficacy of such procedures are firmly established (as noted in its 2015 report on the Human Genome and Human Rights).

Aligned with these recommendations, UNESCO urges researchers, institutions, and governments to uphold globally accepted ethical standards and calls for international cooperation in developing regulations that ensure genome editing is conducted responsibly, with respect for human dignity and rights. UNESCO remains committed to monitoring ethical challenges arising from genome editing and other advancements in life sciences. The organization advocates for ongoing global discussions on the broader ethical implications of these technologies for individuals, societies, and humanity as a whole.

The Data Privacy, Ethics, and Protection: Guidance Note on Big Data for Achievement of the 2030 Agenda (2017) provides guidelines for the ethical and responsible use of big data in supporting sustainable development goals. It emphasizes the importance of data privacy, security, and ethical considerations when using real-time data from private sector sources. The document outlines key principles such as informed consent, risk mitigation, transparency, and accountability to prevent potential harm, including discrimination and misuse of personal information. It also highlights the need for regulatory frameworks and international collaboration to ensure that big data initiatives align with human rights and ethical standards while maximizing their benefits for social and economic development [8].

### 4.3 Nanotechnology

Nanomaterials in food packaging offer promising benefits, yet their widespread adoption faces significant hurdles. Key challenges include inconsistent regulations, safety concerns regarding human and environmental exposure, and low consumer acceptance due to potential health risks [9]. A major issue is the possible migration of nanoparticles from packaging into food, with long-term effects still not fully understood. The rapid pace of nanotechnology development has also outstripped regulatory frameworks, leading to gaps in safety assessments. Ethical responsibility demands rigorous risk assessments and well-defined regulations to mitigate potential hazards and ensure safe application to safeguard public health and the environment while fostering consumer confidence. To foster responsible innovation, proactive policy development and stringent safety measures are essential [10, 11].

## 5. Healthcare disparities and underserved population

Healthcare disparities refer to differences in health outcomes and access to medical services across various populations, often influenced by social, economic, and environmental factors. Underserved populations—such as racial and ethnic minorities, low-income groups, rural communities, and individuals with disabilities—frequently experience these disparities, leading to significant ethical concerns within the field of bioethics.

### 5.1 Understanding healthcare disparities

Healthcare disparities manifest in various forms, including unequal access to preventive services, diagnostic tools, and treatment options. These inequities often result from systemic issues such as socioeconomic status, geographic location, and discrimination. For instance, the integration of genetic testing into clinical practice holds promise for personalized medicine but risks exacerbating existing health disparities if underserved populations lack access to these advancements.

The Just Biomedicine Third Street Project, initiated by the Science and Justice Research Center at the University of California, Santa Cruz, critically examines the juxtaposition of San Francisco's burgeoning biotechnology hub in Mission Bay with the historically underserved Bayview-Hunters Point community. While Mission Bay thrives with substantial investments in biomedical infrastructure, the adjacent Bayview-Hunters Point neighborhood continues to grapple with significant socioeconomic and health disparities. Residents of Bayview-Hunters Point have long faced environmental challenges, including pollution from industrial activities, contributing to elevated rates of asthma, cancer, and other health issues. The Just Biomedicine Third Street Project collaborates with local activists and healthcare workers to document these inequities, aiming to foster narratives that question the allocation of resources and advocate for inclusive health and wealth benefits that encompass all communities along Third Street [12].

### 5.2 Factors contributing to healthcare disparities

1. *Socioeconomic status*: Individuals from low-income backgrounds frequently encounter financial obstacles that impede their ability to obtain quality healthcare services. These challenges encompass limited access to insurance coverage, prohibitive out-of-pocket expenses, and a scarcity of healthcare facilities in economically disadvantaged regions. Such financial constraints often result in delayed medical consultations, underutilization of preventive services, and poorer health outcomes.

   *Geographic barriers*: Rural and remote areas often suffer from a shortage of healthcare providers and facilities, making it difficult for residents to receive timely and appropriate care. The lack of transportation infrastructure further exacerbates this issue, isolating communities from essential health services. This geographic isolation contributes to delayed diagnoses and limited access to specialized treatments.

2. *Ethnicity and race*: Ethnic and racial minorities frequently experience systemic biases and discrimination within healthcare systems. These prejudices can lead to misdiagnoses, inadequate treatment plans, and a general mistrust of medical institutions. For instance, studies have shown that Black women are more likely to die from breast cancer compared to their white counterparts, partly due to delayed diagnoses and limited access to quality care.

3. *Educational attainment*: Limited health literacy, often stemming from inadequate educational opportunities, can hinder individuals' understanding of medical information and their ability to navigate complex healthcare systems. This lack of knowledge may result in non-compliance with treatment regimens, mismanagement of chronic conditions, and reduced utilization of preventive services.

### 5.3 Impact on specific populations

- *Maternal health*: Underserved communities, particularly among ethnic minorities, face alarmingly high rates of maternal mortality. Factors such as inadequate prenatal care, implicit biases among healthcare providers, and socioeconomic hardships contribute to these disparities. Efforts to address these issues include community-based health education programs and systemic policy reforms aimed at improving access to quality maternal care.

- *Cancer outcomes*: Research indicates that individuals residing in impoverished neighborhoods are more susceptible to aggressive forms of cancer and have higher mortality rates. Socioeconomic barriers, including limited access to screening and early detection services, play a significant role in these outcomes. Addressing these disparities requires targeted interventions, such as mobile health clinics and expanded insurance coverage, to ensure timely and equitable cancer care.

### 5.4 Bioethical principles and healthcare disparities

Bioethics provides a framework to address these disparities through core principles:

1. *Justice*: This principle emphasizes fairness in the distribution of healthcare resources. Bioethicists advocate for policies that ensure equitable access to medical services, aiming to reduce disparities affecting underserved communities [13].

2. *Autonomy*: Respecting patient autonomy involves acknowledging individuals' rights to make informed healthcare decisions. Ensuring that underserved populations have access to accurate information and medical options is crucial for true autonomous choice.

3. *Beneficence and non-maleficence*: Healthcare providers are obligated to act in the best interest of patients (beneficence) and avoid causing harm (non-maleficence). Addressing disparities aligns with these principles by striving to improve health outcomes and prevent harm caused by inequitable care.

### 5.5 Ethical challenges in addressing disparities

Several ethical challenges arise when confronting healthcare disparities [14]:

- *Resource allocation*: Deciding how to distribute limited healthcare resources fairly among diverse populations requires careful ethical consideration to avoid perpetuating existing inequities.

- *Cultural competence*: Healthcare providers must understand and respect cultural differences to deliver effective care. Lack of cultural competence can lead to miscommunication and mistrust, further widening disparities.

- *Policy development*: Creating policies that address social determinants of health—such as housing, education, and employment—is essential. Bioethicists play a role in shaping these policies to promote health equity.

### 5.6 Strategies for promoting health equity

To mitigate healthcare disparities, several strategies can be employed:

- *Community engagement*: Involving community members in healthcare decision-making fosters trust and ensures that interventions are culturally appropriate and effective [15].

- *Telemedicine*: The expansion of telemedicine has the potential to increase access to care for underserved populations, especially in remote areas. However, ethical considerations regarding technology access and privacy must be addressed [14].

- *Integrated care models*: Combining physical and behavioral health services can effectively address health disparities in underserved communities. By coordinating primary care and behavioral health professionals within a unified system, these models offer comprehensive, patient-centered care that is both systematic and cost-effective [16]. Such collaborative approaches are particularly beneficial for individuals with complex health needs, as they streamline access to diverse services, thereby improving overall health outcomes [17]. Moreover, integrated care models have been shown to reduce healthcare disparities across various socioeconomic and ethnic groups, enhancing access to quality care for populations that have historically been marginalized [13, 18].

Addressing health disparities in rural populations is not only a matter of public health but also a significant bioethical concern. The unique challenges faced by rural communities—including limited access to healthcare services, underinvestment in health infrastructure, and adverse social determinants—raise critical ethical questions about justice, equity, and the right to health. Bioethics emphasizes the principle of justice, which demands fair distribution of healthcare resources and services. In rural settings, this principle is often compromised due to systemic neglect and urban-centric policies that overlook the needs of rural populations. This oversight leads to inequities that are both unjust and ethically indefensible. Scholars have highlighted the necessity for bioethical discourse to address these rural-specific issues, advocating for a more inclusive approach that considers the unique contexts of rural healthcare delivery [19].

Moreover, the concept of "geographic narcissism," which privileges urban perspectives over rural experiences, exacerbates these disparities. This bias manifests in policy-making and resource allocation, further entrenching health inequities. Bioethicists argue for a conscious effort to recognize and rectify this bias, ensuring that rural communities receive equitable attention and resources [19]. Ethical deliberations in rural healthcare must also consider the social and environmental determinants that disproportionately affect these communities. Factors such as economic deprivation, educational deficits, and environmental hazards contribute to poorer health outcomes. Addressing these determinants is an ethical imperative, requiring policies that go beyond healthcare access to encompass broader social justice issues [20]. From a bioethical standpoint, rectifying rural health disparities necessitates a multifaceted approach that upholds the principles of justice and equity. This involves not only improving healthcare services but also addressing the underlying social determinants and systemic biases that perpetuate inequity. By integrating these ethical considerations into policy and practice, we can move toward a more just and equitable healthcare system for all.

## 6. Cross-cutting ethical considerations

Adapting bioethical principles to diverse cultural contexts highlights a critical discourse in global bioethics. The interplay between universal ethical standards and local cultural values often presents challenges, notably the risks of moral relativism and moral imperialism. Moral relativism suggests that all cultural practices are equally valid, potentially excusing harmful traditions, while moral imperialism involves imposing one culture's moral framework onto another, disregarding local values and autonomy. Navigating between these extremes requires a balanced approach that respects cultural diversity without compromising fundamental human rights.

Engaging with local communities and respecting indigenous knowledge systems are pivotal in this endeavor. The UNESCO Universal Declaration on Bioethics and Human Rights underscores the importance of grounding bioethical principles in respect for human dignity, human rights, and fundamental freedoms. This framework advocates for the integration of diverse cultural perspectives into ethical guidelines, ensuring they are both globally relevant and locally resonant [21].

Incorporating indigenous knowledge into bioethical deliberations not only enriches the ethical discourse but also fosters more inclusive and effective practices. Collaborative models that engage indigenous communities in co-creating scientific and ethical frameworks exemplify this approach. Such partnerships ensure that bioethical guidelines are informed by a multitude of cultural insights, promoting practices that are respectful and beneficial to all stakeholders involved [22].

### 6.1 Challenges in implementing cross-cultural ethics

While the integration of cross-cultural ethics is essential, it presents several challenges:

1. *Balancing universalism and relativism*: A key debate in bioethics is whether universal moral principles can be applied across all cultures or if ethical standards should be relative to cultural contexts. Striking a balance between these perspectives is complex but necessary to respect cultural diversity while upholding fundamental human rights.

2. *Avoiding cultural stereotyping*: There's a risk of oversimplifying or misrepresenting cultural practices. Ethicists and healthcare providers must engage deeply with communities to understand the nuances of cultural beliefs, avoiding assumptions and generalizations.

3. *Addressing power dynamics*: Historically marginalized cultures may distrust external interventions. Building equitable partnerships requires acknowledging past injustices and working collaboratively to empower these communities.

### 6.2 Strategies for fostering inclusivity in bioethics

To navigate the complexities of cross-cultural ethics, the following strategies can be employed:

- *Cultural competency training*: Educating healthcare professionals about different cultural practices and belief systems enhances their ability to provide respectful and effective care. Such training promotes empathy and reduces cultural misunderstandings.

- *Community engagement*: Involving community members in the development and implementation of health policies ensures that interventions are culturally appropriate and accepted. This participatory approach empowers communities and fosters trust.

- *Developing inclusive ethical frameworks*: Ethicists should strive to create models that incorporate diverse cultural values, moving beyond Western-centric paradigms. This inclusivity enriches bioethical discourse and leads to more globally applicable solutions.

- *Continuous dialog and education*: Encouraging ongoing conversations between cultures allows for the exchange of ideas and the evolution of ethical standards that are both universal and context-sensitive.

## 7. Frameworks for ethical decision-making

To navigate these complex issues, several frameworks can be employed:

- *Population-level bioethics*: This approach emphasizes societal obligations to ensure health equity, advocating for resource distribution that accounts for varying needs across different communities.

- *Principle of solidarity*: Particularly relevant in the context of global health, solidarity focuses on collective responsibility and mutual support, promoting policies that address global inequities and support underserved populations.

- *Human rights-based approach*: Grounding bioethical considerations in human rights ensures that dignity, respect, and justice are central to policy development and implementation.

## 8. Future directions

The trajectory of global bioethics must prioritize inclusivity and equity. This involves:

- *Policy development*: Creating regulations that ensure equitable access to medical innovations and protect against exploitation and misuse.

- *Community engagement*: Involving underserved populations in bioethical discussions to ensure their voices and concerns shape the development and application of new technologies.

- *Education and capacity building*: Empowering communities with knowledge about emerging technologies and their implications fosters informed decision-making and advocacy.

As the field of bioethics continues to evolve, it must adapt to emerging challenges and innovations in healthcare, technology, and society. The future of global bioethics will likely be shaped by several key trends and considerations.

### 8.1 Emphasis on diversity and inclusivity

Historically, bioethical discourse has been dominated by Western perspectives, often overlooking the voices and experiences of diverse populations. Future bioethics aims to rectify this by:

- *Incorporating diverse cultural perspectives*: Engaging with ethical frameworks from various cultures, including African and Indigenous philosophies, to enrich bioethical analysis and decision-making.

- *Promoting inclusive dialogue*: Ensuring that underrepresented communities have a platform in bioethical discussions, leading to more equitable and culturally sensitive healthcare policies.

### 8.2 Addressing emerging technological challenges

Rapid advancements in technology present novel ethical dilemmas that bioethics must proactively address:

- *Genetic editing and reproductive technologies*: The rise of services offering embryo screening for traits like intelligence raises concerns about eugenics and genetic inequality.

- *De-extinction and synthetic biology*: Efforts to revive extinct species, such as the wooly mammoth, prompt debates about ecological impacts and the moral implications of such interventions.

- *Stem cell-derived embryo models*: Creating embryo-like structures from stem cells without using eggs or sperm challenges existing ethical frameworks and necessitates a reevaluation of research guidelines.

### 8.3 Strengthening global collaboration

Bioethical issues often transcend national borders, requiring coordinated international efforts:

- *Global forums and committees*: Organizations like the Global Forum on Bioethics in Research (GFBR) provide platforms for discussing ethical issues affecting research practices worldwide, especially in low- and middle-income countries.

- *Harmonizing ethical standards*: Developing universally accepted ethical guidelines can facilitate collaborative research and ensure consistent protection of human subjects globally.

### 8.4 Integrating bioethics into policy and practice

To remain relevant, bioethics must influence real-world applications:

- *Policy development*: Bioethicists should actively participate in crafting policies that govern emerging technologies, ensuring they align with ethical principles and societal values.

- *Public engagement*: Educating and involving the public in bioethical debates fosters transparency and democratic decision-making, leading to more robust and accepted policies.

### 8.5 Focusing on environmental and global health ethics

The interconnectedness of human health and the environment calls for a broader bioethical perspective:

- *Sustainability*: Ethical considerations should include the long-term impacts of medical practices and technologies on the environment, promoting sustainability in healthcare.

- *Global health equity*: Addressing disparities in healthcare access and outcomes requires a commitment to social justice and the ethical distribution of resources.

## 9. Conclusion

As technological advancements continue to reshape healthcare, global bioethics faces the critical task of ensuring these innovations benefit all populations equitably. By addressing ethical challenges, embracing cross-cultural perspectives, and prioritizing the needs of underserved communities, bioethics can guide the responsible and just integration of new technologies into global healthcare systems.

As bioethics progresses, it must adapt to the dynamic interplay of cultural diversity, technological innovation, and global interconnectedness. Embracing diverse cultural perspectives enriches ethical discourse, ensuring that bioethical principles resonate across different societies. Concurrently, the rapid advancement of technologies such as genetic editing, de-extinction, and stem cell-derived embryo models presents unprecedented ethical challenges that require proactive and nuanced responses. Strengthening global collaboration is essential to harmonize ethical standards and address issues that transcend national boundaries. Integrating bioethics into policy-making and public engagement ensures that ethical considerations are embedded in real-world applications, fostering transparency and societal trust.

Finally, a holistic approach that considers environmental sustainability and global health equity is crucial for addressing the complex interdependencies of modern healthcare and ecological systems. By focusing on these areas, bioethics can navigate future challenges with resilience and inclusivity, ensuring that ethical deliberation remains central to the advancement of science and medicine.

## Author details

Rispah Torrorey-Sawe
Immunology Section, Department of Pathology, School of Medicine, College of Health Sciences, Moi University, Eldoret City, Kenya

*Address all correspondence to: torrorey@gmail.com

## References

[1] Muzur A, Rincic I. Fritz Jahr (1895-1953) - The man who invented bioethics a preliminary of european bioethics. Synthesis Philosophica (Niš, Serbia: Faculty of Philosophy, University of Niš). 2011;**51**(1):133-139

[2] Jonsen AR. Virtual Mentor. 2012;**14**(3):264-268

[3] European Medicines Agency (EMA). Guideline good clinical practice E6(R2). Committee for Human Medicinal Products. 2018;**6**(December 2016):1-68. Available from: https://www.ema.europa.eu/en/documents/scientific-guideline/ich-e-6-r2-guideline-good-clinical-practice-step-5_en.pdf

[4] Schenker Y, Meisel A. Informed consent in clinical care: Practical considerations in the effort to achieve ethical goals. Journal of the American Medical Association. 2011;**305**(11):1130-1131. DOI: 10.1001/jama.2011.333

[5] Childress JF. 15 methods in bioethics. In: The Oxford Handbook of Bioethics. Chicago, Illinois, USA: The American Medical Association (AMA), Oxford University Press; 2009. DOI: 10.1093/oxfordhb/9780199562411.003.0002

[6] Davies R, Ives J, Dunn M. A systematic review of empirical bioethics methodologies. BMC Medical Ethics. 2015;**16**(1):1-13

[7] Cheong BC. Transparency and accountability in AI systems: Safeguarding wellbeing in the age of algorithmic decision-making. Frontiers in Human Dynamics. 2024;**6**. DOI: 10.3389/fhumd.2024.1421273

[8] United Nations Development Group (UNDG). Data Privacy, Ethics and Protection Guidance Note on Big Data for Achievement of the 2030 Agenda. Geneva, Switzerland: International Council for Harmonisation of Technical Requirements for Pharmaceuticals for Human Use (ICH); 2017

[9] Kumah EA, Fopa RD, Harati S, Boadu P, Zohoori FV, Pak T. Human and environmental impacts of nanoparticles: A scoping review of the current literature. BMC Public Health. 2023;**23**(1):1059. DOI: 10.1186/s12889-023-15958-4

[10] Xia T, Zhang H, Wang S, Xin W, Liu S. Environmental health and safety of engineered nanomaterials. In: Gu N, editor. Nanomedicine. Singapore: Springer Nature Singapore; 2020. pp. 1-47. DOI: 10.1007/978-981-13-9374-7_23-1

[11] Ghosh M, Kumar R. Regulatory issues in nanotechnology. In: Prasad M, Kumar R, Ghosh M, Syed SM, Chakravarti S, editors. Nanotechnology Theranostics in Livestock Diseases and Management. Singapore: Springer Nature Singapore; 2024. pp. 765-788. DOI: 10.1007/978-981-16-1610-5_31

[12] Reardon J. Toward Justice: A Modest Proposal. Amsterdam, Netherlands: European Medicines Agency (EMA); 2020

[13] Lewis CL, Yan A, Williams MY, Apen LV, Crawford CL, Morse L, et al. Health equity: A concept analysis. Nursing Outlook. 2023;**71**(5):102032. Available from: https://www.sciencedirect.com/science/article/pii/S0029655423001379

[14] Hassan L. The Role of Bioethics in Addressing Healthcare Disparities and Access. 2024;7(5):5-6

[15] Erku D, Resham Khatri AE, Wolka E. Community Engagement Initiatives in Primary Health Care to Achieve Universal Health Coverage: A Realist Synthesis of Scoping Review. Chicago, Illinois, USA: American Medical Association (AMA); 2023. pp. 1-17

[16] Myerholtz L, Sowa NA, Lombardi B. Integrated behavioral health care. In: Daaleman TP, Helton MR, editors. Chronic Illness Care: Principles and Practice. Cham: Springer International Publishing; 2023. pp. 431-445. DOI: 10.1007/978-3-031-29171-5_33

[17] Hudon C, Bisson M, Chouinard MC, Moullec G, Del Barrio LR, Angrignon-Girouard É, et al. Opportunities of integrated care to improve equity for adults with complex needs: A qualitative study of case management in primary care. BMC Primary Care. 2024;**25**(1):391

[18] Ee C, Lake J, Firth J, Hargraves F, de Manincor M, Meade T, et al. An integrative collaborative care model for people with mental illness and physical comorbidities. International Journal of Mental Health Systems. 2020;**14**(1):1-16

[19] Couch DL, Mayes C. Lead essay—Rural bioethics. Journal of Bioethical Inquiry. 2023;**20**(2):177-180

[20] Mann S. Health inequalities. In: Bioethics in Perspective: Corporate Power, Public Health and Political Economy. Cambridge, United Kingdom: Cambridge University Press; 2010. pp. 96-116

[21] UNESCO's Bioethics Programme. Universal declaration on bioethics and human rights. Revista de derecho y genoma humano = Law and the Human Genome Review. UNESCO. 2005;**23**:227-237

[22] Venkatesan A, Begay D, Burgasser AJ, Hawkins I, Kimura K, Maryboy N, et al. Towards inclusive practices with indigenous knowledge. Nature Astronomy. 2019;**3**(12):1035-1037. DOI: 10.1038/s41550-019-0953-2

Chapter 3

# Responsibility, Trust, and Hope in Medical Ethics

*Franz Staudt*


## Abstract

Due to the Corona crisis, medical ethics has received increased attention. Advances in medicine have also created new ethical dilemmas. This chapter is dedicated to concepts that previously have had less significance in the context of medical ethics: Responsibility, Autonomy, Hope, and Trust. In 1919, Max Weber introduced the concept of moral responsibility for politicians ("Politics as a Profession"). But this also applies to physicians. Responsibility has become a new basic term increasingly replacing the ethical concept of Duty. Weber distinguishes between ethics of conviction and ethics of responsibility. Both complement each other. The principle of Hope plays an essential role in the patient's recovery. For the principle of autonomy, a relationship of trust between doctor and patient is a basic requirement. Trust is therefore particularly important for the doctor-patient relationship.


**Keywords:** ethics of medicine, responsibility, autonomy, hope, trust

## 1. Introduction

The coronavirus crisis has brought medical ethics special and increased attention. It suddenly became clear that hospitals were only partially able to cope with the influx of critically ill patients due to overburdened intensive care units and insufficient personnel resources, especially in the nursing sector. Economic or commercial aspects were the subject of much discussion and recognized as a particular challenge for hospitals [1]. The media frequently brought the handling of the pandemic to the attention of the public. The topic of "triage" gave rise to a law being passed by the German Bundestag. In this law, it was made clear "that no one should be disadvantaged when decisions are made about allocation, especially not because of a disability, degree of frailty, age, ethnic origin, religion or belief, gender or sexual orientation."[1]

[1] www.dbk.de/presse/aktuelles/meldung/triage-gesetz-des-deutschen-bundestages [Accessed: November 28, 2022].

The German Ethics Council, with its then chair[2] in November 2022, presented an ad hoc recommendation [2] highlighting the psychological stress experienced by young people during the pandemic.

This shows how difficult it can be to make ethical judgments or give ethical advice in borderline situations. It would be all the more important to raise the profile of ethical issues as early as medical school. As a rule, there is a lecture on the topic of "Ethics and History of Medicine," and in a few lectures (e.g. neonatology or neuropediatrics), ethical questions are also discussed, but they are not relevant to the exam, which naturally limits the motivation of the students. It is therefore obvious that medical ethics has so far also received little attention in the interests of practicing doctors.[3]

Advances in medicine, which give rise to new ethical dilemmas, also argue in favor of a stronger emphasis on medical ethics in medical school. Examples include organ transplantation with the question of the criteria for death, euthanasia, preimplantation, or prenatal diagnostics, in particular the non-invasive prenatal test [3], human genetics, and the discussion about the so-called "informed consensus." A multidisciplinary expertise (philosophy, research, clinical practice, legislation, politics, etc.) is necessary for an ethical consideration of these topics [4]. In addition, there is the question of whether doctors or the medical profession should comment on general topics that are important for the population's health, such as climate change [5].

In the following, the different approaches of medical ethics, the Hippocratic Oath, the Geneva Declaration, bioethics according to Beauchamp and Childress, and other declarations will be briefly addressed under these aspects. Then special attention will be paid to concepts that have so far been given too little importance in the context of medical ethics: responsibility, attitude, hope, autonomy, trust, and sincerity.

## 2. Medical ethics, a branch of philosophical ethics

### 2.1 Ethics, as a branch of philosophy

Ethics, as a branch of philosophy, is the science that deals with ethos or morals [6]. The term medical ethics first dates back to 1803, when Thomas Percival wrote an early code of medical ethics [7]. There are three main types of ethical argument:

- virtue ethics (Plato and Aristoteles),
- the ethics of duty (deontological ethics), as represented by Kant and ecclesial ethics (moral theology), and
- utilitarianism (teleological ethics) [8].

*Virtue ethics* asks, for example, whether a person acts well or virtuously on the basis of the cardinal virtues of wisdom, courage, moderation, and justice. Its

---

2 www.tum.de/studium/lehre/36050 [Accessed: November 28, 2022].

3 Personal communication from medical students.

goal is human happiness (eudaimonia) based on what is to be done in a specific situation [6]. However, it does not provide solutions to current practical issues such as abortion or the death penalty, and does not evaluate the consequences of actions [9].

According to *deontological ethics (duty ethics)*, an action should be taken out of duty. Kant formulated the categorical imperative for this, whereby the so-called human purpose formula is particularly important for medicine: "*Act in such a way that you treat humanity,* whether *in your own person* or in the *person* of any *other, never merely as a means* to an *end,* but *always at the same time as an end*" [10]. In this way, Kant emphasizes the unique "dignity" of the human being, who is "an end in himself" and has an immeasurable value that cannot be replaced by anything and has an immeasurable value that cannot be replaced by anything.[4]

*Utilitarianism* only considers the consequences of an action and asks what the best possible overall benefit is [11]. It is criticized for not attaching value to other ethical goods such as dignity, equality, justice, freedom, or virtue.[5] The *teleological ethics* emphasizes the basic idea that living beings pursue predetermined goals or purposes by nature.[6]

There is a relationship between the *ethics of responsibility,* which emphasizes the question of accountability for the actual results, and the *ethics of conviction,* which assesses the intention behind the action and the personal motives according to given values.[7] In part, the various theories are mutually exclusive. In part, they emphasize different aspects.

Laws, professional regulations, medical licensing boards, and guidelines from the Association of the Scientific Medical Societies in Germany (AWMF)[8] increasingly restrict physicians' personal freedom of decision. Thus, in addition to the classic basic types, there is a further type of ethics, the *heteronomous or legalistic ethics*.

However, there is no congruence between law and ethics. Laws differ from country to country, whereas ethics can be applied equally across national borders [12]. According to Marckmann, it is impossible to solve conflicts in medical ethics in a universally valid and definitive way [13].

Medical ethics is a specialized area of general ethics and is therefore considered an applied branch of ethics [14]. First of all, it is about a general ethical orientation. The (presumed) will of the patient and, thus, his autonomy plays a special role.

Applied ethics in medicine as a field of ethics represents a combination of philosophical thinking and concrete medical practice [12]. Thus, each case or patient can present the doctor with an independent ethical problem.

---

[4] https://www.schule-bw.de/faecher-und-schularten/gesellschaftswissenschaftliche-und-philosophische-faecher/ethik/unterricht-materialien-und-medien/ethik_11_12/moralphilosophie/kant_pflichtethik_deontologie/ki_formeln [Accessed: February 06, 2023].

[5] Utilitarismus: https://de.wikipedia.org/wiki/Utilitarismus [Accessed: February 2, 2023].

[6] Teleologische Ethik: https://de.wikipedia.org/wiki/Teleologische_Ethik [Accessed: February 2, 2023].

[7] Verantwortungsethik: https://de.wikipedia.org/wiki/Verantwortungsethik [Accessed: February 2, 2023].

[8] AWMF-Leitlinien: www.awmf.org/leitlinien.html [Accessed: February 2, 2023].

## 3. Exemplary course setting for medical ethics

### 3.1 The legendary Hippocratic oath

The legendary *Hippocratic Oath*[9] is the first example of medical ethics developed primarily from the medical professional ethos in ancient Greece. The medical profession's reputation is primarily shaped by this text, which is more than 2500 years old. The public is firmly convinced, and rightly so, that every doctor has sworn this oath, at least to the extent that its provisions are still up to date or adapted to today's requirements. However, only a few doctors have seriously considered its content.

### 3.2 The Nuremberg code

During the Nuremberg Military Tribunal (1946–1949),[10] a decision that includes what is now called the Nuremberg Code was made[11] [2]. This ten-point statement delimits permissible medical experimentation on human subjects. According to this statement, humane experimentation is justified only if its results benefit society and it is carried out according to basic principles that "satisfy moral, ethical, and legal concepts." The voluntary consent of the person involved is essential [3, 15].

The *Declaration of Helsinki* is a set of ethical principles regarding human experimentation developed originally in 1964 for the medical community by the World Medical Association (WMA). It is widely regarded as the cornerstone document on human *research ethics*[12] [1].

*Human rights* work at the socio-political level, while medical ethics is more at the level of the doctor-patient relationship [1, 16]. Human rights place a duty on the state and on healthcare providers to comply with minimum standards. Medical ethics place a duty on individual doctors to comply with parallel standards. Human rights and medical ethics complement each other, maximizing the protection available to the vulnerable patient. "Human rights in bioethics have become indispensable" [2, 17].

*Child rights* such as non-discrimination, best interests, right to life, right to express his or her opinion and to have that opinion respected will expand pediatric ethics [18]. They provide a framework for medical and ethical analysis and decision-making that complements other bioethical principles and theories. They are congruent with global human rights principles [2, 19].

---

[9] Hippocratic oath – ethical code: https://www.britannica.com/topic/Hippocratic-oath [Accessed: February 5, 2023].

[10] "Permissible Medical Experiments." Trials of War Criminals before the Nuremberg Military Tribunals under Control Council Law No. 10. Nuremberg October 1946 – April 1949, Washington. U.S. Government Printing Office (n.d.), vol. 2., pp. 181-182.

[11] The University of North Carolina: Nuremberg Code https://research.unc.edu/human-research-ethics/resources/ccm3_019064 [Accessed: February 4, 2025].

[12] 75th WMA General Assembly: *WMA* Declaration of Helsinki – Ethical Principles for Medical Research Involving Human Participants (2024), https://www.wma.net/policies-post/wma-declaration-of-helsinki [Accessed: February 4, 2025].

### 3.3 The declaration of Geneva

Doctors all over the world refer to the *Declaration of Geneva* by the World Medical Association in 1948, which is a modern version of the Hippocratic Oath [12]. The declaration has been revised several times, most recently in 2017. The new declaration [20] now focuses more strongly than before on patient autonomy, which is surprising given how long it took for this to happen. Doctors are now also obliged to share medical knowledge with their colleagues to benefit patients. In this context, the oath also appeals to doctors to take care of their own health. All physicians should be familiar with the Declaration of Geneva, to which the professional code of conduct binds them [21]. However, multiple surveys of doctors have shown that only a few are familiar with this code. As a rule, they have not read its preamble, which is the Declaration of Geneva.

### 3.4 The international code of medical ethics

Based on the Declaration of Geneva, the *International Code of Medical Ethics* adopted [22] by the General Assembly of the World Medical Association in London in 1949 and amended in 1968, 1983, and 2006 has the main goal of establishing the ethical principles of the physicians worldwide.

### 3.5 Principles of biomedical ethics of Beauchamp and Childress

How the Hippocratic Oath, the other settings, and the Declaration of Geneva can be practically applied is illustrated in the four-step model of Beauchamp and Childress [23], which they first published in their book "Principles of Biomedical Ethics" in 1979. The two US medical ethicists have contrasted their principles of ethics with philosophical-ethical theories and have identified four key principles among general principles:

- respect for autonomy,
- doing good (beneficence),
- non-maleficence, and
- justice.

These principles remained relevant over the past 40 years. Many medical ethical questions can be answered well with their help. Therefore, they are an essential aid for medical ethical decisions.

### 3.6 The Belmont report

At the same time, the Belmont Report was written by the National Commission for the Protection of Human Subjects of *Biomedical and Behavioral Research* in 1979 [24]. The Commission was created to examine and identify comprehensive ethical principles that should underlie the research involving human subjects and developing guidelines to ensure that such research is conducted in accordance with those principles. The fact that the balance between the principles was lacking had been criticized, but the three principles were created in such a way that their implications would overlap with the protection of socially vulnerable groups in mind: Respect for Persons, Beneficence, and Justice and their specific applications (Informed Consent, Assessment of Risks and Benefits, and Selection of Subjects) [25]. Beauchamp and Childress included non-maleficence. The two documents actually grew up simultaneously [26].

### 3.7 The principle of proportionality

The two principles of beneficence and non-maleficence often give rise to the problem of deciding between harm and benefit. This also shows the ambivalence of every human action when a decision is shaped by the respective good or benefit, but at the same time, evil and damage are also caused and allowed [27]. This is where the *principle of proportionality* becomes important. A decision is proportionate if the benefit outweighs the harm. This can be the case if, for example, a cytostatic treatment leads to significant side effects, but is carried out with consent because it is hoped that it will combat a malignant tumor. A simpler example is a fire of a house, when the fire department extinguishes the fire, the extinguishing water completely destroys the entire house. This question of the risk-to-benefit ratio also arises for every surgical procedure and for every individual patient. The decision should take into account the patient's autonomy and, if he is no longer able to make decisions, his relatives or healthcare representative [28].

## 4. Ethics of responsibility

### 4.1 When doctors are asked about their sense of responsibility

When doctors are asked about their *sense of responsibility*, they often dismiss the question by saying that it is self-evident and does not need to be addressed. Today, however, the attitude and responsibility of the physician are playing an increasingly prominent role in medical ethics [29]. Physicians' task is to protect and promote health and practice "evidence-based medicine." (**Figure 1**) [31].

The word "responsibility"[13] originally comes from the field of law. In this context, "to answer" means "to defend oneself in court" or "to justify oneself." In the religious sense, there is justification before the judgment seat of God. In addition to the legal and religious sense, the *moral concept of responsibility* [32] was only added in the twentieth century. Before that, the concept of "responsibility" had not yet played a major role in the development of ethical theory. According to the subject index, the term "responsibility" is mentioned twenty-five times in Maio's pioneering textbook [33], but there is no detailed discussion of the term. The term was introduced into the discussion by the sociologist Max Weber (1864–1920) in his remarkable lecture on "Politics as a Vocation," which he gave in a Munich bookshop in 1919 [30], provided food for thought that is not only important for politicians, but also for industry leaders [34, 35] and, to date, has received little attention, for doctors and, finally, for journalists. Responsibility became a new basic word in our language, increasingly replacing the ethical concept of duty. Thus, responsibility has taken on a special

[13] Verantwortung: https://www.ethik-lexikon.de/stichwort/verantwortung [Accessed: February 3, 2025].

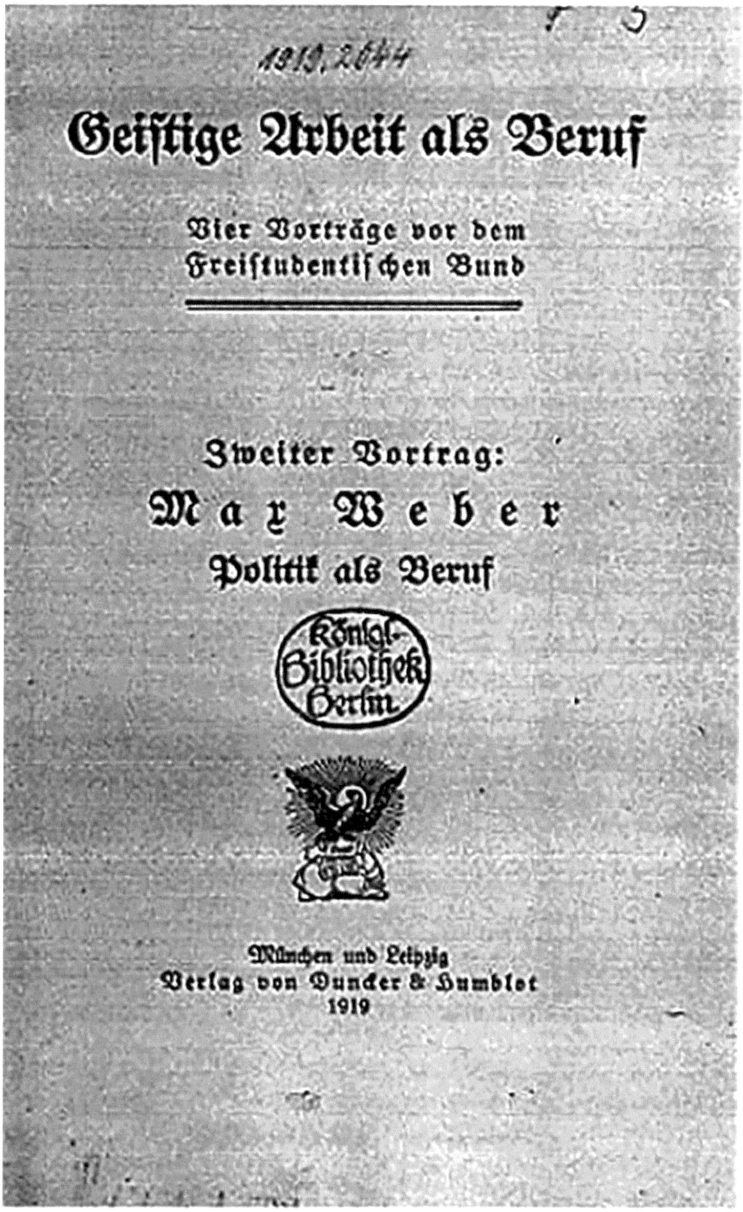
Geistige Arbeit als Beruf

Vier Vorträge vor dem
Freistudentischen Bund

Zweiter Vortrag:
Max Weber
Politik als Beruf



München und Leipzig
Verlag von Duncker & Humblot
1919

**Figure 1.**
*Title page of the second lecture on "Politics as a profession" from the lecture series "Intellectual work as a profession" before the Freistudentischer Bund, Königliche Bibliothek Berlin, published by Duncker & Humblot, Munich and Leipzig [30].*

significance in public discourse and is now considered the guiding concept of an ethic concerned about the future of humanity [36, 37].

Weber first identifies three qualities (passion, sense of responsibility, and sense of proportion) that always belong together. By *passion*, he understands passionate devotion to a cause, but always in conjunction with *responsibility and a sense of proportion*, "the ability to let realities affect you with inner composure and calm, that is, to keep your distance from things and people." In this context, Weber warns against vanity as the "mortal enemy of all dispassionate devotion and all distance, in this case, distance from oneself" [38].

He distinguishes between two types of ethics [35, 39]: *moral philosophy* makes one's convictions, i.e., one's fundamental beliefs and values, the yardstick for action, albeit without considering the consequences of an action or taking responsibility for them. The moral philosopher is the center of attention as the person acting. He assumes that loyalty to principles frees him from responsibility for the consequences, which would be seen as God-given [40]. He shares this approach with virtue ethics [41].

On the other hand, the ethics of responsibility act in a calculating, weighing, and deliberate manner. It primarily considers the longer-term consequences, i.e. the success and effect of the action or decision, whereby one's own fundamental convictions are not in the foreground. Here, there is an overlap with utilitarianism.

Weber does not see these two arguments as absolute contradictions, but rather as complements that make up the genuine human being [42]. Passion and a sense of proportion must also be in an appropriate relationship and maintain a balance [40].

The responsibility ethicist needs and usually has their own good attitude. The deontologist will and must also be aware of the consequences of his actions. Ultimately, a doctor must act responsibly and base his actions entirely on the patient's well-being. The consequences of this are dialog and compromise.

### 4.2 Conflicts of interest

*Conflicts of interest* between responsibility and attitude can arise in a particular way in intensive care units. From the perspective of preserving life, the pure deontologist would be more likely to decide in favor of intensive care treatment, for example, in the case of a geriatric end-stage COPD patient with acute respiratory failure. In contrast, the pure responsibility ethicist would be more concerned about the consequences of his actions and would, therefore, be more likely to opt for conservative or palliative treatment [43].

Analogous decisions have to be made in pediatric intensive care medicine, for example, for extremely premature newborns with pronounced brain damage, for those with encephalitis, or for those who have "almost drowned" [44]. In these cases, the primary concern is often not the continuation or termination of therapy, such as mechanical ventilation, but rather a "change in the treatment goal."

The term intensive care is associated more with maximum therapy, life-saving, or resuscitation and less with a change in treatment goals, treatment discontinuation, or palliative care. Suppose it is recognized that a curative approach is no longer possible. In that case, the use of intensive care measures must be critically questioned to avoid exposing patients to the danger of "over-treatment at the end of life." At this point, at the latest, aspects of palliative medicine should, therefore, be integrated into intensive care medicine [45].

On this topic, the German Medical Association participated in the Pontifical Academy "pro-Vita" of the Vatican in 2017 [46]. Pope Francis referred to a speech by Pope Pius XII on the topic *"Accepting Death"* and called for the prudent use of maximum therapy at the end of life. He explicitly mentioned the withdrawal of treatment as a possible option in hopeless situations. In such cases, therefore, it is not a matter of inducing death but of accepting that it cannot be prevented, and thus subjecting the patient to pointless treatment shortly before his death [47]. When life is needlessly prolonged in intensive care units—perhaps even for commercial reasons or with a misunderstood sense of ethics—the highly equipped hospital is no longer oriented toward the patient's needs, but perhaps toward an ultimately unethical profit. The attempt to prolong human life "at any cost," i.e., for commercial reasons, has also been experienced as a disaster [48]. A commercially induced undersupply is just as reprehensible.

### 4.3 Medical futility

"Medical futility draws a contrast between physician's authority and patients' autonomy and it is one of the major issues of end-of-life ethical decision-making." [49]. In this context, the term futility takes on a special meaning and it is often considered unclear and controversial. It is therefore difficult to achieve a clear consensus over the concept of medical futility. Accordingly, it should be defined and determined at the individual level and based on each unique case. A distinction is made between ineffective therapeutic strategies (Futility type 1), contraindicated therapeutic strategies, and therapeutic strategies with a very unfavorable benefit-to-harm ratio (Futility type 2). This distinction makes it clear when certain measures must or may be avoided from the outset and which considerations should be brought into the doctor-patient discussion for joint decision-making. However, the situation is ethically and communicatively challenging when patients want a therapy that their treating doctors no longer consider to be useful, because there is no reasonable hope of cure or benefit despite continued medical care or treatment [50].

### 4.4 Dying and death

The fight against death should not exclude the possibility of dying and the consequences that arise from it [51]. Unfortunately, dealing with the dying is not yet included in the medical training curriculum or the remuneration paid by the health insurance funds [52].

Dying and death are inextricably linked with life. Medical progress is increasingly making it possible to prevent illnesses or successfully treat potentially fatal illnesses through new treatment options. As a result, life expectancy is constantly increasing. Even if there is a tendency for society to make dying and death taboo, it is necessary to deal with one's mortality. This makes it necessary to appoint a *proxy for healthcare* or to draw up a *living will.*[14]

Often, a doctor has to make a decision on the course of treatment. This situation poses a significant challenge due to both the complexity of modern therapy options and the intellectual demands [51]. For example, the question may arise as to whether chemotherapy should be continued even if a cure is no longer expected and the therapy is also associated with the risk of a deterioration in the general condition and a number of other side effects. The decision is therefore to either accept the adverse effects in the hope of extending life or to prioritize quality of life without wanting to extend life and to end the therapy. An early integration of palliative care can support

[14] Patientenverfügung (living will) https://www.bmj.de/DE/themen/vorsorge_betreuungsrecht/patientenverfuegung/patientenverfuegung_node.html; Gesetz zur Änderung des Betreuungsrechts vom 29. Juli 2009 (BGBl. I S. 2286) eingefügt und zum 1. Januar 2023 in § 1827 BGB verschoben durch Art. 1 des *Gesetzes zur Reform des Vormundschafts- und Betreuungsrechts.*

patients and their relatives in this process [53]. However, there are no generalized answers to these questions; it is always a decision on a case-by-case basis.

### 4.5 Palliative care or hospice care

An early integration of palliative care or hospice care can support patients and their relatives in this process [53]. Although these two forms of care are similar in some ways, they can differ regarding when and where care is received and which treatment options are available. "Palliative care is focused on improving the quality of life for people with serious illnesses. The major elements of palliative care include managing a person's symptoms effectively and ensuring that their care is coordinated. Palliative care is interdisciplinary, which means that it involves multiple types of doctors, nurses, and other care providers, such as social workers, nutritionists, and chaplains. Palliative care improves quality of life and is a resource for anyone living with a serious illness. Organized services may be helpful to any person having general discomfort and disability very late in life. Hospice care is a specific type of palliative care that is provided at the end of life. It is available to people of any age who need it, not just older adults. Like palliative care, hospice provides comprehensive comfort care as well as support for the family, but, in hospice, attempts to cure the person's illness are stopped. The illness runs its natural course" [54].

### 4.6 Palliative care for children

This "represents a small and highly specialized field of healthcare that is different from, albeit closely related to, adult palliative care. Ideally, support for children with palliative care needs starts at diagnosis, and for many children with life-limiting conditions, this can be at birth. It is the active total care of the child's body, mind, and spirit, and also involves supporting the family" [55].

### 4.7 Concept of shared decision-making

It is not uncommon for patients to feel overwhelmed by the exercise of their autonomy and to want to make a decision together with their relatives or doctors. This wish is an essential aspect of the concept of *shared decision-making*, but the process itself can be overwhelming or lead to a feeling of being left alone. If positive experiences with medical and nursing expertise have been made and trust has been established as a result, patients and their relatives can be freed from the "burden" felt with autonomy, exercise their right not to know, and then confidently hand over responsibility for the decision [56]. It has been shown to be helpful to speak of a "change of treatment goal," [57] i.e., away from the cure and toward the alleviation of complaints and dignified accompaniment, if necessary, until death. When dying is allowed, the treatment goal and the situation change fundamentally. The physician's responsibility for preserving life comes to an end [58]. However, this does not mean that the physician should turn away from the dying patient and leave the relatives standing cold. Ethical, compassionate behavior requires the necessary empathy and respect, even after the patient's death. If the doctor cannot provide the necessary attention due to other pressing tasks, for example, it should be ensured that the nursing staff or the hospital chaplain takes over this task. These also serve to maintain and cultivate the relationship of trust between relatives and society in human medicine and in the practice of hospitals.

### 4.8 Economics of medicine

Responsibility also extends to the *economics of medicine*. The demand for the best possible *patient care* in modern medicine puts doctors and nurses under pressure. They take responsibility for their patients, the quality of the care processes, and their results. However, they can only do this within the framework of economic interests and remuneration systems [59].

In hospitals, there is a *division of tasks* between economic optimization of operations (administration) and patient care (doctors, nurses, and therapists), which can lead to conflicts. However, the patient's well-being should be at the forefront, i.e. *responsibility for patient care*. This applies to all professional groups involved.

Everyone working in a hospital is also responsible for *the organization* they work for. However, this should also be aimed at the well-being of the patient and the well-being of the employees, but not primarily at the advantage of those involved in the profit, as is, unfortunately, the case with many institutions run by corporations. Although economic activity is a prerequisite for maintaining the healthcare system, the principle of profit orientation and commerce is increasingly being questioned [60]. Suppose moral responsibility is understood as the pursuit of the good and the common good. In that case, it violates these moral principles when corporate executives in the healthcare sector assume responsibility [61].

### 4.9 Population-related distributive justice

Finally, there is also a responsibility for p*opulation-related distributive justice.* In this context, it is often difficult for employees to distinguish between public health aspects and the economic interests of the company or hospital operator. These interests cannot be based on the availability of public resources. Marckmann explains that the various professional groups in the healthcare system (administration, medical and nursing staff, and other personnel) have different tasks and degrees of freedom of action but emphasizes that there is no difference in responsibility concerning the effects of their actions on patient care and economic efficiency [62, 63]. It is helpful for all involved, especially the business person, to be familiar with and guided by simple biomedical norms and principles (e.g., the principles of Beauchamp and Childress).

### 4.10 The quality of responsibility

The quality of responsibility in the various professional groups and management levels of the healthcare system distinguishes between autonomous action and delegated responsibility, as well as between nursing and medical responsibility for orders. However, there is an intrinsic connection between these terms and the concept of a shared ethics of responsibility for medical professions [29, 64].

In cases of conflict, bearing responsibility can also mean that one must seek justifiable alternatives, contrary to regulations, laws, or guidelines given, if these are not conducive to the good, in particular, the welfare of the patient [65, 66].

There is also a *responsibility for students* in training and junior doctors. This has now been included in the revised version of the Declaration of Geneva 2017: "I will [...] show my students the respect and gratitude they deserve." Finally, *responsibility for one's own health* was also enshrined: "I will take care of my own health, well-being and abilities in order to provide treatment at the highest level" [67].

During the coronavirus pandemic, the *triage* was discussed [36, 68]. Conflicts of interest arose from the scarcity of medicines. But also in organ transplantation, when the well-being of one patient has to be weighed against that of another patient, there is no doubt that the principles of *human rights* (equality and dignity of human beings) must determine the respective decisions.

There is also a *collective responsibility* of the entire medical profession [69]. Here, for example, medical associations or societies and organizations are called upon to express their views on topics such as dealing with pandemics, hunger in the world, vaccinations, climate change, and migration, even if it is not to be expected that a consensus can always be reached among all doctors here.

### 4.11 Hope and responsibility

The *principle of hope* [70] plays an important role in the recovery process and the relationship between patient and doctor (or treatment team). The patient goes to the doctor hoping to be cured or to find relief, and they do not want this hope to be taken away. This is not a problem for harmless illnesses, but it becomes a central issue when a serious diagnosis is made, such as cancer. In the case of a genetic disease or, for example, extreme prematurity, a conflict arises between the duty to inform and the *right not to know* [71].

As the saying goes: "You don't have to understand everything; sometimes it's enough to believe, hope and trust." Faith and hope address the theological virtues [65, 72] and it is also evident that faith and trust are very close. So, people are more likely to believe in God and more likely to trust a doctor.

In this context, hope is scientifically challenging to classify or measure and defies any norms. The spectrum ranges from hoping that threatening family events will pass to eternal life in the Kingdom of Heaven. It includes a lot of justified hopes but also irrational ones [73].

It should not be overlooked that there is no hope without fear, but also no fear without hope. In the Pandora saga of Greek mythology, Pandora opens her box, and all imaginable evils come upon humankind: disease, sorrow, hunger, and distress. Out of compassion, Zeus prevents hope from escaping in time, as it was also counted among the evils and regarded as deceptive and powerless. Nietzsche also regards hope as the greatest evil that has befallen man because it prevents him from dealing truthfully with himself and prolongs his agony [74].

With the third Kantian question, "What may I hope for?" Kant also sees hope more positively and recognizes it as a fundamental question of philosophy. It is precisely the suffering person, the patient, who needs hope. A person needs hope, just like Sisyphus; otherwise, he would not be able to accept the challenge of repeatedly hauling the stone up the mountain. The important thing is that every person has a right to hope, rather than that hope should be given to them [75]. Thus, when providing medical information, it is always a challenge not to take away the patient's hope, but not to give false hope—and for this, the doctor takes responsibility and becomes a bearer of hope for the patient [76].

One example of a measure in which hope plays an important role is the *prenatal examination* using non-invasive prenatal testing (NIPT) [77] to detect chromosomal abnormalities, which would also require a (time-consuming) explanation and, thus, the assumption of responsibility. The assumption of costs by health insurance companies has made the examination considerably easier and suggests something useful and positive to many pregnant women. In practice, however, this has led to the creation of a further screening examination. Ideally, there should be an indication for the examination, but the pregnant woman undergoes the examination in the hope that she will not be found to have a problem. False positive results are then problematic. Even more so, however, is the fact that this has led to the introduction of a screening test for disabilities that, particularly in the case of trisomy 21 (Down syndrome), leads to a termination of pregnancy in 90 percent of cases due to the initial shock or counseling to that effect.

This raises ethical questions about how to treat mentally disabled people, particularly with regard to their perspective and that of their families. Apart from the right to life of every sick person, the unbiased friendliness and cheerfulness of children with Down syndrome also mean a great deal for the affected families and society in many cases, as experience shows. Therefore, parents should always be given time to obtain detailed information and advice.

## 5. The autonomy and trust in the context of medical ethics of responsibility

### 5.1 The principle of autonomy

The *principle of autonomy* represents a significant development for the position of the patient [78]. For a long time, the Hippocratic Oath determined the moral orientation of medicine: the doctor decided what was good for the patient. The medical experts held the decision-making authority; the doctor-patient relationship was more of a patriarchal relationship. Patients had to trust their doctors. Trust meant handing over control and surrendering oneself [79]. In contrast to this, as early as 1977, Beauchamp and Childress added respect for the autonomy (self-determination) of the patient to the principle of care and trust as a paradigm shift and new ethos in their concept of biomedical principles. It was only 40 years later that it was enshrined in the Geneva Declaration [80].

On the one hand, this principle demands freedom from coercion or manipulative influence over the patient *(negative freedom).* Respect for autonomy also avoids (seemingly) well-meaning patronization with the risk of paternalism. This is particularly the case if a personal, medical, or even purely commercial interest, such as performing an operation, is involved. This also means that the doctor promotes the patient's freedom of choice *(positive freedom)* by consistently informing him. In doing so, it must be taken into account that many patients have already obtained a great deal of information independently, mainly from the internet ("Dr. Google") or from other doctors [81].

In practice, the principle of autonomy is expressed in the concept of *informed consent*, which should precede every medical intervention. Before any intervention, the patient must be provided with sufficient information in a language he understands. The patient should have understood the information, be capable of making a decision, make the decision voluntarily, and actively give his consent [82].

By enshrining the doctor-patient relationship as a separate contract in the German Civil Code, informing the patient is now less of an ethical problem. With the German Patients' Rights Act [83] of 20 February 2013, it has also become a legal duty, as the law codifies essential rights of patients, such as the right to comprehensive and timely information. In a compensation process, it is, together with detailed documentation, the focus of the investigations.

Akashe-Böhme and Böhme supplement the abstract concept of autonomy with sovereignty [36]: "A person is sovereign when they can allow something to happen to them and accept dependencies." [84].

Critical questions regarding the absolute principle of autonomy led to a modified concept of so-called *"relational autonomy"* [85], in which one can realistically only ever exercise one's self-determination in the context of social relationships and dependent on the support of others. This compensates for the weaknesses of the concept of autonomy without negating its significance.

The difference in knowledge between doctor and patient also presents a moral challenge, the so-called "moral hazard," [68] which always arises when there is an unequal distribution of information. In addition, there is the so-called "right not to know" [86], which is discussed because telling a patient, for example, that the prognosis is particularly poor can cause the patient's current medical condition to worsen. In this case, the patient, without wanting to know everything, relies entirely on the responsibility of his doctor.

## 5.2 Autonomy and trust

Nowadays, *autonomy and trust* are key concepts and central principles of modern medicine. In 2013, a research project on "Autonomy and Trust in Modern Medicine" was conducted at the University of Göttingen [87].

The principle of *autonomy* requires a *relationship of trust* (or confidentiality) between doctor and patient [88]. In this context, medicine is characterized by an exceptionally high level of trust in doctors among the population. According to a survey conducted in Germany in 2022, around 81 percent of respondents stated that they trust medical and healthcare personnel [89].

Trust therefore has a special significance for the doctor-patient relationship and is indispensable. A contract cannot replace it, and so the medical profession sees itself as a trust-based profession. Trust is also not something that can be calculated; it arises when there is a lack of information that could create mistrust. Something interpersonal must happen for the patient to open up, such as looking into each other's eyes. Only in this way can he develop the certainty that the doctor will take care of him [66].

This includes an examination of the relationship between trust and the principle of patient autonomy, which is central to modern medicine. It is a characteristic of personal integrity and means that the doctor stands by his own values and ideals [63].

## 5.3 Informed consent

In practice, the principle of autonomy is expressed in the Informed Consent, which should precede every medical intervention. This means that the patient must be informed sufficiently and informed in a language they can understand. The patient should:

- understand the information,
- be capable of making a decision,
- make a voluntary decision, and
- actively give his consent (3)

The knowledge asymmetry between doctor and patient will always persist. This gap can be narrowed by a transparent and respectful approach and by taking time for discussions. Unfortunately, the necessary time is usually lacking in the daily routine of a medical practice, but perhaps the necessary training is also missing.

By implementing *teach-back, shared decision-making* in the Informed Consent process may be enhanced [90]. The teach-back method [1] is a dynamic, interactive, and patient-centered process that may require multiple repeated sequential explanations, checks for comprehension, and clarifications. Finally, the question is asked, "tell me back, what I told you." The teach-back method is therefore a valuable tool to significantly improve patient safety and understanding.

The concept of informed consent in medicine is criticized, because Informed consent is experienced as a product of autonomy-dominated medical ethics which neglects intersubjective factors such as trust, concern, and care. The principle of Informed Consent also has two other aspects. On the one hand, there is a risk that doctors will no longer take responsibility for an action because the patient wanted it that way. Conversely, many patients are happy when, especially in difficult situations that are not understood anyway, the doctor takes the decision out of their hands and they can trust in his expertise.

### 5.4 Informed consent in decision-making in pediatrics

A special case is the autonomy of underage children. The experience, perspective, and power of children in the collaboration between pediatricians, their patients, and parents remain essential guide for modern ethical pediatric practice [1]. In the pediatric setting, most patients either lack the ability to act independently or have limited or no capacity for medical decision-making. Parental rights play a central role here. Nevertheless, Informed Consent means a child's agreement to medical procedures in circumstances where he or she is not legally authorized or lacks sufficient understanding to give consent competently. All children have a right to receive information given in a way that they can understand and give their assent or dissent. Doctors have the responsibility to determine the ability and competence of the child to give his or her consent or assent [91, 92]. Children may effectively refuse treatment or procedures that are not necessary to save their lives or prevent serious harm [2, 91, 92].

Trust and autonomy complement and reinforce each other. What primarily matters here is the doctor's moral integrity, sincerity, and veracity [64], which is the main statement in the middle of the Hippocratic Oath: "But I will keep pure and holy both my life and my art."[15] A lack of honesty, reliability, and integrity undermines any relationship of trust. But to do that, medicine needs supportive conditions and, above all, time. In addition to specialist knowledge, doctors must also have learned relationship-building skills. They should not be placed in a moral conflict, having to choose between the patient's well-being and the economic well-being of the clinic and become servants of two masters. This calls into question trust in medical decisions, which is why dealing with trust is so important [66].

[15] Hippocratic oath – ethical code: https://www.britannica.com/topic/Hippocratic-oath [Accessed: February 5, 2023].

### 5.5 Further aspects of trust

Trust is a phenomenon with many aspects of social interaction and is, thus, a valuable social good. It is not just a matter of deliberate, controlled human behavior that one has decided on for rational reasons; rather, it is shaped above all by tacit, often unconscious expectations. Those who trust accept their vulnerability in principle and believe in the ability and will of the other person to act in their interest.

Trust is based on the optimistic expectation that it will be fulfilled, but the trust recipient has sufficient scope for action and decision-making to disappoint this expectation under certain circumstances. Trust can also be broken or abused. In this case, the relationship of interaction is violated, even beyond legally guaranteed safeguards.

The hopes and expectations can be institutionalized in certain social roles (e.g., of parents or doctors) or institutions (e.g., the hospital, doctors, or health insurance companies) and thus enable a special form of social commitment and reliability. However, medicine has become so complex that not every single process can be understood by the patient, let alone controlled. However, this should not be used as a pretext for paternalistic tutelage.

At first glance, autonomy and trust seem to point in different directions. However, they are interdependent. Autonomy, in the sense of individual self-determination, requires control over one's actions. By contrast, trust presupposes the delivery of control. Without trust, we would have much less freedom of action. However, lasting trust is only possible for people who do not have to trust. On the one hand, trust can be earned by the physician; on the other, it can be voluntarily bestowed by the patient.

Autonomy and trust go hand in hand, even if this can lead to friction. The respect for the patient that is necessary for autonomy is not given simply by respecting his decisions; instead, a climate must be actively created in which patients feel taken seriously as unique individuals and can be sure that action is being taken in their interest. For these reasons, trust also has significance for the sphere of morals and, thus, of ethics.

However, the trust that has been acquired can also be undermined by too much information and regulation to obtain consent. On the other hand, blind trust poses a danger to the patient's autonomy [93].

Particularly concerning medical practice, it makes sense to distinguish between "personal" and "institutional" trust [80] Personal trust refers to trust in persons, while institutional trust refers to trust in institutions and institutional processes. Even a highly technical and professionalized medical system depends on personal trust between patients and physicians or medical personnel. However, this trust must also be complemented by trust in the institutions and processes of medicine through reliable regulations.

## 6. Consequences for medical training

Medical ethics has become increasingly important in recent decades, especially with the advances in intensive care medicine. Ethical questions increasingly arise at the beginning of life with premature infant medicine, abortion, prenatal diagnostics, preimplantation, and, in particular, non-intensive prenatal testing with all the consequences of human genetics. At the end of life, questions arise about euthanasia on demand, criteria for death, and organ transplantation. This results in the need for multidisciplinary expertise involving philosophy, research, clinical practice, jurisprudence, politics, ideology, etc. It is therefore all the more important to have knowledge of medical ethics for ethical action and decision-making. So it is necessary for medical ethical issues to be addressed during medical studies and the training of young physicians.

For a competence-orientated restructuring of medical studies, five moral-ethical competencies were specified by the Institute for Ethics, History, and Theory of Medicine at the Ludwig-Maximilians-Universität Munich [94]. They should be present for morally appropriate, ethically reflected actions by future physicians:

- the ability to form a professional moral compass,
- the willingness to align oneself with professional ethical norms and values,
- the ability to perceive moral dimensions of medical action,
- the ability to make moral judgments based on ethical considerations about the right action, and
- the willingness to realize ethically justified action.

These moral-ethical competencies can be used to design a curriculum for medical ethics in medical schools.

## Author details

Franz Staudt
Formerly, Kinderklinik Dritter Orden, Passau, Germany

*Address all correspondence to: franz.staudt@t-online.de

## References

[1] Staudt F. Economy in medicine – Ethical aspects. Monatsschrift für Kinderheilkunde. 2020;**168**:828-833. DOI: 10.1007/s00112-019-00824-8

[2] German Ethics Council. Ad hoc recommendation: Pandemic and Mental Health. Attention, support and assistance for children, adolescents and young adults in and after social crises. 2022. Available from: www.ethikrat.org/publikationen/kategorie/ad-hoc-empfehlungen [Accessed: November 30, 2022]

[3] Rehmann-Sutter C, Timmermans DM, Raz A. Non-invasive prenatal testing (NIPT): Is routinization problematic? BMC Medical Ethics. 2023;**24**:87. DOI: 10.1186/s12910-023-00970-5

[4] Lo B, Malina D, Pittman G, Morrissey S. Fundamentals of medical ethics – A new perspective series. The New England Journal of Medicine. 2023;**389**(25):2392-2394. DOI: 10.1056/NEJMe2308472

[5] Jameton A. The importance of physician climate advocacy in the face of political denial. AMA Journal of Ethics. 2017;**19**(12):1222-1237. DOI: 10.1001/journalofethics.2017.19.12.sect1-1712

[6] Maio G. Mittelpunkt Mensch: Ethik in der Medizin – Ein Lehrbuch. Vol. 58ff. Stuttgart: Schattauer Verlag; 2012

[7] Sara P, Giada GC. Thomas Percival. Discussing the foundation of medical ethics. Acta Biomed. 2018;**89**(3):343-348. DOI: 10.23750/abm.v89i3.7050

[8] Singer P. Praktische Ethik. Stuttgart: Reclam; 1994

[9] Tugendethik: https://de.wikipedia.org/wiki/Tugendethik [Accessed: February 2, 2023]

[10] Gerhardt V. Immanuel Kant. Vernunft und Leben, Stuttgart. 2002;**2002**:222

[11] Moskopp W. Der (Präferenz-) Utilitarismus Peter Singers, Federal Agency for Civic Education. 2018. Available from: http://dx.doi.org/http:/www.bpb.de/gesellschaft/umwelt/bioethik/208812/standpunkt-der-praeferenz-utilitarismus-peter-singers [Accessed: February 2, 2023]

[12] World Medical Association. WMA – Medical Ethics Manual. 2005. pp. 7-13. Available from: https://www.wma.net/what-we-do/education/medical-ethics-manual/

[13] Marckmann G. Was ist eigentlich prinzipienorientierte Medizinethik? Ärzteblatt Baden-Württemberg. 2000;**56**(12):499-502

[14] Staudt F, Schockenhoff E, editors. Ethics in Medicine. Freiburg: Publication of the Cadenabbia Academy of the Konrad Adenauer Foundation; 2016. Available from: https://www.altstipendiaten.de/wp-content/uploads/2017/07/Cadenabbia-Akademie-Ethik-in-der-Medizin-2016.pdf

[15] Shuster E. Fifty years later: The significance of the Nuremberg code. The New England Journal of Medicine. 1997;**337**:1436-1440

[16] Peel M. Human rights and medical ethics. Journal of the Royal Society of Medicine. 2005;**98**(4):171-173. DOI: 10.1258/jrsm.98.4.171

[17] Gordon J-S. Human rights in bioethics: Theoretical and applied. Ethical Theory and Moral Practice. 2012;**15**(3):283-294

[18] UNICEF. The Convention on the Rights of the Child. New York: UNICEF; 1989. Available from: https://www.unicef.org/child-rights-convention/convention-text [Accessed: February 04, 2025]

[19] Jeffrey GJ, Mercer R, Webb E, Nathawad R, Shenoda S, Lansdown G. Toward a child rights theory in pediatric bioethics. Perspectives in Biology and Medicine. 2015;**58**(3):306-319. DOI: 10.1353/pbm.2016.0014

[20] German Medical Association: World Medical Association Adopts New Medical Oath. 2017. Available from: https://www.aerzteblatt.de/nachrichten/83022/Weltaerztebund-verabschiedet-neues-aerztliches-Geloebnis [Accessed: November 21, 2022]

[21] BLÄK: Professional Code of Conduct for Physicians in Bavaria 2018. Available from: https://www.blaek.de/kammerrecht/berufsordnung-fuer-die-aerzte-bayerns/berufsordnung-fuer-die-aerzte-bayerns-bekanntmachung-vom-09-januar-2012-i-d-f-der-aenderungsbeschluesse-vom-28-oktober-2018-bayerisches-aerztebla-tt-12-2018-s-694 [Accessed: November 21, 2022]

[22] WMA International Code of Medical Ethics. 2006. Available from: https://web.archive.org/web/20100428131219/http://www.wma.net/en/30publications/10policies/c8/index.html [Assessed: February 04, 2025]

[23] Beauchamp TL, Childress JF. Principles of Biomedical Ethics. 6th ed. Oxford: Oxford University Press; 2013

[24] Department of Health, Education, and Welfare. National Commission for the Protection of Human Subjects of Biomedical and Behavioral Research: The Belmont report. Ethical principles and guidelines for the protection of human subjects of research. The Journal of the American College of Dentists. 2014;**81**(3):4-13

[25] Nagai H, Nakazawa E, Akabayashi A. The creation of the Belmont report and its effect on ethical principles: A historical study. Monash Bioethics Review. 2022;**40**:157-170. DOI: 10.1007/s40592-022-00165

[26] Oral History of the Belmont Report and the National Commission for the Protection of Human Subjects of Biomedical and Behavioral Research (Interview). Available from: 2004. https://www.hhs.gov/ohrp/education-and-outreach/luminaries-lecture-series/belmont-report-25th-anniversary-interview-tbeacham/index.html [Accessed: February 04, 2025]

[27] Ernst S. Am Anfang und Ende der Lebens – Grundfragen medizinischer thtik, 2. Auflage, p. 48 ff Herder, Freiburg; 2024

[28] Fins JJ, Miller F. Proportionality, pandemics, and medical ethics (editorial). The American Journal of Medicine. 2020;**133**(11):1243-1244. DOI: 10.1016/j.amjmed.2020.06.008

[29] Körtner UHJ. Grundkurs Pflegeethik (3rd Edition, 2008). Vienna: Fakultas Verlags- und Buchhandels AG; 2017. p. 85

[30] Weber M. Politik Als Beruf. Munich and Leipzig: Verlag von Duncker und Humblot; 1919

[31] Rogers W. The art of medicine – Moral responsibility in medicine: Where

are the boundaries? Lancet, Perspectives. 2020;**396**(10248):373-374

[32] Ashcroft RE. Individual freedom versus collective responsibility: An ethicist's perspective. Emerging Themes in Epidemiology. 2006;**3**:11. DOI: 10.1186/1742-7622-3-11

[33] Maio G. Mittelpunkt Mensch: Ethik in der Medizin – Ein Lehrbuch. Stuttgart: Schattauer Verlag; 2012. p. 422

[34] Erdle F. Politik als Beruf – Zwischen Gesinnung und Verantwortung, Der Geschäftsbericht der Nichteisen-Metallindustrie. 2018. https://wvmgb.s3.eu-central-1.amazonaws.com/18-19/index.html [Accessed: January 23, 2023]

[35] Medicoconsult: Gesinnungsethik und Verantwortungsethik (2023) https://www.medicoconsult.de [Accessed: January 30, 2023]

[36] Körtner UHJ. Grundkurs Pflegeethik. 3rd ed. Vienna: Fakultas Verlags- und Buchhandels AG; 2008. p. 85

[37] Schmidt I. Die Kraft der Verantwortung. Hamburg: Edition Körber; 2021

[38] Weber M. Politik Als Beruf. Munich and Leipzig: Verlag von Duncker und Humblot; 1919. p. 50

[39] Buscher K. Gesinnungsethik und Verantwortungsethik, Medicoconsult. 2023. Available from: https://www.medicoconsult.de/gesinnungsethik__verantwortungsethik/ [Accessed: February 05, 2025]

[40] Endreß M. Ethics (ethics of conviction and ethics of responsibility). In: Müller H, Sigmund S, editors. Max Weber-Handbuch. Stuttgart: J.B. Metzler; 2020. pp. 67-68

[41] Hoffmann AF. Tugendethik, Ethik-Evangelisch 2018. Available from: https://www.ethik-evangelisch.de/lexikon/tugendethik [Accessed: January 27, 2023]

[42] Weber M. Politik Als Beruf. Munich and Leipzig: Verlag von Duncker und Humblot; 1919. p. 65

[43] Gäbler M. Medizinethische Entscheidungen am Lebensende. Wiesbaden: Springer Fachmedien Wiesbaden; 2021

[44] Lampl L. Akutversorgung von Ertrinkungsunfälle. Stuttgart: Thieme Verlag; 2005. Available from: https://www.thieme.de/viamedici/klinik-faecher-notfallmedizin-1539/a/ertrinken-3947.htm

[45] Nauck F. Palliativmedizin in der Intensivmedizin. In: Burchardi´ H, Larsen R, et al., editors. Die Intensivmedizin. Berlin, Heidelberg: Springer; 2011. pp. 135-143. DOI: 10.1007/978-3-642-16929-8_14

[46] Parsa-Parsi R. World medical association: Questions at the end of life. Dtsch Arztebl. 2017;**114**:49

[47] Staudt F. Economy in medicine – Ethical aspects. Monatsschrift für Kinderheilkunde. 2020;**168**:831

[48] de Ridder M, Dißmann W. Vom Unheil sinnloser Medizin. Der Spiegel. 1998;**18**:202-210

[49] Aghabarary M, Nayeri ND. Medical futility and its challenges: A review study. Journal of Medical Ethics and History of Medicine. 2016;**20**(9):11

[50] Richter-Kuhlmann E. Futility: Grenzen der Sinnhaftigkeit (Limits of meaningfulness). Dtsch Arztebl. 2022;**119**(19):A-860/B-712

[51] Grübler B. Therapiebegrenzung bei infauster Prognose: Wann soll das Leben zu Ende gehen? Dtsch Arztebl. 2011;**10**(7):A-346/B-278/C-278

[52] Rössler D. Der Arzt Zwischen Technik Und Humanität. Munich: R. Piper & C0. Verlag; 1977. pp. 76-81

[53] Gerhard C. Praxiswissen Palliativmedizin. In: Thieme Verlag Stuttgart. 2nd ed. 2023. pp. 14-17

[54] National Institute on Aging: What Are Palliative Care and Hospice Care?. p. 62. Available from: https://www.nia.nih.gov/health/hospice-and-palliative-care/what-are-palliative-care-and-hospice-care [Accessed: February 04, 2025]

[55] World Health Organisation (WHO). Palliative Care for Children. Available from: https://www.who.int/europe/news-room/fact-sheets/item/palliative-care-for-children [Accessed: February 04, 2025]

[56] Boakye SO, Marx G, et al. Autonomy needs trust – Decision-making at the end of life. In: Wiesemann C, editor. "Autonomy and Trust" Key Concepts in Modern Medicine. Göttingen: Research Project at the University of Göttingen (brochure); 2014

[57] German Medical Association. Principles of the German medical association for the medical care of the dying. Dtsch Arztebl. 2011;**10**(7):A-346/B-278/C-278

[58] Fre C. Das Konzept der Menschenwürde in der medizinischen Ethik, Medizinische Materialien, Heft 190. Bochum. 2012;**64**

[59] Marckmann G. Praxisbuch Ethik in der Medizin, 2. Auflage, Med. Wiss. Berlin: Verlagsgesellschaft; 2022. p. 64

[60] Staudt F. Economy in medicine – Ethical aspects. Monatsschrift für Kinderheilkunde. 2020;**168**(2020):832

[61] Schmidt I. Die Kraft der Verantwortung. Edition Körber: Hamburg; 2021. p. 41

[62] Marckmann G. Praxisbuch Ethik in der Medizin. 2nd ed, Med. Wiss. Verlagsgesellschaft. Berlin; 2022. pp. 231-232

[63] Sincerity. Available from: https://www.duden.de/suchen/dudenonline/aufrichtig [Accessed: January 30, 2022]

[64] Beier K. Vertrauen in der Medizin. In: Schweer MKW, editor. (Hrsg)Facetten Des Vertrauens Und Misstrauens. Wiesbaden: Springer VS; 2022. pp. 265-285. DOI: 10.1007/978-3-658-29047-4_

[65] Schmidt I. Die Kraft der Verantwortung. Edition Körber: Hamburg; 2021. p. 43

[66] Schäfer I. Die Bedeutung von Vertrauen in der Medizin, Stuttgarter Neue Nachrichten. 2022. Available from: https://www.stuttgarter-nachrichten.de/inhalt.stuttgart-neue-reihe-via-medici-im-hospitalhof-die-bedeutung-von-vertrauen-in-der-medizin.0cdb445c-8511-45fa-8320-5743b0385bd9.html [Accessed: February 03, 2025]

[67] World Medical Association: WMA Declaration of Geneva. Available from: https://www.wma.net/policies-post/wma-declaration-of-geneva [Accessed: February 06, 2025]

[68] Rowell D, Connelly LB. A history of the term 'moral hazard'. Journal of Risk and Insurance. 2012;**79**(4):1051-1075

[69] Newton LH. Collective responsibility in health car. The Journal of Medicine and Philosophy. 1982;**7**(1):11-21. DOI: 10.1093/jmp/7.1.11

[70] Westin A. Despite Circumstance': The principles of medical ethics and the role of Hope. New Bioethics. 2018;**24**(3):258-267. DOI: 10.1080/20502877.2018.1487703

[71] David EO. The 'right' not to know. The Journal of Medicine and Philosophy: A Forum for Bioethics and Philosophy of Medicine. 1984;**9**(3):301-312. DOI: 10.1093/jmp/9.3.301

[72] Paulus: 1. Corintherbrief 13:13. Available from: https://www.oekumenischer-christusdienst.de/glaube-hoffnung-liebe/ [Accessed: January 6, 2025]

[73] Frewer A, Bruns F, Rascher W, editors. Hoffnung Und Verantwortung – Herausforderung für Die Medizin. Würzburg: Verlag Königshausen & Neumann; 2010. p. 9

[74] Nietzsche FW. Die fröhliche Wissenschaft. Gröls Verlag; 2021

[75] Flasspoehler S. Interview, Ottfried Höffe: "I may hope if I do what I am supposed to". 2021. Available from: https://www.philomag.de/artikel/otfried-hoeffe-kant-hoffnung [Accessed: November 6, 2024]

[76] Glaser F. The Doctor as the Sick Person's Beacon of Hope. 2009. Available from: https://www.gemeinschaftskrankenhaus.de/fileadmin/Bilddaten-GKH-Web/Downloads/01-Medizin-Therapie-Pflege/01Fachabteilungen/Chirurgie/GKH.Glaser.Arzt.als.Hoffnungstraeger.pdf [Accessed: December 15, 2024]

[77] Richter-Kuhlmann E. Noninvasive prenatal tests: Possible expansion in focus. Dtsch Arztebl. 2024;**121**(21):A-1368/B-1160

[78] Baden-Württemberg L. Beauchamp and Childress (2013): Principles of biomedical ethics. 1979. 1. Respect for patient autonomy. Available from: https//www.schule-bw.de [Accessed: January 28, 2023]

[79] Rüegger H. Vertrauen in der Medizin – Eine ethische Perspektive, ppt-presentation-handout, Privatklinik Hohenegg, Meilen/ Switzerland. Available from: https://file:///C:/Users/user01/Downloads/rueegger_vertrauen-in-der-Medizin_ethisch_praesentation_symposium-hohenegg_09-18(2).pdf [Accessed: February 03, 2023]

[80] Yuan H, Long Q, Huang GL, Luo S. Different roles of interpersonal trust and institutional trust in COVID-19 pandemic control. Social Science & Medicine. 2021;**293**:114677. DOI: 10.1016/j.socscimed.2021.114677

[81] Tscharke G. Dr. Google is Almost Always Wrong About Illnesses. 2020. Available from: https://www.br.de/nachrichten/wissen/dr-google-liegt-bei-krankheiten-fast-immer-daneben,RzLHgfl [Accessed: December 02, 2022]

[82] Bernat JL. Informed consent in pediatric neurology. Seminars in Pediatric Neurology. 2002;**9**(1):10-18

[83] Federal Law Gazette. Law to improve the rights of patients; Federal law Gazette, 2013. Part I No. 2013;**9**

[84] Akashe-Böhme F, Böhme G. Mit Krankheit leben: Von der Kunst, mit Schmerz und Leid umzugehen. 2nd ed. Munich: C.H. Beck; 2023. p. 62

[85] Fink U. Aspekte einer relationalen Autonomie. 2019. Available from: https://www.erzbistum-koeln.de/export/sites/ebkportal/seelsorge_und_glaube/krankheit_und_pflege/.content/.galleries/ethik-medizin-pflege/2019-10-29-Ethikforum_Fink_Relationale-

Autonomie.pdf [Accessed: December 02, 2022]

[86] Davis B, Savulscu J. The right not to know: Some steps towards to a compromise. Ethical Theory and Moral Practice. 2021;**24**:137-150. DOI: 10.1007/s10677-020-10133-9

[87] Steinfath H, Wiesemann C, editors. Autonomy and Trust. Springer Fachmedien Wiesbaden: Key Concepts in Modern Medicine; 2016

[88] Landesbildungsserver Baden-Württemberg: Beauchamp and Childress: Principles of Biomedical Ethics. (1979) 1. Respect for Patient Autonomy. 2013. Available from: file:///C:/Users/user01/Downloads/vier-medizinethische-prinzipien-karteikarte.pdf

[89] Pawlik V. Survey in Germany on Trust in Medicine and Health Personnel. 2022. Available from: https://de.statista.com/statistik/daten/studie/1182464/umfrage/umfrage-in-deutschland-zumvertrauen-in-die-medizin-und-dasgesundheitspersonal/ [Accessed: March 03, 2025]

[90] Seely KD, Higgs JA, Butts L, Roe JM, et al. The "teach-back" method improves surgical informed consent and shared decision-making: A proof of concept study. Patient Safety in Surgery. 28 Oct 2022;**16**(1):33. DOI: 10.1186/s13037-022-00342-9

[91] American Academy of Pediatrics. Informed Consent in Decision-Making in Pediatric Practice. Policy Statement, Pediatrics. 2016;**138**(2):484. DOI: 10.1542/peds.2016-1484

[92] Levy M, Larcher V, Kurz R. Informed consent/assent in children. Statement of the Ethics Working Group of the confederation of European specialists in paediatrics (CESP). European Journal of Pediatrics. 2003;**162**(9):629-633. DOI: 10.1007/s00431-003-1193-z

[93] Pindur A-M, Steinfath H. Wechselspiel von Autonomie und Vertrauen. In: Wiesemann C, editor. (Hrsg)"Autonomy and Trust" Key Concepts in Modern Medicine. Research project at the University of Göttingen (brochure); 2014

[94] Kühlmeyer K, Wolkenstein A, Schütz M, Wild V, Marckmann G. Kompetenzorientierte Ethik-Lehre im Medizinstudium 2021. Ethik in der Medizin. Heidelberg; 2022;**34**:301-318. Available from: https://epub.ub.uni-muenchen.de/106404/1/s00481-022-00700-2.pdf

Section 2

# Technological Advancements

Chapter 4

# Human Enhancement and Our Future Off-Earth

*Chris Impey*

## Abstract

After over a half century when the Space Race was dominated by the world's only two superpowers, a commercial space industry is emerging. Reusable rockets are lowering the cost to reach Earth orbit, and a growing number of civilians are going into space. In the future, as the first colonies are established on the Moon and Mars, bioethical issues will arise. Space travelers will probably self-select to adopt cutting edge technologies, including biomedical strategies for adapting to and thriving in these alien environments. Colonists are likely to pursue genetic engineering, "hacking" of their own genomes, and 3D printing of tissues, organs, and replacement body parts. There is no existing space law to regulate any of these activities, and there has been little attention to the ethical implications. Human enhancement as people move off-Earth is a rich subject for future study, with a view to understanding the pros and cons and operating in space using the same ethical frameworks we have established on Earth.

**Keywords:** space travel, space exploration, colonization, ethics, space law, human enhancement, gene editing

## 1. Introduction

A profound change is taking place in space travel. The first satellite was put into Earth orbit in 1957. Sputnik was the size of a beach ball and weighed no more than an adult. The first human to orbit the Earth was Yuri Gagarin, who spent about an hour and a half in space in 1961. The rest of the decade saw an intense competition between the world's two superpowers to venture into space [1]. While the Soviet Union had most of the initial landmark achievements—first artificial satellite, first man in space, first woman in space, first spacewalk, first space station, and the first probes sent to Venus and Mars—the United States had a major milestone with the Apollo program [2]. Between 1969 and 1972, twenty-four American astronauts traveled to the Moon and twelve walked on its surface. For the next few decades, space was the hegemony of the United States and the Soviet Union, in a geopolitical rivalry with military implications. America concentrated on the Space Shuttle [3] and the International Space Station (ISS) [4], and dreams of going beyond Earth orbit were set aside.

In the past few years, we have witnessed the dawning of a new Space Age. The catalyst for this was the Ansari XPRIZE, a challenge for privately funded teams to build a spaceship that could travel twice within two weeks to an altitude of 100 km, the formal boundary of outer space [5]. In 2004, the $10 million prize was won with a spacecraft designed by Burt Rutan and financed by Paul Allen [6]. Between 2001 and 2009, seven civilians went into space, traveling to the ISS on a Russian Soyuz spacecraft. They paid $20–25 million per trip, giving little indication of a broader commercial market for space tourism. The innovation that has spurred increased space activity is reusable rockets. In 2015, SpaceX and Blue Origin each successfully recovered rockets that had been in orbit and landed them vertically [7]. The cost to launch a kilogram into Earth orbit is dropping dramatically, see **Figure 1** [8]. Since 2020, there have been a flurry of missions putting civilian astronauts into space. SpaceX and Blue Origin are run by their billionaire CEOs Elon Musk and Jeff Bezos, who have invested some of their personal fortunes in their space startups [9].

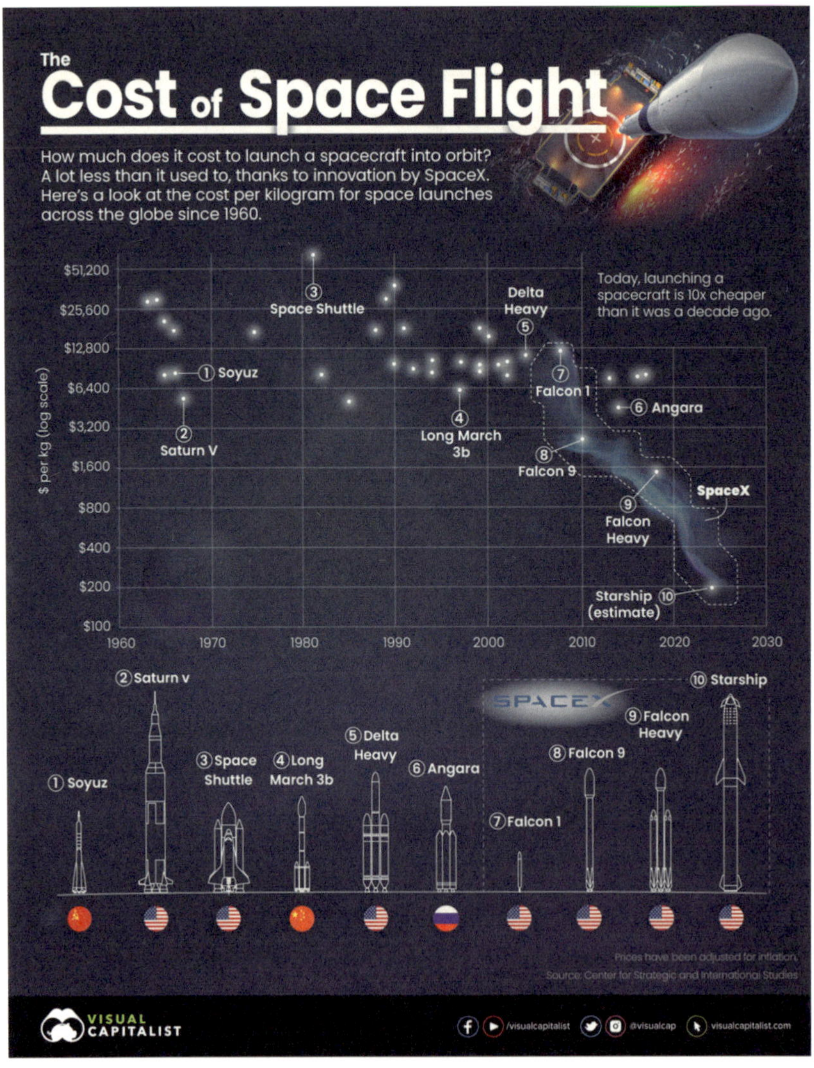


**Figure 1.**
*The cost per kilogram of launching to Earth orbit since 1960. Reusable rockets, especially by SpaceX, have lower the cost by almost a factor of a hundred in fifteen years (Credit Visual Capitalist, https://www.visualcapitalist.com/the-cost-of-space-flight/).*

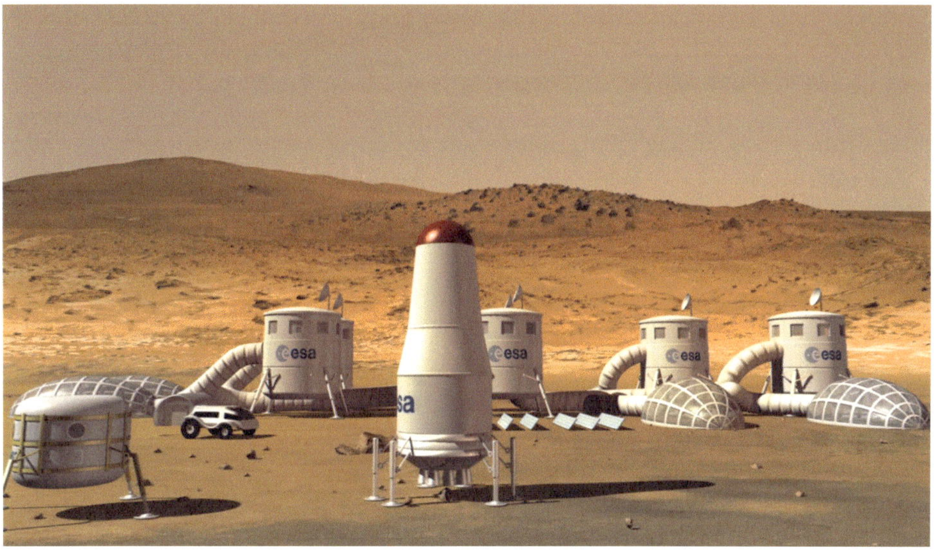


**Figure 2.**
*Concept of a Mars base developed by the European Space Agency; a project unlikely to be realized for 15 to 20 years (Credit ESA/Martin Kornmesser).*

All this activity is in low Earth orbit, at an altitude of 250 to 250 miles. However, NASA plans to return astronauts to the Moon with the Artemis mission [10], and China is a new space rival to the United States, with plans to build a Moon base [11]. Mars is much further than the Moon so even a short-term visit by a few astronauts represents an extremely difficult mission. The very heavy lift capability of SpaceX's Starship is central to Elon Musk's plans to establish a permanent colony on Mars, also see **Figure 2** for concept of a Mars base by the European Space Agency [12]. The motivation is that the long-term survival of humanity may depend on us becoming a multiplanetary species. Another off-Earth activity that might become possible in the next few decades is mining asteroids [13]. To leave the Solar System would require new, nonchemical forms of propulsion, making that a distant prospect [14]. Any long-term habitation off-Earth raises important questions about how humans might adapt to survive the rigors of zero gravity and the challenging space environment.

## 2. Health effects of space travel

If humans are to routinely live and work in space, the health consequences need to be understood. A major hazard for space travelers is radiation [15]. On Earth, the atmosphere and magnetic field provide protection against high energy radiation and particles from space. The three major sources are particles trapped within Earth's magnetic field, energetic particles from the Sun, and galactic cosmic rays. The latter causes the most cellular damage. Radiation exposure increases the risk of cancers and degenerative diseases, such as heart disease and cataracts. The type of radiation in space causes worse health outcomes than the radiation experienced on Earth and once astronauts leave Earth orbit, radiation is the top health risk [16]. Zero gravity or microgravity is the second major risk, with weight-bearing bones losing 1–1.5% of mineral density per month during spaceflight [17]. The microbial ecosystem of a spacecraft can impact astronaut health. Microbes and pathogens travel between people very rapidly in the closed environment, and stress hormone levels are often elevated. Earth-based analogs do not perfectly simulate the spacecraft environment. Last, there are psychological and physiological stress factors resulting from isolation and confinement, which will be amplified for any trip beyond Earth orbit.

The International Space Station has played an essential role in understanding the effects of the space environment, particularly zero gravity, on human physiology. It has been continuously occupied for over 24 years since 2000, by 280 people from 23 countries [18]. Eight NASA astronauts have spent over 200 consecutive days in space, with Frank Rubio holding the record at 371 days. Many astronauts get to fly on multiple missions, and six astronauts have spent over 380 cumulative days in space, with the record held by Peggy Whitson at 675 days [19]. Russian cosmonauts have logged extensive time in the ISS as well as the Russian Mir Space Station, which operated from 1986 to 2001. Eight cosmonauts have logged over 365 consecutive days in orbit, led by Valerie Polyakov with 438 days. Almost all the records for the most cumulative time in space are held by Russians. Seven cosmonauts have been up for more than 700 days, with Oleg Kononenko setting the record in 2024, after his fifth ISS mission, of 1111 days [20].

Of the many medical studies conducted on ISS astronauts, the most interesting was an 11-month research project studying the effects of long-term spaceflight on astronaut Scott Kelly and cosmonaut Mikhail Kornienko [21]. The pair launched on 27 March 2015 in a Soyuz spacecraft and landed in Kazakhstan on 2 March 2016. They were part of the NASA Twins Study, since Mark Kelly, Scott's identical twin, also an astronaut, stayed on Earth, see **Figure 3**. They kept a journal during the experiment, to investigate the psychological effects of living in a confined space. Results of the study demonstrated several long-lasting changes when one twin was compared to the other. They included changes in telomere length, gene regulation, gut microbiome composition, carotid artery dimensions, retina thickness, serum metabolites, and body weight. There was also some eye and bone deformation [22]. Certain factors

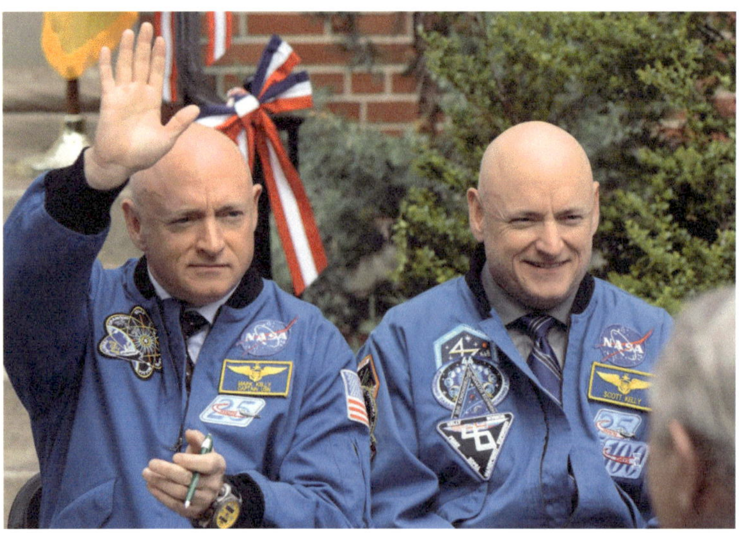

**Figure 3.**
*Mark and Scott Kelly are identical twins and NASA astronauts. In 2015, Scott spent nearly a year in space, while his brother remained on the ground. The physiological effects of long-term spaceflight were documented in the NASA Twins Study, which was published in 2019 (Credit NASA/Derek Storm).*

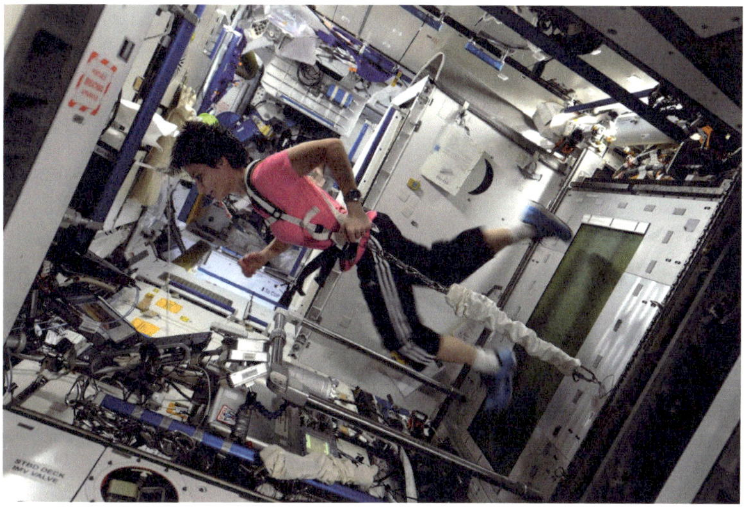

**Figure 4.**
*ESA astronaut Samantha Cristoforetti runs on the International Space Station's T2 treadmill (Credit ESA/NASA).*

were affected by the stress of the return to Earth, like inflammation cytokines and immune response gene networks. Persistent changes were observed even after six months back on Earth. Notably, the astronauts suffered increased DNA damage from chromosomal inversions, an increased number of short telomeres, and attenuated cognitive function. A total of 28 experiments were conducted [23].

The easiest mitigation against loss of bone and muscle tissue in zero gravity is exercise. Early missions used simple elastics bands, but exercise hardware aboard the ISS has become increasingly sophisticated. The challenge is creating resistance in a situation where there is no gravity to give assistance through Newton's third law. To fend off tissue deterioration, astronauts average two hours exercise every day. A weight-lifting system called the Advanced Resistive Exercise Device (ARED) has been in routine use since 2008. Pistons and flywheels mimic weightlifting while weightless. Astronauts use preflight training, just as athletes depend on preseason training to help with later competition [24]. Another system allowed 18 different exercises with up to 300 pounds of resistive force. The ISS cycling machine is called the Cycle Ergometer with Vibration Isolation and Stabilization System (CEVIS). Even with this regimen, 1 in 6 astronauts experienced loss of cardiorespiratory fitness [25]. A treadmill is also used for aerobic training, see **Figure 4**, and research results guided NASA to prefer high-intensity short workouts, letting crew members use the equipment more efficiently. Muscle biopsies identified an enzyme product that was an indicator of muscle health. Current exercise protocols are adequate to maintain health for up to a year [26], but Moon, Mars, and deep space missions will last two years or more, so will need additional research and new protocols.

## 3. Human enhancement off-earth

Space is a brutal and unnatural environment for humans. The physical extremes—total vacuum, high energy radiation, hundreds of degrees of temperature variation from day to night—require protection and climate control. So far, human exposure to space has been limited. Fewer than 700 people have been in Earth orbit, and only 50 have been in space for over a year. They suffered various bodily indignities, but for a limited time [27]. Viable space tourism needs a low enough cost to rival high end vacation experiences on Earth and a vehicle reliability that rivals commercial aircraft [28]. Health consequences for short recreational trips are minimal. But if the space visionaries and billionaire entrepreneurs are right, the time has come to consider long duration spaceflight and our future off-Earth [29]. A one-way trip to Mars would give travelers 700 times the radiation dose of Earth, over a lifetime's worth [30]. A spinning spacecraft with artificial gravity could remove the negative effects of weightlessness [31]. However, in both cases the protection measures will raise costs. Radiation-stopping material like lead would add mass, and a spacecraft large enough to generate artificial gravity will be more massive and complex than a non-spinning spacecraft.

One avenue of human enhancement to consider for future colonists on the Moon and Mars is pharmacological. The issue starts with maintaining a supply or routine drugs and medicines. Even a minimal voyage to Mars will take 2.5 years: 6 months to get there, 18 months to wait for a favorable alignment for the return trip, and 6 months to get home. It would be impossible (and prohibitive in weight) to pack all potentially useful drugs, and limited shelf life means they would become useless partway through a journey. Some drugs will be conventional. For example, the U.S. military uses stimulants and hypnotics to boost performance under duress, regain strength, and facilitate sleep. They have also developed a pancreatic enzyme that accelerates the healing of wounds [32]. NASA is developing an innovative concept called "Astropharmacy," where small quantities of pharmaceuticals can be made in space, on site, and on demand [33]. It centers on a class of therapeutics based on peptides or proteins, used on Earth to treat embolisms, hemorrhages, bone loss, renal stone formation, thrombotic complications, and various inflections. This system will use genetically engineered and pre-programmed cells that are in a space-hardy spore form, then get reconstituted in a sterile medium so the protein can be expressed as a drug. The system would be compact and use microfluidics to not need an external pump [34]. The approach is the opposite of that taken by the pharmaceutical companies on Earth, which produce many doses at a high profit. It could be a model for making "orphan" drugs and delivering personalized medicine.

Genetic engineering is an important tool for human enhancement, since it can potentially ameliorate the effects of both radiation and reduced gravity. Gravity on the Moon and Mars is 16% and 38% of terrestrial gravity, respectively. The least controversial form of gene editing uses somatic cells, since the effects would not be heritable. Tools in this emerging field are developing rapidly. Epigenetic engineering can turn on or off the expression of particular genes [35]. CRISPR has revolutionized genetic engineering, allowing precise and targeted editing of the genomes of living organisms [36], see **Figure 5**. In addition to aiding human adaptation to extreme levels of radiation and low gravity, CRISPR could enable tolerance of low oxygen levels, resistance to muscle and bone atrophy, and even help induce hibernation [37]. However, the technology is not perfect. Off-target effects can occur when CRISPR edits unintended parts of the genome, leading to mutations and health issues. On-target edits can also have unintended results, such as large deletions, translocations, and activation of cancer-causing oncogenes [38]. Another strategy combines the DNA of other species with human cells to enhance a survival trait. Tardigrades are tiny animals that can survive the vacuum and radiation of space [39]. Scientists have identified a protein that protects against radiation damage in tardigrades and have transferred that resistance to human cells [40].

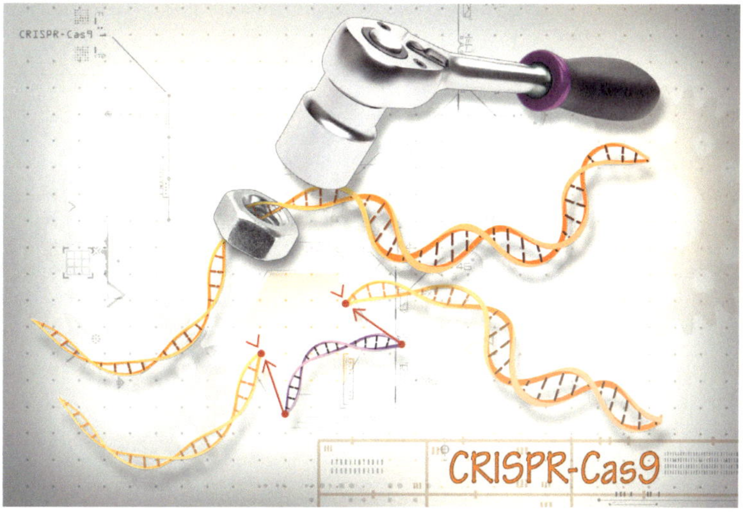


**Figure 5.**
*CRISPR-Cas9 is a tool that lets scientists cut and insert small pieces of DNA at precise areas along a DNA strand. The Cas9 protein acts like the wrench, and the RNA guides, CRISPRs, act as the set of different socket heads. CRISPR can allow for targeted gene editing to allow astronauts to live off-Earth (Credit NIGMS/NIH).*

Gene therapy can only go so far in taking care of human health off-Earth. For routine illnesses and to diagnose more complicated problems, a doctor is needed. The ISS only occasionally has a medical doctor on board; it is assumed that a sick astronaut can quickly return to Earth for treatment. But the Moon and Mars are weeks or months from any hospital. Even if a doctor is among the first colonists, they cannot be experts on all possible conditions, and MRI and CT scanners cannot be miniaturized enough to send them into space [41]. Simple medical equipment could be 3D printed using materials on Mars. Also, the doctor might be the person needing attention. Remote guidance from a terrestrial doctor fails when the communication lag ranges up to 45 minutes. A surgical robot would have to be fully autonomous. Even with a small crew of seven, there will be about one surgical emergency every 2.4 years on Mars [42]. Trauma surgery would be extremely challenging, and even a simple kidney stone could be life-threatening [43]. Useful lessons have been learned from people working at Antarctic bases, the closest analogs to deep space isolation (**Figure 6**). The Antarctic also provides the chilling story of Leonid Rogozov. In 1961, as the polar winter was setting in, the young surgeon diagnosed himself with acute appendicitis. Aided by two assistants, and without anesthetic, since it would dull his senses, Rogozov spent two agonizing hours removing his own appendix and sewing himself up again. He nearly died but was back to normal duties a week later [44].

If an autonomous Martian colony is ever established, enhancement will happen naturally through the process of evolution. The "magic number" to create a viable population for a Mars colony or for multigenerational space travel is 160—the size of a small village [45]. This assumes a judiciously selected gene pool. The population will experience genetic drift, a loss of genetic variation and genetic divergence from the original population. Genetic drift is the change in the frequency of gene variants or alleles due to random sampling [46]. Reduced genetic variation is a double-edged sword. On the one hand, it reduces a population's ability to respond to new selective pressures. On the other hand, genetic drift is a major driver of evolution, and it can lead to new species. How this would proceed is a matter of speculation [47]. Lower

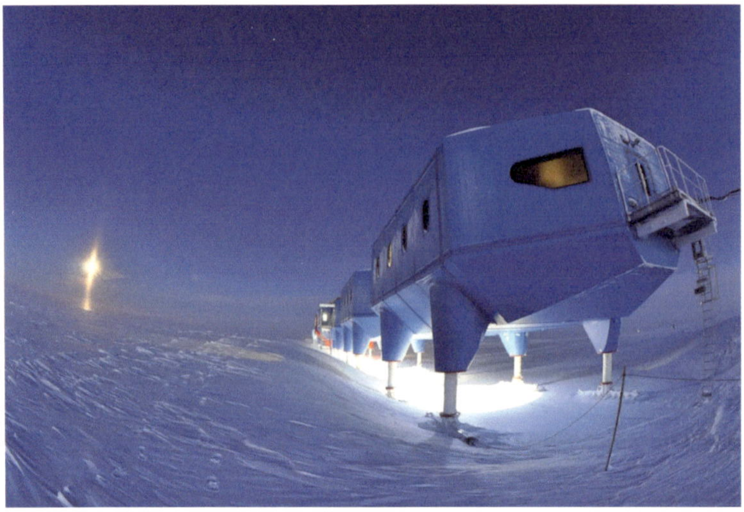

**Figure 6.**
*The Halley VI base of the British Antarctic Survey. Research stations in Antarctica provide the best analogs for the long-term isolation and remoteness from medical facilities that would be experienced by off-Earth colonists (Credit National Environment Research Council/British Antarctic Survey).*

gravity on Mars will alter the cardiovascular system and reduce the cross-sectional area of load-bearing bones and tendons. Trends seen in humans on Earth might be accelerated—toward being taller, and having less body hair, weaker muscles, and smaller teeth. Skin pigment would darken, to protect against the higher radiation even experienced by people who rarely venture outside a protective habitat. The lack of a varied natural environment would weaken immune systems. All of this might lead, after thousands of generations, to a new human species.

Some human enhancement goes beyond the technologies just mentioned. It is routine in medicine to replace hard body parts like hips and knees, soft body parts like livers and hearts, and even complex appendages such as hands [48]. Synthetic blood and tissues have emerged from the lab and are used in clinical settings. Gene therapy will be similarly routine within a decade. Technology can assist or enhance physical capabilities. Powered exoskeletons have been in development for decades, driven by the industrial workplace [49], and the needs of soldiers and firefighters, who carry heavy loads and who must be protected in the field [50]. Think of it as a wearable robot (**Figure 7**). A soft pneumatic exoskeleton has been tested that can prevent muscle atrophy on long-duration space missions [51]. Haptic gloves could also give the colonists an enhanced interface with their environment [52]. These technologies are external and assistive, but brain-computer interfaces can also be implanted. On Earth, brain-computer interfaces restore speech, touch, movement, and other functions to patients with brain damage [53]. Health monitoring can be done with devices that are wearable, ingestible, or implantable [54]. For off-Earth colonists, these interfaces would enable remote control of their health and systems that maintain the safety and smooth functioning of the base.

Radical enhancement strategies start with implants. In 2023, Neuralink became the first company to get FDA permission to perform brain implants to help patients regain speech, sight, or movement [55]. Neuralink's owner, Elon Musk, imagines the technology being part of his plan to colonize Mars [56]. In 1960, Manfred Clynes and Nathan Kline envisaged an eventual merger of human and machine, and they coined

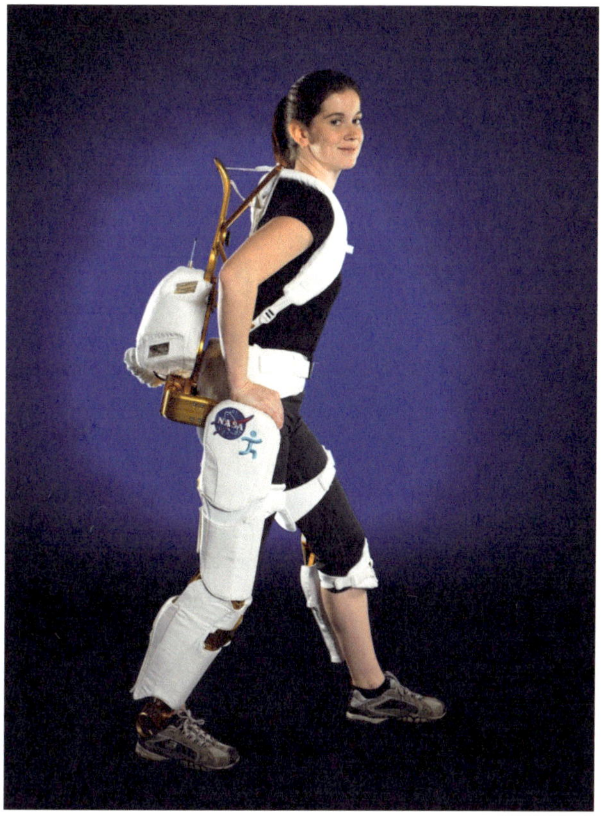

**Figure 7.**
*The NASA X1 Robotic Exoskeleton for resistive exercise and mobility augmentation, with 4 motorized joints and 10 degrees of freedom (Credit NASA).*

the word cyborg to describe this hybrid creature [57]. Cyborgs feature prominently in dystopian science fiction, but the technologies to make them reality are advancing rapidly. As a step along that road, cybernetics professor Kevin Warwick had an RFID chip put in his arm in 1998. Four years later, he had an electrode array implant that let him extend his nervous system over the Internet and control a robotic hand at a remote location. His wife also had a similar implant, and when someone grasped her hand, he was able to feel the same sensation in his hand on the opposite side of the Atlantic, in a bizarre form of cybernetic telepathy [58]. Many promising applications of cyborg technology are emerging when machines are miniaturized to the scale of cells. Tools can be engineered to seamlessly integrate with cells, tissues, organs, or entire animals. Their functions include acting as sensors, actuators, manipulators, assemblers, and drug carriers [59]. For space colonists, these miniature robots will roam within the bloodstream, monitoring vital functions, delivering medicines, and even performing microsurgery.

Neil Harbisson was officially recognized as a cyborg in 2004 after having a radio antenna implanted in his skull. He senses phone calls and satellite signals as audible vibrations. He also uses a head-mounted device to extend his senses by converting ultrasound and wavelengths beyond the visible spectrum into vibrations that he can hear through the bones in his head [60]. This type of experimentation can be seen in research labs, but it has also gone deep underground in the biohacking movement. Biohackers, or "grinders,' do their own implants, often with no anesthetic [61]. A popular starting point is to insert a powerful rare earth magnet into the fingertip. This lets the person sense a variety of electromagnetic fields, as well as subways passing underground and power lines hanging overhead. More advanced biohacks are implanting a sensor that talks to a smartphone or a device that can let fingers "see" by echolocation [62]. The first astronauts in the Mercury, Gemini, and Apollo program formed a monoculture of men with military test pilot backgrounds. They were selected to be disciplined and have a high tolerance for risk. Mars colonists will be more genetically diverse, but they will be technologically savvy and might plausibly share the biohacker ethos of enhancement through physical implants.

Overlying all these mechanistic strategies for human enhancement is the role of computers powered by artificial intelligence (AI). The Apollo Moon landings were carried out using an onboard computer that was far less powerful than a low-end smartphone. AI is transforming every aspect of our personal and professional lives, and it will continue to advance rapidly [63]. By the time colonists will be living off-Earth, it is safe to assume that AI will form an invisible "web" around them, acting to keep them safe and healthy, and advising on suitable means of human enhancement. AI will play an important role in every aspect of a Moon or a Mars colony. It will use geological mapping to help identify optimal sites for a base, including lava tubes that provide protection against radiation and a capacious living volume without needing much excavation [64]. For the journey to Mars, AI can calculate the safest and most fuel-efficient trajectories and mitigate the long communication delays with Earth by making autonomous real-time decisions. It could orchestrate a small army of robots and 3D printers for the construction of the base. 3D printers can also be harnessed to create tissues, organs, and replacement body parts. When the base is operating, AI will coordinate rovers and drones to map local geology, identifying the mineral deposits and areas of subsurface frozen water. It can optimize life support systems and ensure the efficient use of oxygen, water, and food [65]. AI can even monitor mental health, using a sentiment analysis of colonist communications to identify stresses and potential conflicts before they jeopardize the mission.

There is a final aspect of enhancement that moves from science toward science fiction and fantasy. Futurists extrapolate the trajectories of medicine and computers into a movement called transhumanism. Transhumanists believe that a combination of AI, nanotechnology, cryonics, and genetic engineering might enable humans to transcend their current biological limitations and evolve into a "posthuman" species [66]. That would unlock the possibility of travel to the stars. Current rockets still use chemical fuel, so the skyscraper-sized SpaceX Starship is a cousin of the tiny liquid-fueled rocket that Robert Goddard flew in 1926. Even the nearest stars are millions of times further away than Mars. To reach them, we will need new forms of rocket propulsion [67]. The journey would still last longer than a human lifetime, requiring suspended animation with speculative, unproven technologies like cryopreservation and cryonics [68]. Tardigrades achieve metabolic shutdown called cryptobiosis, see **Figure 8**, and it is possible this method might be applied to larger animals [69]. The energy requirements can drop dramatically if the interstellar mission sends frozen embryos rather than adult humans [70]. There has been some success in freezing embryos and growing them for limited periods of time in artificial uteri [71]. The embryos can be unfrozen at the destination, such as an Earth-like planet orbiting a nearby star or created there with frozen sperm and egg cells. Autonomous robots

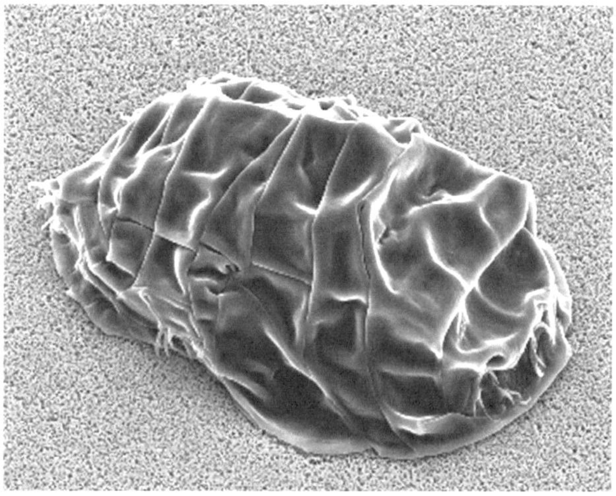

**Figure 8.**
*Scanning electron microscope image of a tardigrade in the tun state, after cryptobiosis reduces metabolic activity almost to zero. This method might eventually be used for humans (Credit Schokraie et al., Creative Commons 2.5 license, https://doi.org/10.1371/journal.pone.0045682.g001).*

would build base infrastructure and raise and educate the newly formed humans. With this remote and chilling—both literally and metaphorically—scenario, we have reached the outer limits of human enhancement.

## 4. Legal and ethical issues

The human enhancement discussed in this article will take place not only in the literal vacuum of space but also in a legal near vacuum. International space law is based on just two pieces of legislation in the past sixty years. The United Nations Outer Space Treaty of 1967 said that no country can claim ownership of planetary or celestial bodies, and that they should only be used for peaceful purposes [72]. Crucially, the treaty prohibited nuclear weapons in space, and it was signed by all the major spacefaring countries. However, the treaty said nothing about companies or individuals, or about the utilization of space resources, so it is not helpful in an era when commercial space activity is surging. Subsequently, the Moon Agreement of 1979 said that the Moon and its natural resources are the common heritage of humanity. However, this treaty is moot since no major spacefaring country has signed it yet [73]. The United Nations also crafted an ancillary "Rescue Agreement" for returning astronauts from deep space, a "Liability Convention" addressing any damage caused by deep space objects, and a "Registration Agreement" to track all objects launched into space. Continuing U.N. oversight comes via the Committee on the Peaceful Uses of Outer Space (COPUS), set up by the General Assembly in 1959 [74]. COPUS has approved 21 nonbinding sustainability guidelines and for the first time in 45 years is considering new treaties. However, none of them address legal and ethical issues associated with human settlements off-Earth.

The framework of statutes and regulations around enhancement is similarly lax. In the vacuum left by international law, countries have acted to protect their own interests. In 2015, Barack Obama signed the U.S. Space Launch Competitiveness Act, recognizing the right of Americans to own any space resources they might harvest and encouraging commercial exploitation of asteroids [75]. In 2020, Donald Trump went further, signing an executive order to say the U.S. does not regard space as a "global commons." Just as shipping companies often register their businesses in a country that lets them avoid tax or regulations, space companies can set up shop in Luxembourg, which has few restraints on their activities [76]. Generally, a country's laws project onto the off-Earth activities of its citizens. A substance that is controlled or illegal in the U.S. keeps that status for any American astronaut. Also, a medical procedure that has not been approved by the FDA is prohibited for a health care provider in space. Germline genome editing is highly controversial and currently prohibited in most countries [77]. The FDA regulates all genetic experiments in scientific labs and can in principle also restrict genetic biohacking by individuals with little or no scientific training, though it has not chosen to do so [78]. If a Moon or Mars colony declares itself independent, with its occupants renouncing their existing citizenships, these inhabitants would not be bound by any national or international laws and they may be emboldened to pursue aggressive and risky enhancement strategies (**Figure 9**).

The field of space ethics is young and evolving; the first conference on the topic was held in 2004 [79]. A broad goal is to define principles for identifying rational compromises between the different stakeholders. For example, deciding whether the Moon and Mars should be protected the way national parks are in the U.S. or companies should use the land and resources without constraint. Space ethics is neither for nor against space exploration. It is a tool for critiquing assumptions that space advocates and space skeptics often fail to realize they are making [80]. One recent

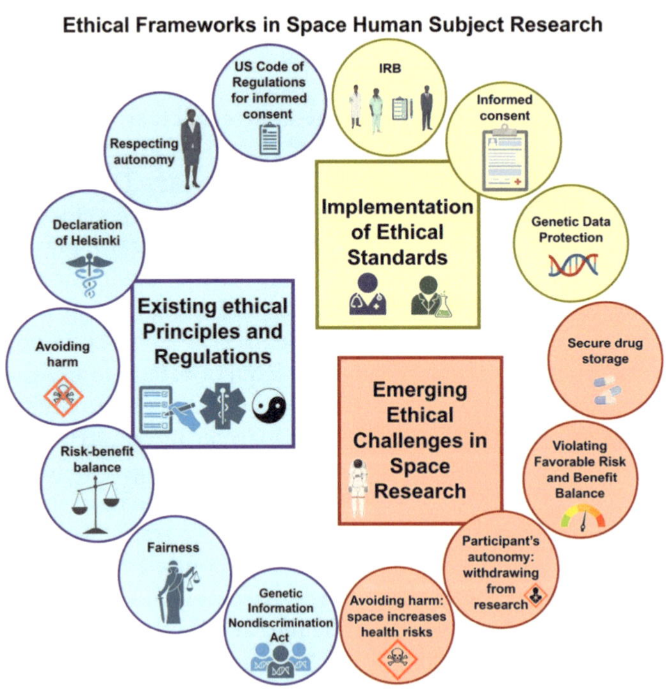


**Figure 9.**
*A schematic ethical framework for human subjects in space, including existing principles and regulations in blue, the implementation of these standards in clinics and research labs in yellow, and ethical challenges in space research in red (Credit Seylani et al., Nature Communications, Creative Commons 4.0 International License, https://doi.org/10.1038/s41467-023-44357-x).*

commentary summarizes the overarching goals: "Space ethics must embrace stewardship of the space environment, the human rights of those endeavoring to extend civilization into space, the rule of law, and how benefits of space can broadly benefit humanity while particularly motivating and rewarding those who risk, dare, invent, and invest" [81]. Ethical arguments must anticipate unpredictable, rapidly evolving technologies, since space companies and those wanting to travel in space are likely to be early adopters of cutting-edge capabilities. When it comes to human enhancement, the lack of regulatory clarity creates risk. Spaceflights sponsored by governments adhere to stringent criteria for research on human subjects, through ethics committees and Institutional Review Boards. U.S. federal rules for informed consent require "a description of any reasonably foreseeable risks or discomforts to the subject" [82]. But the unpredictable risks of a mission to Mars make this type of consent impossible. Colonists engaging in gene editing will be part of an unregulated clinical trial. Human enhancement on Mars is almost inevitable [83]. New rules will need to be worked out that private space companies can agree on to put an ethical framework on the new "Wild West" [84].

To see how the ethical lines can be confusing or blurred, consider this example from the world of sports. In 1999, golfer Tiger Woods was on a long losing streak. He opted for Lasik eye surgery, improving his vision to 20/15, after which he won seven of his next ten events. In 2005, baseball player Mark McGuire had just broken the single season home run record when he was lambasted by a U.S. Congressional committee for using a performance-enhancing steroid that had been legal when he was taking it [85]. Both used enhancements to improve performance, but Woods used a procedure that has since become relatively routine, while McGuire used a drug where abuse carries significant risks. For off-Earth colonists, the risk/reward calculus is different. They are already in a hazardous situation. An argument can be made that they should be encouraged to pursue any means of enhancement that improves performance and increases adaptation to the alien environment. In fact, since the viability of the colony depends on everyone operating at peak efficiency, they might feel obligated to aggressively pursue enhancement. An ethical boundary that will probably be crossed by colonists is going past somatic cell gene therapy to edit germline cells, where any mutations or alterations are passed on to the future generations. To bring the ethics into sharper focus, consider the rights of children born off-Earth, growing up in an alien environment not of their choosing and living with permanent genetic modifications. A new space age is here, and the prospects are equally exciting and frightening [86].

## 5. Conclusions

We are entering a new era in space travel and exploration. An increasing number of countries are pursuing geopolitical ambitions by launching satellites, while China and the United States are using space stations and planning to send astronauts to the Moon and eventually Mars. However, the rapid increase in Earth orbit activity is driven by the private sector, in particular the billionaire-led SpaceX and Blue Origin. The space environment presents profound health challenges for all astronauts, with radiation and reduced gravity at the top of the list. Mitigating these risks with heavy element shielding or artificial gravity add prohibitively to the cost of a mission. As a result, pharmacological approaches are used to help humans cope with space. In the future, humans on long-duration spaceflights or inhabiting colonies on the Moon or

Mars are likely to use gene editing to adapt to their hostile environment. Some will use more radical methods, such as surgical implants and germ line gene therapy. At the moment, there are few legal or regulatory constraints on human enhancement off-Earth. Private space companies have ambitious plans and very few constraints on their activities. New ethical frameworks are needed ensure that space travel is conducted equitably and fairly and that the travelers' well-being is safe-guarded.

## Acknowledgements

I acknowledge useful conversations with my colleagues in the Department of Astronomy, and the feedback on many of these ideas from the Udall Fellows at the University of Arizona. Support from a Udall Fellowship provided teaching release that allowed me to write this article. I appreciate conversations and collaboration with Konrad Szocik, who has thought deeply about issues of off-Earth settlement and human enhancement.

## Author details

Chris Impey
University of Arizona, Tucson, AZ, USA

*Address all correspondence to: cimpey@as.arizona.edu

## References

[1] Cadbury D. Space Race: The Epic Battle between America and the Soviet Union for Dominion of Space. New York, NY: Harper Perrenial; 2007

[2] Cortright E. Apollo Expeditions to the Moon: The NASA History 50th Anniversary Edition. Mineola, NY: Dover Publications; 2019

[3] Jenkins D. A History of the American Space Shuttle. Atglen, PA: Schiffer Military History; 2019

[4] Catchpole J. The International Space Station: Building for the Future. Berlin: Springer Praxis; 2008

[5] Hossain M. Breakthroughs with competition-based innovation: The X-prize foundation. Journal of Organizational Design. 2014;**3**(3):30-36. DOI: 10.7146/

[6] Linehan D, Melvill M. Burt Rutan's Race to Space: The Magician of Mojave and His Flying Innovations. Minneapolis, MN: Zenith Press; 2011

[7] Baiocco P. Overview of reusable space systems with a look to technology aspects. Acta Astronautica. 2021;**189**:10-25. DOI: 10.1016/j.actaastro.2021.07.039

[8] Olsen M. The Future of Space, Part 1: The Setup [Internet]. 2021. Available from: https://futureblind.com/p/the-future-of-space-1 [Accessed: November 21, 2024]

[9] Davenport C. The Space Barons: Elon Musk, Jeff Bezos, and the Quest to Colonize the Cosmos. New York, NY: PublicAffairs; 2018

[10] Creech S, Guidi J, Elburn D. Artemis: An Overview of NASA's Activities to Return Humans to the Moon. IEEE Aerospace Conference; 5-12 March 2022. IEEE: Big Sky, MT; 2022. DOI: 10.1109/AERO53065.2022.9843277

[11] Dahl M, Kups H, Szatkowski M. China's space program and its quest for superpowerhood. In: Dalh M, Szatkowski M, Kups H, editors. China Under Xi Jinping. Leiden, Netherlands: Koninklijke Brill; 2025

[12] Heldmann J et al. Mission architecture using the SpaceX starship to enable a sustained human presence on Mars. New Space. 2022;**10**(3):259-273. DOI: 10.1089/space.2020.0058

[13] Hein A, Mathson R, Fries D. A techno-economic analysis of asteroid mining. Acta Astronautica. 2020;**168**:104-115. DOI: 10.1016/j.actaastro.2019.05.009

[14] Salgado M, Belderrain M, Devezas T. Space propulsion: A survey study about current and future technologies. Journal of Aerospace and Technology Management. 2018;**10**. DOI: 10.5028/jatm.v10.829

[15] Cucinotta F. Space radiation risks for astronauts on multiple international Space Station missions. PLoS One. 2014;**9**(4). DOI: 10.1371/journal.pone.0096099

[16] Chancellor J, Scott G, Sutton J. Space radiation: The number one risk to astronaut health beyond low earth orbit. Life. 2014;**4**(3):491-510. DOI: 10.3390/life4030491

[17] Buckey J. Space Physiology. Oxford: Oxford University Press; 2006

[18] NASA. Station Visitors [Internet]. 2024. Available from: https://www.nasa.

gov/international-space-station/space-station-visitors-by-country/ [Accessed: November 21, 2024]

[19] NASA. Station Record Holders [Internet]. 2024. Available from: https://www.nasa.gov/international-space-station/space-station-astronaut-record-holders/ [Accessed: November 21, 2024]

[20] BBC. Space Crew Returns to Earth after Longest Stay on ISS [Internet]. 2024. Available from: https://www.bbc.com/news/videos/ckgnzr1dx73o [Accessed: November 21, 2024]

[21] Time. Meet the Twins Unlocking the Secrets of Space [Internet]. 2015. Available from: https://time.com/meet-the-twins-unlocking-the-secrets-of-space/ [Accessed: November 21, 2024]

[22] Garrett-Bakelman F et al. The NASA twins study: A multidimensional analysis of a year-long human spaceflight. Science. 2019;**364**:144-165. DOI: 10.1126%2Fscience.aau8650

[23] The Planetary Society, One-Year ISS Mission Preview: 28 Experiments, 4 Expeditions, and 2 Crew Members [Internet]. 2015. Available from: https://www.planetary.org/articles/20150325-one-year-iss-preview [Accessed: November 21, 2024]

[24] Lambrecht G et al. The role of physiotherapy in the European Space Agency strategy for preparation and preconditioning of astronauts before and after long duration space flight. Musculoskeletal Science and Practice. 2017;**1**:S15-S22. Available from: https://www.sciencedirect.com/science/article/abs/pii/S1356689X16307548

[25] Scott J et al. Effects of exercise countermeasures on multisystem function in long duration spaceflight astronauts. Microgravity. 2013;**9**(1):11. DOI: 10.1038/s41526-023-00256-5

[26] Scott J, Weber T, Green D. Introduction to the frontiers research topic: Optimization of exercise countermeasures for human space flight—Lessons from terrestrial physiology and operational considerations. Frontiers in Physiology. 2019;**10**:10173. DOI: 10.3389/fphys.2019.00173

[27] Tinley K. New York Times, the Bodily Indignities of the Space Life [Internet]. 2023. Available from: https://www.nytimes.com/2023/11/12/magazine/space-living.html [Accessed: November 21, 2024]

[28] Penn J, Lindley C. Requirements and approach for a space tourism launch system. Acta Astronautica. 2003;**52**(1):49-75. DOI: 10.1016/S0094-5765(02)00117-0

[29] Impey C. Beyond: Our Future in Space. New York: Norton; 2015

[30] European Space Agency. The Radiation Showstopper for Mars Exploration [Internet]. 2019. Available from: https://www.esa.int/Science_Exploration/Human_and_Robotic_Exploration/The_radiation_showstopper_for_Mars_exploration [Accessed: November 21, 2024]

[31] Braddock M. Artificial gravity: Small steps on the journey to the giant leap. Journal of Space Exploration. 2017;**6**(3):137-145. Available from: https://www.tsijournals.com/articles/artificial-gravity-small-steps-on-the-journey-to-the-giant-leap.pdf

[32] Kamienski L. Brave New Soldier: The Biotechnological Revolution and 21st Century Warfare. Krakow: Jagiellonian Press; 2024

[33] Rothschild L. NASA, an Astropharmacy [Internet]. 2020.

Available from: https://www.nasa.gov/general/an-astropharmacy/ [Accessed: November 21, 2024]

[34] Vine S. The Medicine Maker, the Astropharmacy Concept [Internet]. 2020. Available from: https://www.nasa.gov/general/an-astropharmacy/ [Accessed: November 21, 2024]

[35] Sgro A, Blancafort P. Epigenome engineering: New technologies for precision medicine. Nucleic Acids Research. 2020;**48**(22):12453-12482. DOI: 10.1093/nar/gkaa1000

[36] Liu G, Lin Q, Jin S, Gao C. The CRISPR-Cas toolbox and gene editing technologies. Molecular Cell. 2022;**82**(2):333-347. DOI: 10.1016/j.molcel.2021.12.002

[37] Gouw A. CRISPR challenges and opportunities for space travel. In: Human Enhancements for Space Missions: Lunar, Martian, and Future Missions to the Outer Planets. Switzerland: Springer; 2020. pp. 19-34

[38] Lee H, Kim J-S. Unexpected CRISPR on-target effects. Nature Biotechnology. 2018;**36**:703-704. DOI: 10.1038/nbt.4207

[39] Ledford H. Space suits optional for "water bears.". Nature. 2008. DOI: 10.1038/news.2008,1087

[40] Hashimoto T et al. Extremotolerant tardigrade genome and improved radiotolerance of human-cultured cells by tardigrade-unique protein. Nature Communications. 2016;**7**:12808. DOI: 10.1038/ncomms12808

[41] Lovett L. Mission to Mars: The Healthcare Challenges Facing NASA [Internet]. 2019. Available from: https://www.mobihealthnews.com/news/mission-mars-healthcare-challenges-facing-nasa [Accessed: November 21, 2024]

[42] Summers R, Johnson S, Marshburn T, Williams D. Emergencies in space. Annals of Emergency Medicine. 2005;**46**(2):177-184. DOI: 10.1016/j.annemergmed.2005.02.010

[43] Purvis N. From Floating Guts to "Sticky" Blood—Here's How to Do Surgery in Space [Internet]. 2020. Available from: https://www.kcl.ac.uk/from-floating-guts-to-sticky-blood-heres-how-to-do-surgery-in-space [Accessed: November 21, 2024]

[44] BBC World Service, Lentati S. The Man Who Cut out His Own Appendix [Internet]. 2015. Available from: https://www.bbc.com/news/magazine-32481442 [Accessed: November 21, 2024]

[45] Carrington D. New Scientist, "Magic Number" for Space Pioneers Calculated [Internet]. 2002. Available from: https://www.newscientist.com/article/dn1936-magic-number-for-space-pioneers-calculated/ [Accessed: November 21, 2024]

[46] Pardo L, MacKay I, Oostra B, van Duijn C, Aulchenko Y. The effect of genetic drift in a young genetically isolated population. Annals of Human Genetics. 2005;**69**(3):288-295. DOI: 10.1046/J.1469-1809.2005.00162.x

[47] Freeman D. NBC News, Will Mars Colonists Evolve into this New Kind of Human? [Internet]. 2017. Available from: https://www.nbcnews.com/storyline/the-big-questions/mars-colonists-might-evolve-entirely-new-type-human-n708636 [Accessed: November 21, 2024]

[48] Kupiec-Weglinski J. Grand challenges in organ transplantation. Frontiers in Transplantation. 2022;**1**(5). DOI: 10.3389/frtra.2022.897679

[49] McGowan B. Industrial Exoskeletons: What You're Not Hearing [Internet].

2018. Available from: https://ohsonline.com/articles/2018/10/01/industrial-exoskeletons-what-youre-not-hearing.aspx [Accessed: November 21, 2024]

[50] Laje D. The Rise of the Humanoid: Exoskeletons Revolutionizing Military Readiness [Internet]. 2024. Available from: https://www.afcea.org/signal-media/rise-humanoid-exoskeletons-revolutionizing-military-readiness [Accessed: November 21, 2024]

[51] Marcee A, Treadway E. Self-powered microgravity resistance exercise with soft pneumatic exoskeletons. In: 2022 IEEE Aerospace Conference (Aero). Big Sky, MT: IEEE; 2022. pp. 1-10. Available from: https://ieeexplore.ieee.org/abstract/document/9843743

[52] Ozioko O, Dahiya R. Smart tactile gloves for haptic interaction, communication, and rehabilitation. Advanced Intelligent Systems. 2021;**4**(2). DOI: 10.1002/aisy.202100091

[53] Abrams Z. IEEE Pulse, the Future of Brain-Computer Interfaces [Internet]. 2023. Available from: https://www.embs.org/pulse/articles/the-future-of-brain-computer-interfaces/ [Accessed: November 21, 2024]

[54] Mukherjee S, Suleman S, Pilloton R, Narang J, Rani K. State of the art in smart portable, wearable, ingestible, and implantable devices for health status monitoring and disease management. Sensors (Basel). 2022;**22**(11):4228. DOI: 10.3390/s22114228

[55] Jewett C. New York Times, despite Setbacks, Neuralink's First Brain-Implant Patient Stays Upbeat [Internet]. 2024. Available from: https://www.nytimes.com/2024/05/22/health/elon-musk-brain-implant-arbaugh.html [Accessed: November 21, 2024]

[56] Grind K. New York Times, Elon Musk's Plan to Put a Million Earthlings on Mars in 20 Years [Internet]. 2024. Available from: https://www.nytimes.com/2024/07/11/technology/elon-musk-spacex-mars.html [Accessed: November 21, 2024]

[57] Clynes M, Kline N. Cyborgs and space. Astronautics. 1960:26-76

[58] Warwick K. I, Cyborg. Urbana, IL: University of Illinois Press; 2004

[59] Liu X, Song P, editors. Emerging Micro/Nano Tools for Cyborg and Bionic Systems. Cyborg and Bionic Systems [Internet]. 2021. Available from: https://spj.science.org/page/cbsystems/si/Emerging-Micro-Nano-Tools-Cyborg-Bionic-Systems [Accessed: November 21, 2024]

[60] de Angelis E. Fashion Conscious, Neil Harbisson: The First Human Cyborg [Internet]. 2021. Available from: https://thefashionglobe.com/neil-harbisson/ [Accessed: November 21, 2024]

[61] Mesko B, Dhunnoo P. The Medical Futurist, the Current State and Future of Biohacking [Internet]. 2024. Available from: https://medicalfuturist.com/the-current-state-and-future-of-biohacking/ [Accessed: November 21, 2024]

[62] Popper B. The Verge, Cyborg America: Inside the Strange New World of Basement Body Hackers [Internet]. 2012. Available from: https://www.theverge.com/2012/8/8/3177438/cyborg-america-biohackers-grinders-body-hackers [Accessed: November 21, 2024]

[63] Dellerman D, Calma A, Lipusch N, Weber T, Weigel S, Ebel P. The Future of Human-AI Collaboration: A Taxonomy of Design Knowledge for Hybrid Intelligence Systems [Internet]. 2021. Available from: https://arxiv.org/

abs/2105.03354 [Accessed: November 21, 2024]

[64] Sauro F, Pozzobon R, Massironi M, De Bernardinis P, Santagata T, De Waele J. Lava tubes on earth, moon, and Mars: A review on their size and morphology revealed by comparative planetology. Earth-Science Reviews. 2020;**209**. DOI: 10.1016/j.earscirev.2020.103288

[65] Fowler G. Medium, How AI Will Help Space Missions to Mars [Internet]. 2024. Available from: https://gafowler.medium.com/how-ai-will-help-space-missions-to-mars-7c15c333315d [Accessed: November 21, 2024]

[66] Sorgner S. On Transhumanism. University Park, PA: Penn State University Press; 2020

[67] Nikkisha S, Mankan S, Bose L, Abraham B, Dhanse S. Review on past, present, and future rocket propulsion technologies. International Journal of Scientific Research and Management. 2024;**8**(6). Available from: https://ijsrem.com/download/review-on-past-present-and-future-rocket-propulsion-technologies/

[68] Saey T. Humans Might be Able to Hibernate during Space Travel [Internet]. 2023. Available from: https://www.snexplores.org/article/humans-hibernate-space-travel-cryobiology-suspended-animation [Accessed: November 21, 2024]

[69] Mobjerg N, Neves R. New insights into survival strategies of tardigrades. Comparative Biochemistry and Physiology Part A: Molecular and Integrative Physiology. 2021;**254**:110890. DOI: 10.1016/j.cbpa.2020.110890

[70] Crowl A, Hunt J, Hein A. Embryo space colonization to overcome the interstellar time distance bottleneck. Journal of the British Interplanetary Society. 2012;**65**:283-285. Available from: https://ui.adsabs.harvard.edu/abs/2012JBIS...65..283C/abstract

[71] Shahbazi M et al. Self-organization of the human embryo in the absence of maternal tissues. Nature Cell Biology. 2016;**18**(6):700-708. DOI: 10.1038/ncb3347

[72] United Nations. Treaty on Principles Governing the Activities of States in the Exploration and Use of Outer Space, Including the Moon and Other Celestial Bodies [Internet]. 1967. Available from: https://www.unoosa.org/oosa/en/ourwork/spacelaw/treaties/introouterpacetreaty.html [Accessed: November 21, 2024]

[73] United Nations. Agreement Governing the Activities of States on the Moon and Other Celestial Bodies [Internet]. 1979. Available from: https://www.unoosa.org/oosa/en/ourwork/spacelaw/intromoonagreement.html [Accessed: November 21, 2024]

[74] United Nations. Space Law, United Nations Office for Outer Space Affairs [Internet]. 2024. Available from: https://www.unoosa.org/oosa/en/ourwork/spacelaw/index.html [Accessed: November 21, 2024]

[75] Molloy M. The Telegraph, Asteroid Mining Made Legal after Passing of Historic Space Bill in US [Internet]. 2015. Available from: https://www.telegraph.co.uk/news/worldnews/northamerica/usa/12019740/Who-owns-space-Asteroid-mining-made-legal-in-US-after-passing-of-2015-space-bill.html [Accessed: November 21, 2024]

[76] The Economist. Space Law Is Inadequate for the Boom in Human Activity there [Internet]. 2019. Available from: https://www.economist.com/

international/2019/07/18/space-law-is-inadequate-for-the-boom-in-human-activity-there [Accessed: November 21, 2024]

[77] Baylis F, Darnovsky M, Hasson K, Krahn T. Human germline and heritable genome editing: The global policy landscape. The CRISPR Journal. 2020;**3**(5):365-377. DOI: 10.1089/crispr.2020.0082

[78] Zettler P, Guerrini C, Sherkow J. Regulating genetic biohacking. Science. 2019;**365**(6448):34-36. DOI: 10.1126/science.aax3248

[79] UNESCO. Legal and ethical framework for astronauts on space sojourns. In: A Symposium. United Nations Educational, Scientific and Cultural Organization. Paris, France: UNESCO; 2004. Available from: https://unesdoc.unesco.org/ark:/48223/pf0000139752

[80] Schwartz J, Mulligan T. "Space Ethics" According to Space Ethicists. The Space Review [Internet]. 2021. Available from: https://www.thespacereview.com/article/4117/1 [Accessed: November 21, 2024]

[81] Sergel J, Kwast S. Politico, to Boldly Go... Responsibly [Internet]. 2020. Available from: https://www.politico.com/news/2020/11/20/space-ethics-opinion-438526 [Accessed: November 21, 2024]

[82] U.S. Federal Register. Federal Policy for the Protection of Human Subjects [Internet]. 2017. Available from: https://www.federalregister.gov/documents/2017/01/19/2017-01058/federal-policy-for-the-protection-of-human-subjects [Accessed: November 21, 2024]

[83] Szocik K et al. Future space missions and human enhancement: Medical and ethical challenges. Futures. 2021;**133**:102819. DOI: 10.1016/j.futures.2021.102819

[84] Seylani A et al. Ethical considerations for the age of non-governmental space exploration. Nature Communications. 2024;**15**:4774. DOI: 10.1038/s41467-023-44357-x

[85] Saletan W. Slate, the Beam in your Eye [Internet]. 2005. Available from: https://slate.com/technology/2005/04/if-steroids-are-cheating-why-isn-t-lasik.html [Accessed: November 21, 2024]

[86] Impey C. Unbound: Ethics, law, sustainability, and the new space race. Studia Humana. 2021;**10**(4):1-17. DOI: 10.2478/sh-2021-0020

Chapter 5

# The Ethical Issues of Neurotechnologies

*Susanna Davtyan and Milena Mesropyan*

## Abstract

The main objective of this chapter is to consider the features of neuroethics as an emerging scientific problem. Neuroethics is viewed from several angles. On the one hand, it is presented as a new issue in bioethics and on the other hand, it is studied as a part of social transformations, which in the era of biotechnology has received the name "human enhancement". The social, economic and political consequences of the use of neurotechnologies in different fields of life are also analyzed. The need for critical reflection and ethical regulation of the use of neurotechnologies, especially as directed by organizations, such as UNESCO, is emphasized.

**Keywords:** neurotechnology, bioethics, human improvement, dignity, fundamental rights and freedoms, neurorights, brain imaging, brain enhancement

## 1. Introduction

The actuality of neurotechnologies is due to the fact that the complex and contradictory nature of its progress, social, economic and moral changes require a new understanding of the value foundations of human civilization and life itself.

At the first glance, it seems that neurotechnologies are designed to make human life better, and their development should be supported and encouraged in every possible way. However, like any other scientific and technical achievement, its dissemination and expansion of operation are associated with security, privacy and many other bioethical issues. Every progress may have a regress in it.

Humanity today faces the danger of turning into a self-serving technical machine; as a result, respect and ethical responsibility for all manifestations of life are lost. Under these conditions, all technological achievements in the field of medicine create such problems that are in dire need of ethical analysis.

Throughout history, medical science has recorded many new achievements, but they have never given rise to such confused and conflicting moral opinions as today ([1], p. 89). The reason for all this is the advancement of the latest scientific achievements and new technologies to the level of human life management.

The progress of neurotechnology certainly has its positive aspects, but they are not comparable to the explosive situations that humanity may face in the future because of them. Therefore, we have an obligation to control the progress of neurotechnology, keeping it within moral limits.

It has never been possible to stop the progress of ever-developing science, so it remains to use it wisely for its proper purpose ([2], p. 71). The fundamental criterion of regulation in the above field should be the preservation of the spiritual integrity of the person. The modern developments and researches of neurotechnologies should be carried out and applied for the benefit of the development of the spiritual requirements of a person, emphasizing the protection of human sovereignty, self-determination, dignity, and fundamental rights and freedoms.

Currently, neurotechnologies are developing at a rapid pace. The volume of public and private investments in this sector is steadily increasing. For their development, various international and local initiatives are created; moreover, very often in the form of public-private sector cooperation. At the same time, the significant potential of neurotechnologies is manifested not only in the treatment of a wide range of diseases and disorders of the nervous system but also in various scientific studies aimed at improving human nature in general.

However, the uncontrolled use of these technologies can lead to disastrous consequences in terms of preserving fundamental human freedoms and sovereignty. Therefore, the discussion of the development and application of neurotechnologies requires a wide involvement of the ethics, with further implementation of the principles developed by them in the legal acts regulating the field.

It must be admitted that currently the ethical regulation of the development of science and technology lags behind the development process itself, because it is based on a simple response mechanism to specific situations caused by existing or even widely used technologies. There is no doubt that the introduction of these technologies will lead to drastic changes in society and will also lead to some unintended consequences. International organizations, including UNESCO and its advisory body, the Bioethics Committee, have a major role to play in these processes ([3], pp. 503, 505). The works carried out by the latter's expert group and the draft recommendations based on them are definitely a necessary step in the difficult path of defining moral and legal regulations for the sector.

## 2. What are neurorights

We want to particularly emphasize the definition of the so-called "neurorights" concept and the clarification of its scope. The normative analysis of ethical and legal issues arising from the activities of the sciences engaged in the study of the mind and brain has attracted increased attention in recent years. That happened due to the expansion of philosophical, ethical and legal studies of neurology as a rapidly developing branch of medicine (this particularly concerns research in the fields of neuroethics and neurolaw) from the point of view of the threat of violation of fundamental human rights and freedoms.

The term "neurorights" also arose within the framework of these scientific disciplines and refers to the study of new methods of treatment and research created in neurology and the moral and legal consequences of their application. Although the scope of possible moral and legal violations and abuses caused by them is quite wide, it is especially necessary to single out all those problems that can arise in the event of restriction of the freedom of an individual's intellectual activity and its distortion. Therefore, by neuro-rights, we mean all internationally accepted normative guidelines of an ethical, legal, and social nature that are designed to preserve and protect human freedom of thought in all its manifestations.

These rights are based on the recognition of the right to physical and mental integrity, privacy of personal data, freedom of thought, free will, and access to scientific progress of all people without discrimination, and the need to protect and promote these rights. They also include the right to make free and responsible decisions about the use of neurotechnologies without any discrimination, coercion, or violence. These rights do not simply restate pre-existing human rights frameworks; rather, they offer normative specifications pertaining to the protection of the individual's mental and neurological realm. Furthermore, it supports the idea that the basic freedoms and rights pertaining to the human mind and brain serve as the foundation for all other freedoms and rights. Thus, safeguarding neurorights is a primary responsibility of international human rights law and could help increase the protection of other liberties and rights.

The Republic of Armenia, as a member state of the United Nations, certainly shares the concerns related to the introduction of neurotechnologies and is ready to adopt relevant regulations on the protection of mental health at the state level, as well as ensuring the protection of neurodata as personal data, based on the recommendations of the UNESCO's Bioethics committee ([4], pp. 91, 102).

At the same time, we would like to emphasize that there is almost no mention of the application of neurotechnology in the military field. Of course, the simplest and most "positive" use of neurotechnology in the military is the creation of new types of brain-related prostheses for soldiers who have lost limbs or the treatment of neurological disorders such as post-traumatic stress syndrome. However, these technologies can also be used for offensive purposes on the battlefield, causing various ethical, psychological, political, security and other challenges. For example, a computer device can be injected into a soldier's blood that can be magnetically directed to certain areas of the brain. Such soldiers will be able to control weapons thousands of kilometers away from them using only their thoughts ([5], pp. 271, 272).

The next level may be the use of a device that can directly monitor the behavior of soldiers. In this case, new ethical challenges will arise in connection with the distortion of our classical perceptions of moral and legal responsibility, which may affect the degree of brutality and the expansion of the scope of war crimes.

Neurotechnologies can also bring hybrid warfare to a new level. If today's battlefield confrontations are aided and abetted by electronic media propaganda, then in neurowarfare it will be possible to literally control the brains of people both on the front lines and behind, threatening the political and social stability of the adversary ([6], p. 22).

Responsible use of neurotechnologies should only take place as a result of close cooperation between representatives of science, legal and ethical fields. When developing neurotechnologies, it is also important to take into account the needs and concerns of the people who will be their direct consumers. Therefore, public awareness of what neurotechnologies are and what consequences can be expected from their development and use, is the main mission of the relevant authorities and organizations.

## 3. UNESCO and the development of neuroethics as bioethical problem

UNESCO plays a significant role in the field of neurotechnologies, relying on its rich experience in the field of bioethics. It is logical and encouraging that the principles included in the UNESCO document "Universal Declaration on Bioethics and Human Rights" (2005) should also be used in solving neuroethical issues.

In addressing the moral dilemmas brought up by the application of medicine, life sciences, and related technology to people, the Declaration grounds the values it upholds in the laws governing respect for fundamental freedoms, human rights, and human dignity. The Declaration acknowledges the connection between ethics and human rights in the particular field of bioethics by protecting human life and enshrining bioethics in international human rights ([7], pp. 495, 497, 503).

Neuroethics is a young and promising branch, or rather, an interdisciplinary field of research, the subject of which are ethical problems and issues related to neuroscience and the study of the human brain as a whole. In other words, it combines integral neuroscience, modern technologies, and ethics in different proportions. This discipline appeared only at the beginning of the twenty-first century, in response to modern challenges in the field of neurophysiology, but it already covers a fairly large segment of knowledge and most likely will have a future. The faster the sciences and technologies related to human life and consciousness develop, the more they need an ethical assessment and an ethical view of the ongoing progress.

The emergence of new humanitarian disciplines, especially at the intersection of various fields of scientific knowledge, is a common occurrence today. Among them, neuroethics has a number of features that raise questions of the ultimate methodological level. If we pay attention to the formation of bioethics, to which we will appeal in order to answer the question "How is neuroethics possible?", then in its history it is quite difficult to identify moments and events that would clearly indicate its beginning. We usually consider as its beginning the Nuremberg Trials of Nazi doctors and the development of the Nuremberg Code, which underlies the modern regulation of biomedical research and is the core of research ethics. Also, such key moments are considered to be the publication of the book by V.R. Potter "Bioethics - bridge to the future" or the first successful heart transplant by the South African surgeon K. Barnard and the subsequent discussions about the criteria by which a person can be declared dead in order to legitimize the removal of organs for transplantation, and some other events that are separated by decades.

The beginning of neuroethics, unlike bioethics, can be discussed more clearly. Its formation was facilitated, on the one hand, by the rapid development of various methods of neuroresearch itself and the expansion of the scope of neuroscience. On the other hand, it became increasingly obvious that all scientific projects and innovations implemented in the field of biomedicine needed axiological and ethical study by humanitarian disciplines, which also stimulated the advancement of neuroethics. The first such experience was the ethical review of the human genome project, which was formalized in terms such as "gene ethics" or "ethics of genomics". The Human Genome Project (HGP) was a worldwide scientific project that tried to identify, map, and decode every gene in the human genome from a functional and physical standpoint, as well as to identify the base pairs that make up human DNA. Beginning in 1990, it was completed in 2003 ([8], pp. 48, 49). This collaborative biological project was the largest in the world. Although the initiative has a lot to offer for science and healthcare, some authors emphasized that the potential ethical, legal, and social consequences of mapping the human genome needed to be acknowledged.

When neuroscience started to actively develop in the 1990s, it turned out that a precedent for their humanitarian study had already been established. This was due to the institutional consolidation of the practice of humanitarian examination, which led to the assumption that other scientific trends should also have their own ethics. Since the idea of "neuroethics" had been around since the 1970s, the name did not need to be created. Despite this, it was quite specialized and represented medical ethics in the field of neurology. The location of neuroethics, in most scientists' opinion, is in the field of philosophy, but by studying the mechanisms of morality, neuroethics conquers new territory from the classical philosophical disciplines ([9], pp. 3, 4).

In order to describe the contours of neuroethics, let us consider the main variants of its interpretation. It can be understood, firstly, as a section of bioethics; secondly, neuroethics can be interpreted as applied ethics; thirdly, as an independent type of research or professional ethics in the field of neuroscience and in neurological practice in medicine. Finally, the fourth variant presents neuroethics as the ethics of consciousness or the philosophy of the brain, claiming to declare the final victory of the naturalistic paradigm in understanding morality in the modern society ([10], p. 1897).

Neuroethics can be considered as one of the types of bioethics, which from a certain point of view can act as a structural element of research ethics. The basis for inclusion in this case is the general subject—ethical problems arising in neuroresearch and the application of their results not only in medical and clinical practice but also in other areas: in the penitentiary system, marketing, education, etc. The subject area of bioethics extends to all those areas, if the situation is problematic for a human being—his health, physical and mental integrity, identity, the boundaries of the beginning and end of life. In neuroethics, the question of identity and psychophysical integrity of a person is the most important one ([11], pp. 45, 50).

Neuroethics in the aspect of applied ethics, can probably be viewed as a system of provisions regulating possible moral and legal issues in the field of neuroscience, for which the principles enshrined in the main bioethical documents (for example, the European Convention on Human Rights in Biomedicine (1997), the Universal Declaration of Bioethics and Human Rights of UNESCO (2005)), can serve as a theoretical basis ([12], pp. 29, 36).

However, in addition to the above-mentioned international regulations, neuroethics can certainly develop certain norms, principles, and methods for managing and solving problems within its own framework, which will be a significant step toward specifying the permissible boundaries of practical research activities in the field of neuroscience in general, which, in turn, is a weighty argument for many specialists to develop neuroethics as a new and important section of applied ethics ([13], pp. 281, 284).

The many specific issues that neuroethics includes are still poorly studied. Their clear description and systematization is very important theoretical and methodological task. We would like to specifically dwell on the two main ethical issues of neurotechnologies, which are brain imaging and brain enhancement related moral and social problems.

## 4. Neuroethics of brain imaging and brain enhancement

Brain imaging is a crucial technology of modern neuroscience, and its dissemination creates several ethical concerns, particularly when the results are used for non-medical objectives such as marketing, investigative and judicial practice, and so on. The application of brain imaging techniques began in the 1920s. Initially, oxygen was employed as a source to excite the brain while pneumoencephalography was recorded. Then electrical impulses were recorded using EEG. If earlier investigations revealed knowledge about the brain's broad shapes and structural aspects, following ones delved deeper, examining tissues, cells, and intracellular substances.

The search for an observable substance, a breakdown that could explain the etiology or character of psychoneurological illnesses, prompted neuronogenetic study. Pneumo- and electroencephalography paved the path for today's high-precision tomographic (layer-by-layer) brain studies. In 1976, computed tomography, which uses X-rays, was introduced. The introduction of electromagnetic waves in MRI, which, by the way, was invented by Raymond V. Damadian—Armenian-American scientist, however, enabled a true breakthrough into the depths of brain matter. In the twenty-first century, brain imaging technologies allowed for the accurate assessment of the cortex and subcortical components of the brain, as well as its white and gray matter ([14], pp. 90, 91).

Computerized and magnetic resonance imaging, which records the structural properties of the brain at the cellular level, has created fundamentally new options for neurophysiologists and neurologists. Special cognitive exams were introduced to supplement some of these study possibilities. The development of brain imaging methods today is aimed at further immersion: functional (fMRI) and magnetic resonance spectroscopy (MRS), positron emission tomography (PET), and single-photon emission tomography (SPET), which use high-weight atomic isotopes with a short lifespan as gamma emitters. Multidimensional penetration into brain structures has helped to identify complex morphological changes, which are being studied not only to understand pathogenesis but also to investigate the possibility of influencing normal brain function and recreating it in neural networks. Diagnostic complication provides a more thorough understanding of the brain's function as a physiological organ, and it is accompanied by the creation of therapeutic impact approaches, which are not always therapeutic in nature, with the goal of improving brain function. Immersion at the molecular-genetic level aligns with a certain epistemic paradigm in the study of mental diseases, which is based on the reduction of behavior and consciousness to neurological bases ([15], p. 170).

In addition to the issues inherent in bioethics, such as the risks of radiation exposure and obtaining informed consent from the incompetent patients, the medical use of brain imaging raises new problems. For example, drug use, depression, and other pathological processes in the brain alter its morphology, which can be detected in a neuroimaging study, increasing the importance of confidentiality and exacerbating the problem of non-interference in the subject's privacy.

Therefore, respecting research subjects' privacy and maintaining their confidentiality are an ethical duty for investigators. Without the data subjects' consent, an investigator should never use test results, identifiable records, or other patient data. Researchers that study neuroimaging must be aware of the regulations pertaining to the protection of human subjects, particularly the changing guidelines for maintaining confidentiality and disclosing risks in "non-therapeutic" research. New privacy and confidentiality issues are brought up by methods for producing realistic surface renderings from volumetric anatomical imaging data.

But above all, the social use of brain imaging threatens the personal boundaries that delineate the space of the "sovereign ego", thus eroding the established principles of inviolability on which civil liberties are based. The contradiction between the need to protect personal space and to defend the public interest is exacerbated. When this issue is related to public safety, the use of brain imaging is easily sanctioned, for example, to detect deliberate lies. Note that, as in medicine, confidentiality may be violated in cases where medical information is required to solve crimes or to combat the spread of particularly dangerous infections ([16], pp. 145, 149).

The use of brain imaging removes the boundaries of the "sovereign ego", while overcoming ethical barriers, and thus opens wide access to technology through commerce, sports, education and other channels. After this, the spread of technology is difficult to regulate, which entails at least two noticeable consequences: firstly, an increase in the trend of medicalization in society, associated with an increase in dependence on medicine, an increase in expenses on it, which is not converted into an increase in the level of health. Secondly, the risk of discrimination against the individual increases, since neurotechnological effects on consciousness and behavior are presented as an act of consumer choice or a desire for self-improvement, which has a positive-improving connotation. That is, an individual autonomously makes their choice in favor of, for example, the use of psychopharmacological agents that improve cognitive abilities, but as a result, their self-identity is called into question. Which manifestation of personality—under the influence of drugs or without them—is true? Does brain enhancement really unlock a person's potential by maximizing their thinking, memory, ability to concentrate, etc., or does it create an inferiority complex and make a person dependent on means of observation and influence on the brain? ([17], pp. 378, 384).

Ethical and legal regulation in this case turns out to be difficult, first because brain enhancement becomes a matter of personal choice, with no possibility of implementing institutionalized control, and second because the value foundation of social norms that must be protected is undermined. Even if internal autonomy is a fundamental value that underpins self-identity and the concept of individual rights, such as, the right to personal inviolability and mental integrity, interpersonal competition will play an important role when individual qualities, such as creativity, talent, speed, and depth of thinking, are valued. Neurotechnologies provide a quick and modern means to achieve the required state of mind and cognitive capacities, and they have become an appealing instrumental value.

The concept of "brain enhancement" is a concretization of a more general term that has come into widespread use in philosophical and bioethical literature—human enhancement. it implies the improvement, strengthening, and expansion of a person's capabilities as a result of the converging application of various types of technologies, such as genetic, reproductive, orthopedic, and plastic; as well as informational, social, and neuropsychological technologies. Human enhancement is defined as the use of technologies not only to fight diseases but also to increase the capabilities or qualities of normal, healthy people. The greatest attention of scientists and ethicists is focused on technologies for increasing life expectancy, improving mood and cognitive abilities ([18], p. 125).

But from ethical point of view, it is crucial to remember the difference between enhancement and therapy. In many situations, this differentiation can aid in separating the legal and illegal use of different neurotechnologies. Therapy is making something right or repairing something that is wrong, whereas enhancement entails changing something that is not a problem or improving something to a state that we can term better than good. According to this perspective, "therapy," as it is often understood, is the application of neurotechnologies to treat people who have known illnesses, impairments or disabilities in an effort to return them to a normal level of fitness and health. "Enhancement," on the other hand, refers to the focused application of neurotechnologies to directly modify not illness processes, but rather the "normal" functioning of the human body and mind in order to enhance or improve their innate abilities and performances ([19], p. 584).

The shift in medicine and technology from therapy to enhancement is a big one, and it brings up a lot of ethical issues regarding the goals of medicine, human dignity and many other fundamental presumptions about both technological advancement and human rights. The transition from therapy to augmentation should not be taken for granted as the next natural step in the process. Rather, this is an area that necessitates not just analyzing each invention separately but also analyzing the assumptions that underpin this shift. This, of course, can lead to social and ethical injustice and discrimination, meanwhile the goal of any scientific progress should be the exact opposite, which is to be providing fair, equitable and appropriate treatment for everyone.

Intensive brain research, initially motivated by the fight against diseases, creates new ethical problems related to methods of cognitive improvement, since it affects how people think and feel and changes a human's personality. In the context of critical analysis of neurotechnologies, traditional bioethical questions about autonomy, cognitive freedom, personal identity, confidentiality are heard in a new perspective.

Therefore, the focus of bioethics turned out to be a variety of tasks: from the search for answers to fundamental questions about the identity of a person in the light of the transformation of his nature in biomedicine, to the creation of institutional and normative practices in which an attempt is made to determine the permissible limits of the application of technologies. However, their spectrum and social implications are continuously expanding.

## 5. Conclusion

In conclusion, we would like to state that with a new turn in the development of neuroscience, around the 1990s, new ways of observing brain activity and its correlation with behavior began to appear. The new data and perspectives that open up together with these perspectives influence the decisions of a person, their cognitive activity, are used not only in medicine but also in everyday life—in the economy, trade, education, etc., as evidenced by the emergence of new scientific and practical fields, such as neuromarketing, neuropedagogy, neurolaw and neuroeconomics. The need to assess the consequences and permissible limits of technologies, which began to develop with the ability to "look" under the skull of an individual, to study the unconscious patterns of choices made by a person and reaction in various situations and then to use this knowledge to manage and control them, led to the emergence of neuroethics.

The dynamics of brain research, coupled with the rapid growth of neurotechnologies, is constantly expanding the range of problems of neuroethics as a bioethical discipline. The development of neuroresearch and the technological implementation of discoveries are transforming society and actualizing the problems of social and humanitarian expertise in the format of neuroethics. That is why the goal of bioethics and neuroethics should be, first of all, critical. At the same time, humanists should first of all listen to the voice of those scientists who do not so much rely on the successes of neuroscience as they are focused on assessing the consequences of their application, such as, for example, the discoverer of mirror neurons, Vittorio Gallese. "I would say that we should focus on the classical philosophical goal of self-knowledge and follow at least a minimal ethical principle: to reduce and prevent suffering, and not to play with scientific evolution, as with fire, which may well get out of control" ([20], p. 211). The naturalness and immediacy of life cannot be constructed by replacing it with imaginary perfect worlds, therefore neuroethics, in order to preserve its moral principle, must protect these indisputable values.

## Author details

Susanna Davtyan* and Milena Mesropyan
YSMU After M. Heratsi, Yerevan, Armenia

*Address all correspondence to: susannadavtyan47@gmail.com

## References


[1] Davtyan SA. Intradaction to Bioethics, Monography. Yerevan: YSMU after M. Heratsi; 2012. p. 329 in Armenian

[2] Davtyan SA. Bioethics Handout. Yerevan: YSMU after M. Heratsi; 2013. p. 189 in English

[3] Davtyan SA. Experimental course of bioethics upon the bioethics curriculum of UNESCO: Methodology and result of investigation. International Journal Medicine and Law. 2012;**31**(4):495-513 in English

[4] Davtyan SA. Ethical Review System for Biomedical Research in the Republic of Armenia (Historical and Cultural Background, Legal Regulations, Education in Bioethics, Perspectives and Forms of International Cooperation), in Ethical Review of Biomedical Research in CIS Countries (Social and Cultural Aspects). Russia, Saint Petersburg: Licpublish; 2007. pp. 89-103 (in English and in Russian)

[5] Ienca M. From healthcare to warfare and reverse: How should we regulate dual-use neurotechnology? Neuron. 2018;**2**:269-274

[6] Roskies A. Neuroethics for the new millenium. Neuron. 2002;**35**:21-23

[7] Davtyan SA. Experimental course of bioethics upon the bioethics core curriculum of UNESCO: Methodology and result of investigation. Medicine and Law. 2012;**31**(4):495-512

[8] Maloy S, Hughes K. Brenner's Encyclopedia of Genetics. 2nd ed. London: Academic Press; 2013. pp. 48-49

[9] Safire W. Visions for a new field of "Neuroethics". In: Neuroethics: Mapping the Field Conference Proceedings, 13-14 May 2002. San Francisco, California. – New York: The Dana Press; 2002. pp. 3-9

[10] Neuroethics WP. Encyclopedia of Bioethics. 3rd ed. Vol. 3. New York: The Gale Group; 2004. pp. 1895-1898

[11] Fins J. Toward a Pragmatic Neuroethics in Theory and Practice: Debates about Neuroethics Perspectives on its Development, Focus and Future. New York: Springer International Publishing AG; 2017. pp. 45-66

[12] Have HT, Jean MS. The UNESCO Universal Declaration on Bioethics and Human Rights: Background, Principles and Application. Paris: UNESCO Publishing; 2009. pp. 19-33

[13] Levy N. Neuroethics: Challenge for the 21st Century. Cambridge: Cambridge University Press Publ; 2007. p. 364

[14] Ackerman S. Hard Science, Hard Choices: Facts, Ethics, and Policies Guiding Brain Science Today. New York: Dana Press; 2006. p. 152

[15] Hyman SE. The diagnosis of mental disorders: The problem of reification. Annual Review of Clinical Psychology. 2010;**27**(6):155-179

[16] Davtyan SA. Bioethics: Handout. Yerevan: YSMU after M. Heratsi; 2013. p. 257 in Russian

[17] Dees RH. Better Brains, Better Selves? The Ethics of Neuroenhancements. 2007;**17**(4):371-395

[18] Forlini C, Hall W. Navigating the enhancement landscape, ethical issues in research on cognitive enhancers for

healthy individuals. EMBO Reports. 2013;**14**(2):123-128

[19] McMahan J. Cognitive disability and cognitive enhancement. Metaphilosophy. 2009;**40**(3):582-605

[20] Metzinger T. The Ego Tunnel - The Science of the Mind and the Myth of the Self. New York: Basic Books; 2009. p. 288

Chapter 6

# The Decline of *Ordre Public* and Morality in the Regulation of Patented Genetic Materials in the United States

*Dorkina Myrick*

## Abstract

Scholars have long debated if *ordre public* and morality violations are relevant to patent eligibility. *Ordre public* is often linked to public policy exceptions for legal actions pertinent to patented scientific inventions. Adherence to *ordre public* is not a requirement for United States patent issue or regulation. Historical evidence demonstrates that *ordre public* has evolved with changes in societal beliefs, morality, and ethics. Although the United States Constitution omits morality provisions for patentability, the early nineteenth century Moral Utility Doctrine outlined in *Lowell v. Lewis* addressed morality and usefulness in United States patents. Eugenic studies were associated with few late nineteenth century public policy and morality exceptions. Such pseudoscientific studies served as foundations for immorality in and encouraged the regulation of patent awards for unethical studies like phrenology. As time progressed, changes in societal views made scientific pariahs of eugenics practitioners. *Bedford v. Hunt* bolstered the Moral Utility Doctrine in United States patents. Reforms outlined in the Patent Act of 1952 and subsequent court cases signaled the Moral Utility Doctrine's decline. This chapter will engage further discussion of the absence of morality regulation of genetic materials - including gene editing patents - in policy, regulation, and current case law.

**Keywords:** CRISPR, gene editing, genes, genetics, *ordre public*, morality, ethics, patents, intellectual property, law

## 1. Introduction: Defining *Ordre Public*, Morality, Ethics, and Foundations of Eugenics

Currently, there are nearly 100,000 patents containing genes or genetic materials, inclusive of 5,000–9,000 United States human genetic patents [1, 2]. Although human DNA which occurs naturally cannot be patented, several other types of genetic materials can be patented.[1] Patent eligible genetic materials and procedures include

[1] Patent Act §101; *Association for Molecular Pathology v. Myriad Genetics, Inc.*, 569 U.S. 576, 580 (2013).

laboratory-synthesized DNA sequences, methods, and processes of creating or modifying DNA sequences, and man-made complementary DNA (cDNA) sequences.[2] As gene editing technology and patenting become more significant in the advancement of both research and medical applications of gene editing, *ordre public* and morality become integral patentability issues. However, this is not necessarily the case in the United States. This chapter examines how the irrelevance of *ordre public* and morality in the issuance of gene editing patents has impacted government regulation of gene editing patents in the United States.

*Ordre public* can denote principles and decisions made based upon societal standards, also known as public policy, agreed upon by most of the people [4]. As such, laws are made in accordance with public policy [4]. According to the Stanford Encyclopedia of Philosophy, morality can be defined "descriptively to refer to certain codes of conduct put forward by a society or a group (such as a religion), or accepted by an individual for her own behavior, or normatively to refer to a code of conduct that, given specified conditions, would be put forward by all rational people" [5]. Ethics can be envisioned as "...applied to any system or theory of moral values or principles" [6].

The history of the absence of *ordre public* and morality in United States gene editing patents can be traced to eugenics practices, which were legitimized by the United States government through the issue of patents. The United States government issued patents for inventions conceived through phrenology as early as the year 1856.[3] The practice of phrenology bolstered the field of eugenics and legitimized the award of patents for inventions in congruence with the *ordre public* and morality of the day [7]. Phrenology taught that differences in brain and skull size and conformation were correlated with positive and negative physical characteristics [8, 9]. Ethnic distinctions in anatomy were classified in a hierarchical manner, with Caucasian skulls at the top of the anatomical hierarchy of desirability [8]. The United States Patent and Trademark Office even issued a patent entitled, "Apparatus for Teaching Phrenology," in 1856.[4] The patented invention consisted of a bust model with a diagrammed head which aided "lecturers in giving a correct knowledge of phrenology as they can give correct ideas of conformation of brain by giving correct conformations of heads."[5] The questionable issue concerning *ordre public* and morality was the fact that the phrenology patent was issued at all. However, *ordre public* and morality in the mid-1800s did not condemn eugenics and phrenology teachings [10].

## 2. The United States Supreme Court Legally Authorizes Eugenics Practices in *Buck v. Bell*

Germany during World War II provided a characteristic template for the implementation of eugenics practices in the United States, particularly in the American

[2] Patent Act §101; *Association for Molecular Pathology v. Myriad Genetics, Inc.*, 569 U.S. 576, 580 (2013); Ref. [3].

[3] Geo P. Wilcox and WM Butler. United States Patent and Trademark Office. "Apparatus for Teaching Phrenology." Specification of Letters Patent No. 14,685. April 15, 1856.

[4] Geo P. Wilcox and WM Butler. United States Patent and Trademark Office. "Apparatus for Teaching Phrenology." Specification of Letters Patent No. 14,685. April 15, 1856.

[5] Geo P. Wilcox and WM Butler. United States Patent and Trademark Office. "Apparatus for Teaching Phrenology." Specification of Letters Patent No. 14,685. April 15, 1856.

South [11]. As such, eugenics was mainstream scientific practice in the United States through the mid-twentieth century, legitimized with pseudoscientific journals such as the *Annals of Eugenics* and the *Annals of Heredity* [10]. Widespread sterilization campaigns against individuals with disabilities and those of non-Aryan ancestry were implemented in the United States [12]. Many such sterilization campaigns were formalized with the passage of laws ordering the sterilization of individuals considered societal outcasts by eugenics standards [10].

The United States Supreme Court opined on the utility of eugenics sterilization practices in *Buck v. Bell*.[6] Carrie Buck had a tri-generational genetic heritage of mental disability in her family.[7] The Superintendent of the Virginia State Colony of Epileptics and Feeble Minded declared that Ms. Buck was "feeble-minded of the lowest grade, moron class" [13]. The Virginia State Colony of Epileptics and Feeble Minded, where Carrie Buck was a resident, was established in Lynchburg, Virginia in 1910.[8] [13] On March 20, 1924, the state of Virginia enacted a law, the Virginia Sterilization Act of 1924, which sanctioned the eugenic sterilization of its residents.[9] Specifically, the Virginia Sterilization Act of 1924 authorized "the operation of sterilization on any such patient confined in such institution afflicted with hereditary forms of insanity that are recurrent, idiocy, imbecility, feeble-mindedness or epilepsy."[10] In accordance with Virginia state law, a salpingectomy procedure – which is a form of sterilization in which the fallopian tubes are removed, thus impeding the descent of the egg into the uterus – was to be performed on Ms. Buck.[11] The issue raised before the United States Supreme Court in *Buck v. Bell* was whether the Virginia State Colony of Epileptics and Feeble Minded committed a 14th amendment due process violation in deciding to sterilize Ms. Buck.[12] Ultimately, the United States Supreme Court declared that "[t]hree generations of imbeciles are enough."[13] The Supreme Court stated that Ms. Buck's rights of due process and that the "welfare and that of society will be promoted by her [Ms. Buck's] sterilization."[14] Thus, eugenics practices were affirmed by the highest court in the land. Such a decision issued by the Supreme Court indicated that the United States did not oppose human rights violations based upon one's genetic predisposition.[15] The demise of eugenics practices accompanied the end of World War II, the aftermath of the horrors of the Holocaust, and the United States' aid in drafting and supporting the Universal Declaration of Human Rights. As such, eugenics policies were eventually found to be inconsistent with societal tenets of *ordre public* and morality.

[6] 274 U.S. 200 (1927).

[7] 274 U.S. 200, 205 (1927).

[8] 274 U.S. 200, 201 (1927).

[9] Virginia Sterilization Act of 1924.

[10] Virginia Sterilization Act of 1924.

[11] 274 U.S. 200, 201 (1927).

[12] 274 U.S. 200, 205 (1927).

[13] 274 U.S. 200, 207 (1927).

[14] 274 U.S. 200, 207 (1927).

[15] 274 U.S. 200, 207 (1927).

## 3. Absence of United States Regulation of *Ordre Public* and Morality in Patents

### 3.1 Absence of *Ordre Public* and Morality Provisions for Patents in the United States Constitution

Patents are regulated in the United States through the United States Constitution; federal law; federal statutes; federal Supreme Court; federal appellate courts; federal district courts; and federal administrative agencies. The rapid and continued growth of intellectual property creation and rights protections – particularly for patents – was considered when the United States Constitution was drafted in 1789. The Founding Fathers of the United States believed it was important to incorporate federal laws and federal statutes which conferred patent power to the United States Congress.

The US Constitution Article I, Section 8, Clause 8 gives Congress the power "to promote the progress of science and useful arts, by securing for limited times to authors and inventors the exclusive right to their respective writings and discoveries."[16] Article I, Section 8, Clause 18 of the United States Constitution states that Congress can also "make all Laws which shall be necessary and proper for carrying into Execution the foregoing Powers, and all other Powers vested by this Constitution in the Government of the United States, or any Department or Officer thereof."[17] Clause 18 gives Congress the power to make laws establishing and regulating the granting of patents for inventions to inventors, as being a power necessary and proper to support Clause 8.[18]

A patent is a property right granted by the government of the United States of America to an inventor "to exclude others from making, using, offering for sale, or selling the invention throughout the United States or importing the invention into the United States" for a limited time in exchange for public disclosure of the invention when the patent is granted.[19] The first patent in the United States, signed by President George Washington, was awarded to Samuel Hopkins on July 31, 1790, for a new method for making pot and pearl ash.[20] Later, the first pharmaceutical patent, U.S. Patent 111X for "Composition of Bilious Pills," later known as "Dr. Lee's Bilious Pills," – was awarded to Samuel Lee on April 30, 1796.[21] Later, Thomas Hollis was granted a patent for "Balm of America."[22]

16 US Constitution Article I, Section 8, Clause 8.

17 US Constitution Article I, Section 8, Clause 18.

18 US Constitution Article I, Section 8, Clauses 8 and 18.

19 Patent FAQs. United States Patent and Trademark Office. Patent Help – Getting Started – Other. What is a Patent? Published on: Dec 5, 2016, 04:31 PM EST. Last Modified: May 8, 2020. 09:02 AM EDT. [Internet] https://www.uspto.gov/patents/ptab.

20 10 million patents: A Celebration of American Innovation [Internet]. USPTO.gov. 2018 [cited 2025 May 7]. Available from: https://www.uspto.gov/subscription-center/2018/10-million-patents-celebration-american-innovation.

21 Directory of American Tool and Machinery Patents. U.S. Patent: 111X. Composition of Bilious Pills. Granted: Apr. 30, 1796. https://www.datamp.org//patents/displayPatent.php?pn=X111&id=47175.

22 Origin of Patent Medicines. History. Balm of America: Patent Medicine Collection. Behring Center. [Internet]. National Museum of American History. Available from: https://americanhistory.si.edu/collections/object-groups/balm-of-america-patent-medicine-collection/history#:~:text=Origin%20of%20Patent%20Medicines&text=Patent%20medicines%20are%20named%20after,monopoly%20over%20his%20particular%20formula.

While Article 1, Section 8, Clauses 8 and 18 of the Constitution enable Congress to balance granting exclusive (monopoly) rights to the inventor for the sake of the promotion of innovation and progress with public disclosure of the invention, the United States Constitution contains no explicit provision for *ordre public* or morality in these clauses [14].[23]

### 3.2 Moral Utility Doctrine in United States Patent History

#### *3.2.1* Lowell v. Lewis *and the Moral Utility Doctrine*

The United States case *Lowell v. Lewis* delineated the distinction between morality and usefulness concerning patent rights.[24] In *Lowell v. Lewis*, Jacob Perkins was granted a patent for a method of construction of a water pump in 1813.[25] Perkins granted a patent assignment for the water pump invention to Francis C. Lowell (Plaintiff).[26] James Baker cited that he had invented an improvement upon Perkins' method of construction for a water pump.[27] Baker granted a patent assignment to Winslow Lewis (Defendant).[28] Lowell disputed Lewis' claim that Lewis created an improvement for a method of construction of a water pump invented by Lowell.[29] Lowell emphasized the novelty of his invention, while Lewis disputed both Lowell's claims of novelty and usefulness.[30] Lowell brought a patent infringement action against Lewis in 1813.[31] The court in *Lowell v. Lewis* failed to rule that a patent infringement occurred.[32] When considering *ordre public* and morality, *Lowell v. Lewis* stated that "[a]ll that the law requires is that the invention should not be frivolous or injurious to the well-being, good policy, or sound morals of society."[33] Hence, many legal scholars credit *Lowell v. Lewis* for the establishment of the Moral Utility Doctrine.

#### *3.2.2* Bedford v. Hunt: *Solidification of the Moral Utility Doctrine*

The Moral Utility Doctrine was a source of reference for considering patentability concerning *ordre public* and morality after the decision in *Lowell v. Lewis* until at least the early 1900s.[34] *Bedford v. Hunt* solidifies the use of the Moral Utility Doctrine concerning patents in the ruling of Justice Joseph Story of the United States Supreme Court on the case.[35] According to Justice Story:

---

[23] US Constitution Article I, Section 8, Clause 8.
[24] 15 F. Cas. 1018 (C.C.D. Mass. 1817) (No. 8568).
[25] 15 F. Cas. 1018 (C.C.D. Mass. 1817) (No. 8568).
[26] 15 F. Cas. 1018 (C.C.D. Mass. 1817) (No. 8568).
[27] 15 F. Cas. 1018 (C.C.D. Mass. 1817) (No. 8568).
[28] 15 F. Cas. 1018 (C.C.D. Mass. 1817) (No. 8568).
[29] 15 F. Cas. 1018 (C.C.D. Mass. 1817) (No. 8568). Lowell claims a right to the patent via assignment (Perkins). Lewis claims a right to the patent via assignment (Baker).
[30] 15 F. Cas. 1018 (C.C.D. Mass. 1817) (No. 8568).
[31] 15 F. Cas. 1018 (C.C.D. Mass. 1817) (No. 8568).
[32] 15 F. Cas. 1018 (C.C.D. Mass. 1817) (No. 8568).
[33] 15 F. Cas. 1018, 1019 (C.C.D. Mass. 1817) (No. 8568).
[34] 15 F. Cas. 1018 (C.C.D. Mass. 1817) (No. 8568).
[35] 3 F. Cas. 37 (C.C.D. Mass. 1817) (No. 1216).

> *"No person is entitled to a patent under the act of congress unless he has invented some new and useful art, machine, manufacture, or composition of matter, not known or used before. By useful invention, in the statute, is meant such a one as may be applied to some beneficial use in society, in contradistinction to an invention, which is injurious to the morals, the health, or the good order of society. It is not necessary to establish, that the invention is of such general utility, as to supersede all other inventions now in practice to accomplish the same purpose. It is sufficient, that it has no obnoxious or mischievous tendency, that it may be applied to practical uses, and that so far as it is applied, it is salutary. If its practical utility be very limited, it will follow, that it will be of little or no profit to the inventor; and if it be trifling, it will sink into utter neglect. The law, however, does not look to the degree of utility; it simply requires, that it shall be capable of use, and that the use is such as sound morals and policy do not discountenance or prohibit. In the present case there cannot be the slightest doubt upon the evidence, that the patent is for a useful invention, in a very large sense."*[36]

### *3.2.3 Demise of the Moral Utility Doctrine*

The use of the Moral Utility Doctrine eventually declined beginning in the 1950s and 1960s with the Patent Act of 1952 (35 U.S.C. § 101), which did not include provisions for morality for patent eligibility.[37] Notably, in *Juicy Whip, Inc. v. Orange Bang, Inc. and Unique Beverage Dispensers*, a dispute arose as to the patentability of a beverage dispensing machine.[38] The case involved a specific interpretation of 35 U.S.C. § 101, which states that "whoever invents or discovers any new and useful process, machine, manufacture, or composition of matter, or any new and useful improvement thereof, may obtain a patent on the invention or discovery."[39] The drink machine consisted of a transparent mixing container which contained what buyers believed to be the actual beverage they would be purchasing and consuming.[40] However, the visibly mixed beverage in the transparent container merely simulated the actual beverage dispensed to consumers.[41] Juicy Whip, Inc., brought legal action for patent infringement against Orange Bang, Inc. and Unique Beverage Dispensers.[42] The legal issue in *Juicy Whip, Inc. v. Orange Bang, Inc. and Unique Beverage Dispensers* was whether the simulation of the actual drink in the dispenser constituted utility.[43] The district court had previously ruled that the patent for the drink dispenser could not be considered valid because the simulation of the actual drink in the dispenser, being a deception, did not meet the utility requirement as per 35 U.S.C.S. § 101.[44] The Federal Circuit Court disagreed with the district court ruling, stating that just because consumers were misled, it did not equal a lack of utility.[45] Specifically, *Juicy Whip, Inc. v. Orange Bang, Inc. and Unique Beverage Dispenser* stated that "[t]he requirement of 'utility' in patent law is not a directive to the Patent and

36 3 F. Cas. 37 (C.C.D. Mass. 1817) (No. 1216).
37 Patent Act of 1952 (35 U.S.C.S. § 101).
38 185 F.3d 1364-1366 (Fed. Cir. 1999).
39 35 U.S.C. § 101; 185 F.3d 1364-1366 (Fed. Cir. 1999).
40 185 F.3d 1364-1366 (Fed. Cir. 1999).
41 185 F.3d 1364-1366 (Fed. Cir. 1999).
42 185 F.3d 1364-1366 (Fed. Cir. 1999).
43 185 F.3d 1364-1366 (Fed. Cir. 1999).
44 185 F.3d 1364-1366 (Fed. Cir. 1999).
45 185 F.3d 1364-1366 (Fed. Cir. 1999).

Trademark Office or the courts to serve as arbiters of deceptive trade practices. Other agencies, such as the Federal Trade Commission and the Food and Drug Administration, are assigned the task of protecting consumers from fraud and deception in the sale of food products."[46] In language most closely associated with tenets of *ordre public* and morality, *Juicy Whip, Inc. v. Orange Bang, Inc. and Unique Beverage Dispenser* quoted *Webber v. Virginia* in stating that "[c]ongress never intended that the patent laws should displace the police powers of the States, meaning by that term those powers by which the health, good order, peace and general welfare of the community are promoted."[47,48] Patent infringement was found because the deception in *Juicy Whip, Inc. v. Orange Bang, Inc. and Unique Beverage Dispenser* was equivalent to utility in the drink dispenser.[49] The significance of *Juicy Whip, Inc. v. Orange Bang, Inc. and Unique Beverage Dispensers* was that this case set a notable legal precedent for ethical considerations in subsequent patent cases, including those involving genetic engineering and gene editing.

#### *3.2.4 Faux Revival of the Moral Utility Doctrine*

Although the Moral Utility Doctrine is no longer a factor in patentability, this does not mean absolutely anything can be patented. Limitations for patentability have been imposed by other laws [15, 16]. As such, a faux revival of the Moral Utility Doctrine exists. For instance, the 1954 Atomic Energy Act prohibits the issue of patents "for any invention or discovery which is useful solely in the utilization of special nuclear material or atomic energy in an atomic weapon. Any patent granted for any such invention or discovery is hereby revoked, and just compensation shall be made therefor [15, 16]."[50] Later, the use of gene editing for the creation of human beings such as the creation of a baby using gene editing techniques was prohibited [15, 16]. Doing so would not only be questionable regarding reasonable morals and ethics, but also to with regard to international treaties and declarations which eschew tampering with the human germline as deleterious activity for the sake of mankind in general.[51] Thus, "[t]he discretion to consider the wellbeing and good policy of society implicit in the statutory term 'useful' is properly applied when a refusal to grant a patent is necessary to avoid preempting the power of Congress to define essential questions of public policy."[52,53]

## 4. Genetic Foundations of Gene Editing

The human body is composed of organs (*e.g.* heart, brain, liver, kidneys) which perform various functions vital for the sustenance of life. These organs are composed of different types of tissues which form their structure and aid in their function. These tissues are built from billions of cells which nourish, regulate, and maintain homeostasis

[46] 185 F.3d 1364,1368 (Fed. Cir. 1999).

[47] 185 F.3d 1364,1368 (Fed. Cir. 1999); *quoting* 103 U.S. (13 Otto) 344, 347-48, 26 L.Ed. 565 (1880).

[48] 185 F.3d 1364, 1367 (Fed. Cir. 1999).

[49] 185 F.3d 1364, 1367 (Fed. Cir. 1999).

[50] United States Patent and Trademark Office, 42 USC §2181(a) (1961).

[51] Universal Declaration on the Human Genome and Human Rights

[52] Seymore SB. Making Patents Useful. Minnesota Law Review. 2014 [17]; 301:1046–109. Seymore SB, Patently Impossible, 64 Vanderbilt Law Review 1491, 1494, 1507 (2011).

[53] *Lowell v. Lewis*, 15 F. Cas. 1018 (Story, Circuit Justice, C.C.D. Mass. 1817) (No. 8568).

(a balanced and healthy environment for growth and function). The cellular nucleus – a type of structure called an organelle – serves as the control center for all activity within the cell. In addition, the nucleus contains genetic information which acts as a collective memory not only for the cell, but for the entire human body. Genetic material codes for a host of physical, character, and personality traits, along with predispositions for disease traits [18]. This genetic material is carried on somatic chromosomes, also known as autosomes [19]. Each human cell consists of 46 chromosomes, or 23 pairs of chromosomes, which are comprised of genes [19]. The sex chromosomes are determinative for gender – XX for female and XY for male [19]. The Y chromosome is instrumental for gender identification [19]. Genetical material in chromosomes is stored in units called nucleosomes, which consist of structured proteins called histones around which the former chromosomes are wrapped and stored [18].

Several types of information are stored within deoxyribonucleic acid (DNA), including information regarding cellular functions.[54] DNA is housed within the nucleus of a human cell, which serves as a control center for all of the activities conducted within a cell.[55] Deoxyribonucleic acid, or DNA, consists of a double helical structure.[56] DNA is composed of the bases adenine (A), cytosine (C), guanine (G), and thymine (T).[57] When pairing within the double helix, A binds with T, and C binds with G.[58] Thus, many base pairings are possible [20].

The "genetic material" referenced heretofore is also known as a gene or genes. Genes are composed of double-helical DNA [18]. Genes serve as information repositories for the human body. Genetic information also codes for characteristics which are expressed after the DNA is translated – or decoded – typically into amino acids, the building blocks for proteins [18]. Physical traits and/or characteristics are expressed through these proteins [18]. CRISPR edits genes in very much the same manner that a pair of molecular scissors locates a desired gene segment with the aid of cellular molecular machinery and selects the portion of the genetic sequence for editing.[59] Cas9 cuts DNA at the site of the genetic sequence of interest [21]. The undesired genetic information is then removed [22]. After the DNA of interest is removed, the desired genetic sequence is added [23]. The CRISPR-Cas9 system then reconnects the cut ends of the gene segment [24].

[54] MLA CE Course Manual: Molecular Biology Information Resources (Genetics Review: Gene) [Internet]. www.ncbi.nlm.nih.gov. Available from: https://www.ncbi.nlm.nih.gov/Class/MLACourse/Original8Hour/Genetics/gene.html.

[55] MLA CE Course Manual: Molecular Biology Information Resources (Genetics Review: Gene) [Internet]. www.ncbi.nlm.nih.gov. Available from: https://www.ncbi.nlm.nih.gov/Class/MLACourse/Original8Hour/Genetics/gene.html.

[56] MLA CE Course Manual: Molecular Biology Information Resources (Genetics Review: Gene) [Internet]. www.ncbi.nlm.nih.gov. Available from: https://www.ncbi.nlm.nih.gov/Class/MLACourse/Original8Hour/Genetics/gene.html.

[57] MLA CE Course Manual: Molecular Biology Information Resources (Genetics Review: Gene) [Internet]. www.ncbi.nlm.nih.gov. Available from: https://www.ncbi.nlm.nih.gov/Class/MLACourse/Original8Hour/Genetics/gene.html.

[58] MLA CE Course Manual: Molecular Biology Information Resources (Genetics Review: Gene) [Internet]. www.ncbi.nlm.nih.gov. Available from: https://www.ncbi.nlm.nih.gov/Class/MLACourse/Original8Hour/Genetics/gene.html.

[59] CRISPR/Cas9 – Molecular Scissors Made of Enzyme and RNA [Internet]. www.mpg.de. Available from: https://www.mpg.de/11823385/crispr-cas9.

## 5. A New Eugenics movement? *Ordre Public* and Morality Concerns in Direct-to-Consumer Genetics Testing

The development of direct-to-consumer technology has elicited fears of the emergence of a new eugenics movement in the twenty-first century. Direct-to-consumer genetics testing allows consumers to bypass physician and health care provider consultation for the diagnosis and interpretation of genetics testing devices. Patents for direct-to-consumer genetics testing biotechnology have been issued to several companies for exploring DNA databases for the purpose of gleaning information concerning ancestry, heredity, and genealogy through direct-to-consumer testing. These include Ancestry, Nebula Genomics, 23andMe, MyHeritage DNA, Living DNA, Sequencing, and Vitagene. Many of these companies also provide information concerning an individual's nation or continent of origin.

For instance, 23andMe has been issued numerous patents for recombinant DNA technology to compare users' DNA with DNA samples in preexisting DNA databases in anticipation of matches for DNA traits for certain physical characteristics [25]. Ideally, having higher numbers of users in the 23andMe genetic database optimizes the possibility of successful genetic matches. Traits such as eye color and athleticism are of interest in the 23andMe tests [25]. 23andMe also claims the ability to test for genetic traits that increase the likelihood of contracting specific medical diseases or ailments later in life, including cancer, lupus, Crohn's disease, multiple sclerosis, and heart disease [26]. These trait associations are also categorized as "inheritance risk" for developing these ailments later in life. Ethicists are concerned that fertility clinics will be tempted to use information for selecting desirable traits for the creation of "designer babies" with 23andMe patents, including "Gamete donor selection based on genetic calculations [27]."[60] In expressing their concerns, ethicists cite the nineteenth century patent case *Bedford v. Hunt* for positing that the patent(s) granted for 23andMe direct-to-consumer genetics testing violates principles of "sound morals" [28]. Additional questions surrounding privacy and consent issues concerning the vast DNA 23andMe databases have arisen as well, challenging moral and ethical boundary issues of the 23andMe genetics testing patents [28].

## 6. Moral Prohibitions against Gene Editing and Patenting

Scientific innovation in genetic technology has resulted in advances such as assisted reproductive technology, embryo research, stem cell therapy, genetic engineering, and CRISPR gene editing technology. However, like that of direct-to-consumer genetic testing, the development of CRISPR gene editing technology has elicited fears of the emergence of a new eugenics movement for the twenty-first century. Growing worldwide concerns over ethical issues surrounding CRISPR-Cas9 and the ability of those conducting such research to manipulate the genome are very concerning. As such, a regulatory plan or a worldwide consensus on CRISPR-Cas9 was needed to delve more deeply into ethical concerns regarding gene editing technology. The International Summit on Gene Editing conducted by the National Academies of Science at the Institute of Medicine in December 2015 addressed these concerns. There, support for continued exploring of gene editing was voiced [29].

[60] United States Patent 8,543,339.

## 7. United States Legislative and Statutory Regulation of Patents

Statutory law further elaborates on the issue of patentable subject matter at 35 U.S.C. § 101: "Whoever invents or discovers any new and useful process, machine, manufacture, or composition of matter, or any new and useful improvement thereof, may obtain a patent therefor, subject to the conditions and requirements of this title." Here, we ascertain the requirements for patentability under United States law: (1) patentable subject matter, (2) novelty, (3) utility (usefulness), (4) non-obviousness, and (5) written disclosure.[61] Patent owners have exclusive rights, which include rights to make, use, sell, import, or exclude others from profiting from the invention.[62] The inventor or owner of the rights of a patented invention may prevent others from utilizing the patented invention. As per 35 U.S.C. § 271 (a), "whoever without authority makes, uses, offers to sell, or sells any patented invention, within the United States or imports into the United States any patented invention during the term of the patent therefor, infringes the patent."[63]

The Bayh-Dole Act is a government mechanism implemented to encourage the commercialization of patents.[64] The 1970s was an economically stagnant era in which the government sought alternative means for injecting vigor into the economy. Incentivizing research innovation by reexamining the administration of the federal patent system and modifying federal statutes and regulations if needed was one way to accomplish this goal. Before the Bayh Dole Act, the United States federal government assumed intellectual property rights for inventions patented at academic research institutions supported with federal funds. However, these government-issued patents were not widely utilized [30]. The problem with this federal model was that it disincentivized research and innovation by not allowing either inventors or academic institutions to be able to capitalize on potential commercial profits for inventions. Essentially, the inventors had little to no agency regarding the ability to also license the technology to other entities that might benefit from the research. This is not to mention the dampening effect upon the ability of inventors and institutions to create and cultivate research collaborations both nationally and internationally. Government agencies failed to harmonize policies with regard to the issuance and management of federal research and development funding [30]. After the enactment of the Bayh-Dole Act, the number of patents issued to universities in the United States increased from 390 in 1980 to nearly 7000 in 2015 [30].

### 7.1 National Institutes of Health (NIH)

Legal prohibitions against gene editing in human germ cell lines exist in over 40 countries worldwide. The United States National Institutes of Health (NIH) reiterated that gene editing would not be supported by NIH funding [31]. A moratorium on germline gene editing followed [32]. According to the Dickey-Wicker amendment in United States law, congressionally appropriated funds to the NIH are not to be used

[61] 35 U.S.C. §§ 101, 102, 103, 112.

[62] 35 U.S.C. 154 (a) (1).

[63] 35 U.S.C. § 271 (a).

[64] P.L. 96-517.

for research that may lead to the destruction of human embryos.[65,66,67] Leadership at the National Institutes of Health believes that an international moratorium should be instated on germline gene editing [33]. Yet, the term "moratorium" could have a variety of different meanings. One meaning of moratorium could be the placement of all germline gene editing activities on hiatus until countries can further agree on the social and ethical impact of gene editing. Another meaning of a moratorium could mean to cease all germline gene editing activities until a formal assessment of state positions on the matter. Still another meaning could be to temporarily ban all germline gene editing activities. Moreover, a moratorium could mean a more permanent ban on germline gene editing activities until all outstanding controversial issues are resolved. This is a seemingly impossible feat considering the number of stakeholders who likely have divergent opinions on germline gene editing. One issue that is important to distinguish is whether germline editing should be permitted for research purposes only [32]. Yet, the inclination to expand germline editing beyond research purposes plus the additional potential profits from doing so stretches the limits of ethical and societal tolerance. For these reasons, some form of government regulation is advisable.

### 7.2 Food and Drug Administration (FDA)

The Federal Food, Drug, and Cosmetic Act (FD&C Act) regulates CRISPR-Cas9 gene editing in the United States.[68] Concerning CRISPR-Cas9 gene editing, the Federal Food, Drug, and Cosmetic Act (FD&C Act) references "articles intended for use in the diagnosis, cure, mitigation, treatment, or prevention of disease in man or other animals."[69] Diagnostics or therapies may be initially tested in animals with a later purpose of using them to treat diseases in humans on a wide scale. The FD&C Act continues by stating that the Act has jurisdiction over "articles (other than food) intended to affect the structure or any function of the body of man or other animals."[70] The United States Code states that "[i]t shall not be an act of infringement to make, use, offer to sell, or sell within the United States or import into the United States a patented invention (other than a new animal drug or veterinary biological product (as those terms are used in the Federal Food, Drug, and Cosmetic Act and

[65] H.R. 2880, 104th Cong. § 128 (1996).

[66] Consolidated Appropriations Act, 2017, Public Law 115-31, §736, 131 Stat. 135, 173.

[67] Embryos, Pub. L. No. 104-99, § 128, 110 Stat. 34 (1996). "Section 128. None of the funds made available by Public Law 104–91 may be used for— (1) the creation of a human embryo or embryos for research purposes; or (2) research in which a human embryo or embryos are destroyed, discarded, or knowingly subjected to risk of injury or death greater than that allowed for research on fetuses in utero under 45 CFR 46.208(a)(2) and 42 U.S.C. 289 g(b). For purposes of this section, the phrase 'human embryo or embryos' shall include any organism, not protected as a human subject under 45 CFR 46 as of the date of enactment of this Act, that is derived by fertilization, parthenogenesis, cloning, or any other means from one or more human gametes."

[68] 21 U.S.C. 321 *et seq*.

[69] Federal Food, Drug, and Cosmetic Act (FD&C Act), Section 201(g); Draft Guidance #187. Guidance for Industry Regulation of Intentionally Altered Genomic DNA in Animals. 2017. (Revision of Guidance #187, "Regulation of Genetically Engineered Animals").

[70] Federal Food, Drug, and Cosmetic Act (FD&C Act), Section 201(g); Draft Guidance #187. Guidance for Industry Regulation of Intentionally Altered Genomic DNA in Animals. 2017. (Revision of Guidance #187, "Regulation of Genetically Engineered Animals").

the Act of March 4, 1913) which is primarily manufactured using recombinant DNA, recombinant RNA, hybridoma technology, or other processes involving site specific genetic manipulation techniques) solely for uses reasonably related to the development and submission of information under a Federal law which regulates the manufacture, use, or sale of drugs or veterinary biological products."[71]

Genetic manipulation impacts the structure and/or function of living organisms in a manner intended to alter the biology and physiology of genes to achieve an effect desired by the researcher. Often, this effect is to diagnose, prevent, or treat diseases. The Food and Drug Administration (FDA) initially released non-binding draft guidance for the regulation of genetic engineering in 2008 and 2009.[72] The 2008 and 2009 draft guidance were followed by the additional release of draft guidance in 2017 which expanded regulation of genetic engineering to include the oversight and regulation of gene editing in animals [34].[73] FDA standards classify CRISPR-Cas9 or other types of edited genomes as "altered" [35]. Such alterations include genetic deletions, insertions, and other types of changes modulated using recombinant DNA (rDNA) or other types of genetic molecular technology [35].

## 7.3 United States Patent and Trademark Office (USPTO)

Federal provisions for the activities of the United States Patent and Trademark Office (USPTO) are codified at 35 U.S.C. §§ 1–376. The Code of Federal Regulations outlines specific regulations for the activities of the USPTO.[74] Created by the America Invents Act, the Patent Trial and Appeal Board (PTAB) is an administrative board of USPTO Department of Commerce.[75] The PTAB is comprised of federal statutory members, administrative patent law judges, and administrative support staff.[76,77] Federal statutory members of the PTAB include the USPTO Director, who is appointed by President with Senate advice and consent; the Deputy Director, who is appointed by the Secretary of Commerce; the Commissioner for Patents, who is appointed by the Secretary of Commerce; and the Commissioner for Trademarks, who is appointed by the Secretary of Commerce.[78] Administrative Patent Law Judges are appointed by the Secretary of Commerce.[79] Administrative support staff include patent attorneys, law clerks, paralegals, and support staff.[80]

The PTAB has several duties. Primarily, these duties involve patent prosecution. The PTAB conducts (1) trials, including *inter partes review*; (2) post-grant review; (3)

---

[71] 35 U.S.C. § 271 (e).

[72] Draft Guidance for Industry #187: Regulation of Genetically Engineered Animals Containing Heritable rDNA Constructs. September 18, 2008.

[73] Draft Guidance #187. Guidance for Industry Regulation of Intentionally Altered Genomic DNA in Animals. 2017. (Revision of Guidance #187, "Regulation of Genetically Engineered Animals")

[74] 37 CFR (2016).

[75] Patent Trial and Appeal Board [Internet]. USPTO.gov. 2024 [cited 2025 Mar 17]. Available from: https://www.uspto.gov/patents/ptab.

[76] 35 U.S.C. § 6.

[77] Patent Trial and Appeal Board [Internet]. USPTO.gov. 2024 [cited 2025 Mar 17]. Available from: https://www.uspto.gov/patents/ptab.

[78] 35 U.S.C. § 6(a) (b).

[79] 35 U.S.C. § 6(a).

[80] 35 U.S.C. § 6(a).

covered business method patent reviews; (4) and derivation proceedings. In addition to conducting trials, the PTAB hears appeals from adverse examiner decisions in patent applications and reexamination proceedings. Finally, the PTAB renders decisions in interferences.[81] *Inter partes review* (IPR) is a trial proceeding conducted at the PTAB to review the patentability of one or more claims in a patent only on a ground that could be raised under 35 USC §§ 102 (novelty) or 103 (non-obviousness).[82] The IPR is a "hybrid proceeding" with "adjudicatory characteristics."[83]

Patent examiners review patent applications during patent prosecution and issue decisions on the approval of those applications. Patent examiners also aid in evaluating and resolving disputes concerning patent infringement. The Manual of Patent Examining Procedures (MPEP) serves as an aid to patent examiners in executing their patent prosecution duties.[84] Specific protocols concerning the determination of patentability and the patent examination procedure are included in the MPEP.[85] *Public ordre* and morality congruence with potentially patentable subject matter, however, are not required for determination of patentability.

## 8. United States Genetic Engineering and Patent Cases

The United States courts adjudicated several cases which addressed genetic engineering rights. These included *Funk Brothers Seed Co. v. Kalo Inoculant Co., Diamond v. Chakrabarty, Association for Molecular Pathology v. Myriad Genetics, Inc., Ariosa Diagnostics, Inc. v. Sequenom, Inc., and Regents of The University of California v. Broad Institute. Funk Brothers Seed Co. v. Kalo Inoculant Co.* was a United States Supreme Court case that deliberated the patentable qualities of *Rhizobia*, or nitrogen-fixing bacteria.[86] In *Diamond v. Chakrabarty*, the issue brought to the Supreme Court by the petitioners was whether genetically modified bacteria could be patented as a new invention.[87] Scientists attempted to patent predictive markers indicative for breast cancer, BRCA1 and BRCA2, in *Association for Molecular Pathology v. Myriad Genetics*.[88] *Ariosa Diagnostics, Inc. v. Sequenom, Inc.* addressed the patent eligibility of cell-free fetal DNA ("cffDNA") in discarded maternal plasma and serum samples.[89] *Regents of The University of California v. Broad Institute* concerned CRISPR gene editing litigation over patenting rights.

[81] Patent Trial and Appeal Board [Internet]. uspto.gov. 2024 [cited 2025 Mar 17]. Available from: https://www.uspto.gov/patents/ptab.

[82] 35 USC §311–319; Inter Partes Review [Internet]. www.uspto.gov. [cited 2025 Mar 17]. Available from: https://www.uspto.gov/patents/ptab/trials/inter-partes-review.

[83] *Saint Regis Mohawk Tribe v. Mylan Pharms*, 896 F.3d 1322, 1326 (Fed. Cir. 2018).

[84] US Patent and Trademark Office. *Manual of Patent Examining Procedure*. 9th ed. October 2019. Last Revised June 2020, https://www.uspto.gov/web/offices/pac/mpep/index.html. Last visited June 15, 2021.

[85] 2100. Patentability. US Patent and Trademark Office. *Manual of Patent Examining Procedure*. 9th ed. October 2019. Last Revised June 2020, https://www.uspto.gov/web/offices/pac/mpep/mpep-2100.html. Last visited June 15, 2021.

[86] 333 U.S. 127 (1948).

[87] 447 U.S. 303, 305 (1980).

[88] *Association for Molecular Pathology v. Myriad Genetics, Inc.*, 569 U.S. 576 (2013).

[89] 788 F.3d 1371 (Fed. Cir. 2015).

### 8.1 *Funk Brothers Seed Co. v. Kalo Inoculant Co.*, 333 U.S. 127 (1948)

The question before the court in *Funk Brothers Seed Co. v. Kalo Inoculant Co.* concerned whether mixing and presenting for sale different types of *Rhizobia* bacteria characterized by differences in their ability to enhance the growth of legumes constituted patentable subject matter.[90] *Rhizobia* bacteria colonize plant roots through the root hairs of certain species of plants, particularly legumes (*e.g.* peanuts, peas, beans, soybeans, lentils, chickpeas) [36, 37]. Nitrogen coexists freely with oxygen in the earth's atmosphere [36, 37]. The process of nitrogen fixation occurs in the roots of the legume plants [38].[91] Nitrogen fixing bacteria extract nitrogen from the air and convert the nitrogen to ammonia, a nitrogen-containing chemical, that is used by the legumes [36, 37]. However, nitrogen-fixing bacteria are not created equally. When various species of nitrogen-fixing bacteria are mixed and combined in close contact with the roots of legume plants, different *Rhizobia* species may cancel or inhibit the nitrogen-fixing characteristics of others.[92] *Funk Brothers Seed Co. v. Kalo Inoculant Co* states that "[t]he qualities of these [nitrogen-fixing] bacteria, like the heat of the sun, electricity, or the qualities of metals, are part of the storehouse of knowledge of all men. They are manifestations of laws of nature, free to all men and reserved exclusively to none. He who discovers a hitherto unknown phenomenon of nature has no claim to a monopoly of it which the law recognizes."[93]

### 8.2 *Diamond v. Chakrabarty*, 447 U.S. 303 (1980)

General Electric Company scientist Ananda Chakrabarty used plasmids to create a genetically engineered bacteria, *Pseudomonas putida*, which was designed to break down crude oil.[94] Chakrabarty filed a patent claim for the genetically modified bacterium in 1972, along with a process claim for the construction of the bacteria and a carrier material.[95] The Patent and Trademark Office rejected the initial patent claim for the genetically engineered *Pseudomonas putida* bacteria. Chakrabarty appealed the decision all the way to the United States Supreme Court. The Supreme Court ruled that a "human-made, genetically engineered bacterium [that was] capable of breaking down multiple components of crude oil" is patentable.[96] More generally, the Supreme Court found in *Diamond v. Chakrabarty* that "anything under the sun that is made by man" could be patented.[97] Chakrabarty was victorious, and his patent for genetically engineered bacteria was issued.

As for ethics and morality, *Diamond v. Chakrabarty* is mostly silent.[98] *Diamond v. Chakrabarty* defers to elected officials and independent decision-making bodies for decision-making concerning the morality of patenting genetic materials. Specifically,

---

[90] *Funk Brothers Seed Co. v. Kalo Inoculant Co.*, 333 U.S. 127 (1948).

[91] Wagner S. Biological Nitrogen Fixation [Internet]. www.nature.com. 2011 [cited 2025 Mar 18]. Available from: https://www.nature.com/scitable/knowledge/library/biological-nitrogen-fixation-23570419/.

[92] 333 U.S. 127, 130–131 (1948).

[93] 333 U.S. 127, 130 (1948).

[94] 447 U.S. 303, 306 (1980).

[95] 447 U.S. 303, 306, 307 (1980).

[96] 447 U.S. 303, 305 (1980).

[97] 447 U.S. 303 (1980).

[98] 447 U.S. 303 (1980).

*Diamond v. Chakrabarty* "involve[d] the balancing of competing values and interests, which in our democratic system is the business of elected representatives."[99] Balancing competing values and interests does not necessarily mean making moral or ethical decisions on those competing values and interests. Nor does balancing competing values and interests mean the denial or approval of a patent for a somatic gene edited product. Thus, many legal scholars conclude that the approach of *Diamond v. Chakrabarty* is to indiscriminately approve patents for "anything under the sun that is made by man" without regard for ethics and morals concerning patents.[100,101]

In other words, "[p]atent first. Ask questions later."[102] Ultimately, Dale Hoeschit, Chakrabarty's attorney in *Diamond v. Chakrabarty*, summarized the prevailing view regarding the morality of the genetic modification of bacteria in the case (*Diamond v. Chakrabarty*) [39]. Hoeschit stated, "The patents for these innovations are limited only by the skill of the individuals drafting the claims. Although there are moral and ethical issues involved in the manufacture of living things, patents themselves are not designed to address such issues. The role of the Patent Office is to determine novelty and nonobviousness; issues of morality and ethics are best left to other organizations specifically tasked to deal with those issues" [39].

### 8.3 *Association for Molecular Pathology v. Myriad Genetics, Inc.*, 569 U.S. 576 (2013)

The goal in *Association for Molecular Pathology v. Myriad Genetics* was to isolate genetically coding regions of BRCA1 and BRCA2 from non-coding regions of BRCA1 and BRCA2. In this case, synthetically created cDNA, a copy of the original DNA sequences for BRCA1 and BRCA2, was proposed as a newly created genetically material. The Association for Molecular Pathology claimed that "[t]he nucleotide sequence of cDNA is dictated by nature, not by the lab technician." Consequently, the Association for Molecular Pathology argued that a patent could not be obtained for the cDNA sequence. The Supreme disagreed by ruling on behalf of Myriad Genetics, Inc., ultimately stating that human genetically engineered cDNA was patentable [39]. In ruling on behalf of Myriad Genetics, Inc., the Supreme Court relied partly upon the reasoning of *Parke-Davis & Co. v. H.K. Mulford Co.* in which a new man-made synthetic compound was created based upon a naturally occurring substance in the adrenal gland.[103] The Court stated that the inventors successfully attempted to patent synthetic complementary DNA ("cDNA").[104] The Supreme Court referred to Section 101 of the Patent Act in its ruling in *Association for Molecular Pathology v. Myriad Genetics*, stating that the "Patent Act permits patents to be issued to '[w]hoever invents or discovers any new and useful...composition of matter,' §101, but 'laws of nature, natural phenomena, and abstract ideas' 'are basic tools of scientific and technological work' 'that lie beyond the domain of patent protection.'"[105] The

[99] 447 U.S. 303, 317 (1980).

[100] 447 U.S. 303 (1980).

[101] Margo A. Bagley. Patent First, Ask Questions Later: Morality and Biotechnology in Patent Law. 45 Wm. & Mary L. Rev. 469 (2003–2004).

[102] Margo A. Bagley. Patent First, Ask Questions Later: Morality and Biotechnology in Patent Law. 45 Wm. & Mary L. Rev. 469 (2003–2004).

[103] *Parke-Davis & Co. v. H.K. Mulford Co.*, 189 F. 95, 103 (C.C.S.D.N.Y. 1911).

[104] *Association for Molecular Pathology v. Myriad Genetics, Inc.*, 569 U.S. 576, 582–585 (2013).

[105] *Association for Molecular Pathology v. Myriad Genetics, Inc.*, 569 U.S. 576 (2013).

Supreme Court determined that the DNA claim in *Association for Molecular Pathology v. Myriad Genetics* qualified as a "law of nature exception."[106]

## 8.4 *Ariosa Diagnostics, Inc. v. Sequenom, Inc.*, 3d 1371 (Fed. Cir. 2015)

The scientists in *Ariosa Diagnostics, Inc. v. Sequenom, Inc.* who discovered the cffDNA claimed patents for both the cffDNA and for methods of use of the cffDNA for prenatal diagnostic medical testing.[107] The Court ultimately determined that the patent claims were ineligible.[108] The patent claims were rendered ineligible because the claims were directed to natural aspects of the cffDNA.[109] Therefore, the patent claims did not meet patentability requirements as per 35 U.S.C. § 101.[110]

## 8.5 *Regents of the University of California v. Broad Institute* (2017)

*Regents of The University of California v. Broad Institute* (2017) concerned CRISPR gene editing litigation. Jennifer Doudna of the University of California at Berkeley and Emmanuelle Charpentier of the University of Vienna (now at Max Planck Institute in Germany) filed a United States patent for CRISPR applications in bacteria (prokaryotic cells).[111] Doudna and Charpentier claimed that CRISPR-patented applications in prokaryotic cells would also work in eukaryotic (animal or human) cells.[112] Doudna and Charpentier were the first to file a CRISPR patent application for use in prokaryotic cells.[113] In December 2012, Broad Institute scientist Feng Zheng filed a fast-track CRISPR patent application for gene editing in eukaryotic (animal and human) cells at the United States Patent and Trademark Office.[114] Although Zheng was not the first to file, he was the first to receive the CRISPR patent.[115] The Broad argued that a person having ordinary skill in the art (PHOSITA) would not infer animal and human cell CRISPR applications from the UC Berkeley patent application.[116] The Leahy-Smith America Invents Act (AIA) changed the criteria for awarding patents from a first to invent to a first to file system.[117] In the Pre-Leahy-Smith America Invents Act (AIA), before March 16, 2013, the first to invent was awarded the patent.[118] In the Post-Leahy-Smith America Invents Act (AIA), after March 16, 2013, the first to file as per the effective filing date wins the patent.[119] In the *California v. Broad Institute* patent dispute, Zheng was awarded the patent for being the first to

[106] *Association for Molecular Pathology v. Myriad Genetics, Inc.*, 569 U.S. 576 (2013).

[107] 788 F.3d 1371 (Fed. Cir. 2015).

[108] 788 F.3d 1371 (Fed. Cir. 2015).

[109] 788 F.3d 1371 (Fed. Cir. 2015).

[110] 788 F.3d 1371 (Fed. Cir. 2015).

[111] *Regents of The University of California v. Broad Institute (2017).*

[112] *Regents of The University of California v. Broad Institute (2017).*

[113] *Regents of The University of California v. Broad Institute (2017).*

[114] *Regents of The University of California v. Broad Institute (2017).*

[115] *Regents of The University of California v. Broad Institute (2017).*

[116] *Regents of The University of California v. Broad Institute (2017).*

[117] *Regents of The University of California v. Broad Institute (2017).*

[118] *Regents of The University of California v. Broad Institute (2017).*

[119] *Regents of The University of California v. Broad Institute (2017).*

invent.[120] The United States Patent and Trademark Appeals Board declared that the Broad Institute invention was patentable, not the Berkeley invention, based upon dates of filing and invention.[121] The United States Court of Appeals of the Federal Circuit upheld the United States Patent and Trademark Appeals Board decision in September 2018, stating that the Broad Institute invention was patentable.[122]

## 9. Balancing Gene Editing Patents with *Ordre Public* and Morality

Prioritization and balancing of research, clinical, ethical, and societal goals is important to maintain a healthy marketplace for innovation in gene editing patents. However, as inventors increase their pursuit of gene editing patents, the likelihood of monopoly behavior may increase, as well [40]. Financial gains for companies and industry from CRISPR technology have been significant [41]. Tens and hundreds of millions of dollars have been invested in companies involved with CRISPR technology, including Caribou, CRISPR Therapeutics, Vertex, and Editas [41]. A pharmaceutical deal between CRISPR Therapeutics and Vertex was valued at billions of dollars [41]. Vast socioeconomic disparities among those able to afford to invest in and utilize CRISPR-Cas9 technology and those who cannot is purportedly inevitable [40]. Owners of CRISPR patents may engage in horizontal conduct, in which pharmaceutical competitors gain competitive advantages for all by working together as a pact [42]. For example, several pharmaceutical companies which manufacture and own COVID-19 vaccine CRISPR-patented technologies may form pacts in order to monopolize the vaccine market. Mergers and cartels may accompany horizontal pact activity through collusion, which may result in detrimental consequences for competitors.[123] Thus, gene editing technology proprietors who are economically strongest have the best possibility for survival. This could make smaller-scale gene-editing inventors more susceptible to failure to achieve their patenting and business goals.

Before government regulation of genetic engineering technology, pharmaceutical and biotechnology stakeholders usually make their marketing, licensing, and business practices amenable to distribution to larger numbers of consumers from all socioeconomic backgrounds. Several mechanisms are available for ensuring that patented genetic technology is available to all. In this manner, both large and small companies could earn revenue and profit from the licensing system. This means the exercise of flexibility in licensing arrangements. One way is licensing of patented genetic engineering technology in a non-exclusive manner. Another means is through graduated royalties for patented genetic engineering. Still other ways are through the absence of licensing for non-profit use and flexibility in licensing agreements.

Compulsory licensing of patented inventions is one mechanism governments can use to ensure gene editing technology remains accessible to all [43]. Compulsory licensing can be a viable means for making more of a patented product available. CRISPR-Cas9 diagnostic testing can be made available to patients in need by freeing intellectual property pharmaceutical licensing and marketing to greater numbers of

---

120 *Regents of The University of California v. Broad Institute (2017).*

121 *Regents of The University of California v. Broad Institute (2017).*

122 *Regents of The University of California v. Broad Institute (2017).*

123 Glossary of Industrial Organization Economics and Competition Law, compiled by R. S. Khemani and D. M. Shapiro, commissioned by the Directorate for Financial, Fiscal and Enterprise Affairs, OECD, 1993.

individuals on an international scale [44, 45]. The United States government could negotiate fair compensation for compulsory licensing. Specifically, "(a) Whenever an invention described in and covered by a patent of the United States is used or manufactured by or for the United States without license of the owner thereof or lawful right to use or manufacture the same, the owner's remedy shall be by action against the United States in the United States Court of Federal Claims for the recovery of his reasonable and entire compensation for such use and manufacture.... For the purposes of this section, the use or manufacture of an invention described in and covered by a patent of the United States by a contractor, a subcontractor, or any person, firm, or corporation for the Government and with the authorization or consent of the Government, shall be construed as use or manufacture for the United States."[124] This would enable patented product availability "for the purpose of enabling the Government to purchase goods for the performance of its functions without the threat of having the supplier enjoined from selling patented goods to the Government."[125]

## 10. Conclusion

The USPTO does not adhere to specific prohibitions on patents for gene editing beyond those outlined by United States statutes, laws, and administrative regulations. Specifically, "[u]nder current law, there is no morality determination made at the USPTO and a patent examiner may not reject a patent application on moral grounds" [46]. As gene editing methods are introduced, patented, and marketed, accessibility to greater numbers of people in need of the technology should increase as well. In the interim, the legal system must do more to prepare for a continued tsunami of patent infringement cases involving gene editing. Staffing legal personnel who are adequately experienced in matters of law pertinent to gene editing would help tremendously in both passing regulatory legislation and adjudicating cases. More importantly, however, an overall shift in legal culture which embraces, rather than fears, the exponential progression of genetic patent litigation would be immensely helpful in striking the right balance when regulating gene editing technology.

[124] 28 U.S.C. § 1498.

[125] *Coakwell v. United States,* 372 F. 2d 508, 511 (Ct. Cls. 1967).

## Author details

Dorkina Myrick[1,2,3,4,5]

1 Public Policy (MPP), University of Oxford, UK

2 Laws (LLM) in Intellectual Property, University of Turin/World Intellectual Property Organization/International Training Centre of the International Labour Organization, Italy

3 Laws (LLM) in European Law, Université Paris II Panthéon-Assas, France

4 Boston University School of Law, USA

5 Brown University School of Medicine, USA

*Address all correspondence to: dcm776@gmail.com

## References


[1] Wadhwa R, Yu J, Parikh A. eP277: Exploring the landscape of genetics patents in the United States from 2005 to 2020. Genetics in Medicine. Mar 2022;**24**(3):S174-S175

[2] Cook-Deegan R. Gene patents. Hastings center bioethics briefings. In: From Birth to Death and Bench to Clinic: The Hastings Center Bioethics Briefing Book for Journalists, Policymakers, and Campaigns. New York: Hastings Center; 2015. pp. 69-72

[3] Kesselheim AS, Cook-Deegan RM, Winickoff DE, Mello MM. Gene patenting—The supreme court finally speaks. New England Journal of Medicine. 2013;**369**(9):869-875. DOI: 10.1056/nejmhle1308199

[4] Husserl G. Public policy and ordre public. Virginia Law Review. 1938;**25**(1):37-67. DOI: 10.2307/1068114

[5] The definition of morality (Stanford encyclopedia of philosophy) [Internet]. 2025. Available from: https://plato.stanford.edu/entries/morality-definition/ [Accessed: March 10, 2025]

[6] Singer P. Ethics | definition, history, examples, types, philosophy, & facts [internet]. Encyclopedia Britannica. 2025. Available from: https://www.britannica.com/topic/ethics-philosophy [Accessed: March 10, 2025]

[7] Turda M. New perspectives on race and eugenics. The Historical Journal. 2008;**51**(4):1115-1124. DOI: 10.1017/S0018246X0800722X

[8] Bank A. Of 'native skulls' and 'Noble Caucasians': Phrenology in colonial South Africa. Journal of Southern African Studies. 1996;**22**(3):387-403. DOI: 10.1080/03057079608708501

[9] Hilts VL. Obeying the laws of hereditary descent: Phrenological views on inheritance and eugenics. Journal of the History of the Behavioral Sciences. 1982;**18**:62-77

[10] Kevles DJ. From eugenics to patents: Genetics, law, and human rights. Annals of Human Genetics. 2011;**75**(3):326-333. DOI: 10.1111/j.1469-1809.2011.00648

[11] Larson EJ. Sex, Race, and Science: Eugenics in the Deep South. Baltimore, Maryland: Johns Hopkins University Press; 1996

[12] Larson EJ, Reilly PR. The surgical solution: A history of involuntary sterilization in the United States. Journal of American History. 1992;**79**(1):300. DOI: 10.2307/2078572

[13] Emma SJ, Carrie V. How a family became a test case for forced sterilizations. NPR [Internet]. 2018. Available from: https://www.npr.org/2018/04/23/604926914/emma-carrie-vivian-how-a-family-became-a-test-case-for-forced-sterilizations

[14] Barrett M. Intellectual Property. Emanuel Law Outlines. 3rd ed. 2012. p. 29

[15] Is gene editing patentable? AMA Journal of Ethics [Internet]. 2019;**21**(12):E1049-E1055. DOI: 10.1001/amajethics.2019.1049

[16] Myrick D. Perspective chapter: Ethical implications and international human rights protections of gene editing of DNA sequences [Internet]. Genome Editing - Recent Advances and Applications [Working Title]. London, UK: IntechOpen; 2025. DOI: 10.5772/intechopen.1009025

[17] Seymore S. Making patents useful. Minnesota Law Review. 2013;**98**:1046

[18] National Human Genome Research Institute. A brief guide to genomics [Internet]. Genome.gov. National Human Genome Research Institute. 2022 . Available from: https://www.genome.gov/about-genomics/fact-sheets/A-Brief-Guide-to-Genomics

[19] Introduction to genomics [Internet]. Genome.gov. Available from: https://www.genome.gov/About-Genomics/Introduction-to-Genomics#one

[20] Bates S. Deoxyribonucleic acid (DNA) [Internet]. Genome.gov. National Human Genome Research Institute. 2024. Available from: https://www.genome.gov/genetics-glossary/Deoxyribonucleic-Acid

[21] Sternberg SH, Redding S, Jinek M, Greene EC, Doudna JA. DNA interrogation by the CRISPR RNA-guided endonuclease Cas9. Nature. 2014;**507**(7490):62-67. DOI: 10.1038/nature13011

[22] Ledford H. Five big mysteries about CRISPR's origins. Nature. 2017;**541**(7637):280-282. DOI: 10.1038/541280a

[23] National Library of Medicine. What are genome editing and CRISPR-Cas9? [Internet]. Medlineplus. 2022. Available from: https://medlineplus.gov/genetics/understanding/genomicresearch/genomeediting/

[24] Sander JD, Joung JK. CRISPR-Cas Systems for Editing, regulating and targeting genomes. Nature Biotechnology [Internet]. 2014;**32**(4):347-355. DOI: 10.1038/nbt.2842

[25] Rojahn S. Should you worry about 23andMe patenting "designer babies"? MIT Technology Review [Internet]. 2013. Available from: https://www.technologyreview.com/2013/10/03/176244/should-you-worry-about-23andme-patenting-designer-babies/

[26] Pray L. DTC genetic testing: 23andme, DNA direct and Genelex. Nature Education [Internet]. 2008;**1**(1):22. Available from: https://www.nature.com/scitable/topicpage/dtc-genetic-testing-23andme-dna-direct-and-674/

[27] Sterckx S, Cockbain J, Howard HC, Borry P. "I prefer a child with …": Designer babies, another controversial patent in the arena of direct-to-consumer genomics. Genetics in Medicine. 2013;**15**(12):923-924. DOI: 10.1038/gim.2013.164

[28] DeFrancesco L. 23andMe's designer baby patent. Nature Biotechnology. 2014 Jan;**32**(1):8-8

[29] Gene editing summit committee statement offers support for basic research, continued discussion [Internet]. GenomeWeb. 2015. Available from: https://www.genomeweb.com/policy-legislation/gene-editing-summit-committee-statement-offers-support-basic-research-continued

[30] Schacht W. CRS report for congress. The Bayh-Dole Act: Selected issues in patent policy and the commercialization of technology [Internet]. 2012. Available from: https://sgp.fas.org/crs/misc/RL32076.pdf

[31] Statement on NIH funding of research using gene-editing technologies in human embryos [Internet]. National Institutes of Health (NIH). 2025. Available from: http://www.nih.gov/about-nih/who-we-are/nih-director/statements/statement-nih-funding-research-using-gene-editing-technologies-human-embryos

[32] Lander ES, Baylis F, Zhang F, Charpentier E, Berg P, Bourgain C, et al.

Adopt a moratorium on heritable genome editing. Nature. 2019;**567**(7747):165-168. DOI: 10.1038/d41586-019-00726-5

[33] Wolinetz CD, Collins FS. NIH supports call for moratorium on clinical uses of germline gene editing. Nature. 2019;**567**(7747):175. DOI: 10.1038/d41586-019-00814-6

[34] Medicine C for V. Q&A on FDA regulation of intentional genomic alterations in animals. FDA [Internet]. 2020. Available from: https://www.fda.gov/animal-veterinary/animals-intentional-genomic-alterations/qa-fda-regulation-intentional-genomic-alterations-animals

[35] Docket No. FDA-2008-D-0394. Heritable intentional genomic alterations in animals: Risk-based approach; Guidance for Industry; Availability [Internet]. 2024. Available from: https://www.federalregister.gov/documents/2024/05/02/2024-09278/heritable-intentional-genomic-alterations-in-animals-risk-based-approach-guidance-for-industry

[36] Poole P, Ramachandran V, Terpolilli J. Rhizobia: From saprophytes to endosymbionts. Nature Reviews Microbiology. 2018;**16**(5):291-303. DOI: 10.1038/nrmicro.2017.171

[37] Wang Q, Liu J, Zhu H. Genetic and molecular mechanisms underlying symbiotic specificity in legume-Rhizobium interactions. Frontiers in Plant Science. 2018;**9**:313. DOI: 10.3389/fpls.2018.00313

[38] Beijerinck MW. Über oligonitrophile Mikroben. Zbl. Backt. 1901;**7**:561-582

[39] Robinson D, Medlock N. Diamond v. Chakrabarty: A retrospective on 25 years of biotech patents. Intellectual Property & Technology Law Journal. 2005;**17**(10)

[40] Capps B, Chadwick R, Joly Y, Mulvihill JJ, Lysaght T, Zwart H. Falling giants and the rise of gene editing: Ethics, private interests and the public good. Human Genomics. 2017;**11**(1)

[41] World KM. Money from genes: CRISPR Goes commercial [Internet]. Scientific American. 2016. Available from: https://www.scientificamerican.com/article/money-from-genes-crispr-goes-commercial/

[42] Leary T. A structured outline for the analysis of horizontal agreements [Internet]. Federal Trade Commission. 2003. Available from: https://www.ftc.gov/sites/default/files/documents/public_statements/structured-outline-analysis-horizontal-agreements/chairsshowcasetalk.pdf

[43] Thomas J. Compulsory Licensing of Patented Inventions. Washington, DC: Congressional Research Service; 2014 Jan. pp. 1-14

[44] Bond E, Saggi K. Compulsory licensing, price controls, and access to patented foreign products [Internet]. 2012. Available from: https://www.wipo.int/edocs/mdocs/mdocs/en/wipo_ip_econ_ge_4_12/wipo_ip_econ_ge_4_12_ref_saggi.pdf

[45] Reinsch W, Tuljapurkar S, Caporal J. Compulsory licensing: A cure for distributing the cure? [Internet]. www.csis.org. 2020. Available from: https://www.csis.org/analysis/compulsory-licensing-cure-distributing-cure

[46] McCallum J. The reality of restricting rights on morally controversial subject matter. New Eng L R. 2005;**39**:517-518

Chapter 7

# A Narrative View on Drug Development and Its Ethical Aspects

*Matthias Klüglich*


## Abstract

Historically, searching for new drugs evolved from a trial-and-error paradigm toward a more science-based approach. The driving force behind it has always been dual headed, as altruistic principles went hand in hand with hope for profit. Constraints of budget, time and quality necessitate constant validation along ethical standards and practical feasibility. Hoping to find a formula for predicting success, the digital, virtual and artificial intelligence revolution provides a tentative answer to the quo vadis of drug research. When altruistic and economic goals are aligned, focus can increasingly be set on rare diseases and vulnerable populations, which, however, creates new ethical challenges.


**Keywords:** drug development, ethical standards, pediatric clinical research, rare diseases, medical progress

## 1. Introduction

The 2019 issue of the National Geographic Magazine was dedicated to the Future of Medicine [1]. Medical research is at its highest. Humanity's effort to overcome disease, suffering and health decline is unfaltering. At the same time, trust in science and medicine is on the decline [2]. Fake news are omnipresent [3]. It is important to understand where drugs come from.

For thousands of years, searching for drugs meant: try it out. Drug development by design took a long time to evolve. Today, technological progress improves patient care if embedded in a humane, respectful setting. Vulnerable populations deserve specific consideration. While the market largely sets the conditions, drug research needs rules, laws and control. History has witnessed the horrors when it gets out of control [4].

Basic sciences lay the ground to identify disease-relevant drug targets. During the preclinical phase of drug development, drug candidates are identified. The elucidation of their pharmacological, pharmacokinetic and toxicological profile goes in parallel with chemical and pharmaceutical development. If the results of preclinical studies allow, the drug is tested in humans. Clinical development is a sequence of pharmacological-pharmacokinetic (phase 1), exploratory (phase 2) and confirmatory (phase 3) trials, followed by submission and approval. A fourth phase ensues with clinical trials conducted while the drug is marketed.

In the following, drug development is presented from a holistic perspective. In a first section, the role of chance, observation and purposeful design is explored. The second section describes the dynamics of business and altruism. How budget, time and quality go along are discussed in a third section, and the hurdles of clinical trials in a fourth section. In a fifth part, the future of drug development is tentatively outlined. The final section describes the challenges of investigating new drugs in minors.

## 2. Drug development and its ethical aspects

### 2.1 Trial and error

Prior to searching for a new drug, it must be clear which target it should be directed at. The prerequisite of drug treatment is the knowledge of the human biology. Only by starting from normal functionality can disorders be described. Without a sound pharmacological hypothesis, the selection of drugs to target disease makes little sense. Benefits must outweigh potential risks; therefore, drug candidates are thoroughly explored before being used in clinical trials [5].

Unlike a diagnosis, which covers all aspects of a disease including signs, symptoms and complaints, a pharmacological target represents a limited sub-process. The receptor model implies an effect on a single signal transmission step. Thus, it is all about finding the central player. Simultaneous intervention at multiple receptors in a system that has gone out of balance is unrealistic. Even in monocausal situations, for example. Hormone replacement, drugs are short of the functional precision achieved by nature [6]. That plant medicine offers more precise, or multi-target treatment is a popular thought but lacks scientific understanding [7].

For thousands of years, shamans and healers relied on experience and speculation. They tried it out and observed. What helped once should help again. Drugs were a secret. Democratization of medicine came when treatment rules were established. With a system and the teaching of it, medical knowledge—even if not based on science—could be acquired by whoever wanted to. Since their advent in the late Middle Ages, universities in Europe taught medicine. Examples of attempts to set up a diagnostic-therapeutic system include Humoral Pathology, the Doctrine of Signatures, and, more lately, Homeopathy. Humoral Pathology was the standard of Western medicine from the times of Hippocrates (460-370 BC) [8] until a few centuries ago. The Doctrine of Signatures [9] is deeply anchored in folk medicine. Homeopathy was developed in the nineteenth century and is still immensely popular [10].

According to Humoral Pathology, bodily functions run smoothly if the humoral system, composed of four or more fluids, is in equilibrium. Disorder appears when the fluids fall out of balance. Countermeasures are taken to re-establish the equilibrium. Humoral Pathology relies on diets and applications that relate to the quantity (blood, stool), type (blood, yellow bile, black bile, mucus), or properties (sour, sweet, bitter, salty, spicy) of the fluids. Due to its somewhat oversimplified explanatory concept, it has always remained challenging to strictly apply Humoral Pathology [11, 12].

The Doctrine of Signatures believes nature to send messages. The logic behind the Doctrines' anthropocentric interpretation is obscure. Selection of therapeutic principles is based on their phenomenological appearance. A fungus that resembles the human ear helps against ear problems. The parasitic mistletoe contains an antidote to cancer. The rough, spotty cucumber is believed to render the skin soft and smooth and drive away spots. Remedies are based on the adept's interpretation of nature's message [13].

Homeopathy was developed by Samuel Hahnemann in the nineteenth century. The concept seems to be influenced by vaccination. Vaccines prevent "like" (e.g., smallpox infection) by treating with "like" (e.g., cowpox virus). The observation that someone who survived an infection is hitherto protected against it goes long back in history. Immunological mechanisms, however, were unknown. Samuel Hahnemann developed a universal concept of treating like with like. Homeopathy postulates a force or potency present in each substance. The potency can be liberated from its molecular attachment and enriched by sequential dilutions and agitations. At the end of the potentiation series, the potency is present in high concentration with little substance left. Its effects are antagonistic to those of the substance [14]. For the individual patients' symptoms, the homeopath selects the matching substance and prescribes its potency. Homeopathy is stringent in itself but lacks insight into what causes disease.

Such systematic approaches were pioneering at the time. In the absence of scientific evidence, they remain constructs of thought. Still, alternative medical concepts remain popular. There are arguments for them. In the absence of pharmacological efficacy, patients draw benefit from the placebo effect [15]. Patients want to be seen as individuals. The selection of the right antidot in Homeopathy requires in-depth anamnesis. An hour of empathy will have a positive health impact [16].

Historically, non-scientific treatments often did more harm than good. Aggressive bloodletting accelerated the death of Wolfgang Amadeus Mozart [17]. Paracelsus fatally poisoned himself at age 46 through excessive use of mercury [18]. What comes out of nature must not necessarily be good for health. Also, patients may forego efficacious therapy while using alternative medicines. Interestingly, adepts of populistic movements and conspiracy tend to prefer alternative medicines [19]. Scientific medicine, to the contrary, stands for openness in a democratic society. Its know-how is publicly available.

Research has been on a constant rise since the sixteenth century and is accelerating from decade to decade in the twenty-first century. Insight into cellular, biochemical, molecular, genetic and epigenetic mechanisms offers the basis for drug development that is no longer dependent on trial-and-error. As more and more is understood, drugs can be developed by-design. Still, drugs aim to restore an equilibrium. Somewhere in the depths of physiology, a process is running hot, a signal circuit is broken, triggers remain constantly switched on or off, or a feedback loop fails. It is here that drugs try to kick in.

Many diseases take decades to develop. Senescence and disease are driven by environmental and genetic factors and need time. Acute disorders are the final stage of a long process. Drugs rarely address etiology, the ultimate cause of a disease. Monogenic causality addresses etiology [20] as do antibiotics. In most instances, however, pharmacology is about pathophysiology. By attacking defined targets, medicine proceeds from trial-and-error to design. Targets are identified in disease models using cells, tissues or animals.

Once a target is defined, a suitable drug must be found. Molecules are tested in assays that represent the target structure. Substance pools contain hundreds of thousands of molecularly defined substances, which were specifically synthesized, collected from nature, or derived from combinatorial chemistry. High-throughput screening (HTS) assays can test up to 100,000 substances within 24 hours. Using pattern recognition from virtual databases, digital technology amends HTS. Computational chemistry and AI-based modeling simulate the chemical-physical interactions and identify lead structures. Molecular components indicating a risk of side effects are digitally identified and replaced. Structures that impact duration and strength of receptor binding, potency of effect or absorption behavior are added. In repetitive cycles, information from chemical-synthetic or biological experiments is introduced into the design process. Target interaction is represented in three-dimensional models. X-ray structure analysis, magnetic resonance imaging, resonance spectroscopy and other molecular imaging techniques support spatial structure elucidation.

The art of developing biologicals does not rely on selection. Biologicals are constructed based on the understanding of their role. The concept is by design, only the technical process—like screening of hybridoma cells for the cell that produces most antibodies—depends on trial-and-error. Genetically engineered human insulin was the first biosynthetic drug approved by FDA [21]. Already during the 1970s, monoclonal antibodies were produced with recombinant DNA technology [22]. Many of today's antibodies originally stem from rodent cells but are nearly human because of numerous gene transfers. Some are directly developed from human B-cell lymphocytes [23]. Coding the Fab fragment region directs the antibody to defined targets. By fusing peptides to the Fc structure, properties such as stability can be achieved. It is done by design.

The spectrum of synthesized biologicals has expanded from monoclonal antibodies to antibody fragments, fusion proteins, non-antibody binding protein (NABPs), cytokines, small-interfering ribonucleic acid (sRNAs) and gene therapies including engineered viruses. The concern that Covid-19 may have inadvertently left a laboratory illustrates the risky downside [24]. Even worse, technological advances may be misused for military purposes [25]. The ability to create by design forces to re-think the purpose of research.

## 2.2 Altruism and economy

Business must ensure return on investment. The longer development takes or the riskier it is, the higher the profit expectation. Successful projects cover failed ones. Profit is essential. Hans Roslund, mathematician and physician, illustrates the mechanism [26]: After a long working life, an old lady depends on her private pension which is financed by equity funds. The funds are driven by pharmaceutical stocks. Their profitability ensures a decent life for the pensioner.

The top priority for Managing Directors is the annual balance sheet. Jobs, salaries, pensions and dividends must be secured. Bills must be paid and financial obligations fulfilled. Reinvestment in research is crucial to secure sustainability. There is little room for charitable investments other than promotional donations.

Probability of success must be weighed against the monetary investment. The forecasted profit, after deducting all expenses, must be at least as high as the same financial means if otherwise invested. The Net Present Value (NPV) must be positive at any given point in time, with some room for maneuver as NPV calculation is not standardized [27]. Once on the market, the drug generates sales, but further profiling—often medically desirable—is limited. Clinical trial programs during the marketing phase are subject to the same NPV restrictions as during development. If approval of an additional indication falls into the period after patent expiry, the NPV slips into the negative. As a consequence, among generic drugs, unrecognized treatment opportunities are lurking. In the absence of return on investment, sponsors cannot finance a clinical trial.

Somewhat unrealistically, public opinion tends to expect altruistic behavior from the pharmaceutical industry. The objective should be the well-being of patients, not making profit. Drug development is thought to be embedded in a tradition of charity. Aiming for profit appears unethical. The public wants to see more research into sensitive populations and neglected diseases.

In the EU and the US, drug development must include a pediatric clinical trial program. Incentives make the programs economically attractive. Waivers are only granted if the drug cannot be used in minors. Pediatric clinical trials with generics are incentivized by an 8-year data protection period [28, 29].

Consequently, politics supports drug development in rare, or orphan, diseases. The European Medicines Agency (EMA) classifies a disease as orphan if no more than 5 in 10,000 people in the EU are affected [30]. To be considered orphan in the US, no more than 200,000 people in the US must suffer from the disease [31]. An orphan drug is granted 10 years of market exclusivity in the EU, subject to regular review of orphan status [32]. Orphan drug designation by the US FDA offers similar incentives, including tax credits for clinical trials, exemption from user fees and 7-year market exclusivity [31].

Tropical diseases are primarily dealt with by foundations such as the Melinda and Bill Gates [33] or the Clinton Foundation [34]. Tropical countries cannot ensure a return-on investment. The give priority to prevention, community-based primary care and medical education [35]. Rarely, a pharmaceutical company may develop drugs or vaccines for a tropical disease with the aim of achieving positive publicity. Theoretically, profitability would be expected if the tropical country is in economic upswing. However, with economic growth, urbanization, hygiene, air-conditioning and proper housing, non-communicable diseases like ischemic heart disease, stroke, or diabetes outpace tropical diseases [36]. The country becomes interesting for pharmaceutical industry, but not as a market for drugs against tropical disease.

However, an ethically driven focus in industrial drug research needs not be prematurely dismissed. Amidst constraints and business limitations, room for maneuver remains. The trick is to do it right. Identifying medical gaps and patients' needs build an overarching category. A drug that makes a difference for patients will ensure a return on investment. With a game-changer, willingness to pay comes like for Hepatitis C [37]. The tyrosine kinase inhibitor nintedanib was developed as an orphan drug for idiopathic pulmonary fibrosis (IPF). It reached €3.5 bn sales in 2023 [38]. For highly prevalent diseases, breakthrough drugs are high-hanging fruit. Not necessarily so in rare and neglected diseases. Even if sales do not always soar, a higher number of successful projects may cover investments.

Business principles need not be abandoned if focus is put on medical needs. This applies all the way down to neglected and tropical diseases. When selecting targets, the question arises as to which aspect priority should be given. Does one blindly aim for profit or follow wisdom: seek first the kingdom of God, and all these things shall be added unto you [39]. Alleviate the suffering and you will win the market. Adopt altruism as a value. Focus on neglected disease. Accept budget constraints and uncertainty. Financial success will come as a bonus where core values are realized (adapted from behavioral psychology [40]). Anxiously looking for profit while disregarding the true health gaps is unlikely to yield economic stability and growth.

Patients are not only customers of drugs. No new drug will come to the market without the contribution of thousands of patients. Trial complexity is constantly rising, requiring them to become experts. Physiological tests, biomarkers from plasma, sputum or biopsy, complex tasks ranging from exercise performance to facial expression analysis: What is a tick box in the flowchart of a protocol represents a half-day of work for the patient. The patient is an active member of the study team. The patient's accurate engagement is key for success.

In planning a trial, patient-centricity is crucial. Patient organizations are important consultants during drug development [41, 42]. They advise on practical details: A questionnaire on well-being, filled out after an exercise test, rather reflects the state of exhaustion than satisfaction with life. A pediatric protocol must consider that children who suffer from chronic illness already miss too many schooldays. Lung function testing in scleroderma patients requires child-sized mouthpieces.

Patient centricity ensures that design, methodology, objectives, endpoint selection and data analysis reflect reality and address the needs. As a bonus, the clinical trial becomes more attractive, facilitating recruitment. Among trial endpoints, patient-reported outcomes (PRO) are increasingly considered meaningful. A mere improvement of physiological parameters may impress scientists but in isolation is worthless. Unfortunately, PRO measurement tends to be rather variable, pushing the hurdle for significance. On the other hand, it is exactly this hurdle that gives proven PRO efficacy strong evidence [42].

### 2.3 Budget, time, quality

When building a highway, each extra mile costs around 10 million dollars [43]. During drug development, money lost for each extra week is in the same ballpark. Patent expiry fixes the end of profitable marketing. Protection ends 20 years after patenting, of which 14 years are eaten up by development. Once generics come to the market, sales collapse. The sooner a new drug comes onto the market, the better.

Front loading is one option to save time. If, for example, initial toxicology studies are carried out according to Good Laboratory Practice (GLP) standards, time can be saved. However, if the project must stop prematurely, it would have been better to explore toxicity in a non-GLP study that is inexpensive and less demanding in terms of animal welfare. Drug interaction potential can be clarified at an early development stage. This saves time because critical decisions are taken early. However, budget is then spent on several candidates, even though only one goes on.

Much time can be saved during clinical development. Recruitment is a key factor in determining the duration of a clinical trial. The more countries and sites are involved, the faster the sample size is reached. Also, proceeding from one development phase to the next can be shortened. Regulators may approve the start of a pivotal phase 3 program based on promising, but rather limited data from a small phase 2. However, aside from the money at risk, ethical aspects need to be considered. With less information available, the risk of lack of safety issues is higher.

For good reasons, aviation and pharmaceutics are strictly regulated industries. They must comply with the highest quality standards. Adding detail to law and regulation, guidelines like those of ICH provide advice on quality management in drug development. They do not have normative character but are used by regulatory authorities as a basis for their quality review. Any deviation must be explained and documented, and the deviation must not violate applicable law. There is little flexibility left for business once it comes to quality management. Negligence and fraud in quality end with regulatory sanctions, scandal and fines [44].

However, careful risk assessment and regulatory consensus may allow flexibility. A frequently cited example is the FDA's approval of the first HIV drugs prior completion of a full Phase 3 clinical trial program [45]. Regulatory agencies and patients accepted the risk and won as drugs became quickly available.

Below what is defined by laws, regulations and guidelines, the careful weighing of quality extend is daily life. The third Good Clinical Practice (GCP) revision advises that resources be spent with consideration. The guideline proposes risk-based approaches instead of, for example, working strictly to the 100% source data verification rule [46]. Bringing safe and efficacious drugs to market as quickly as possible is an ethical demand. Quality can drive costs to a level where a project is stopped. Drug development will stagnate unless the trend of skyrocketing costs [47, 48] is reversed.

Only by working as partners, industrial sponsors, investigators, patients, ethics committees and regulatory authorities will master the magic triangle of budget, cost and quality.

### 2.4 From hurdle to hurdle

The development of antibiotics is a striking example of science-based drug development. Its final success built on the progress of bacteriological research. Sulfonamide antibiotics came first. They were developed based on an idea by Paul Ehrlich (1854-1915). Ehrlich had postulated that a chemical compound used for staining bacteria accumulates in the cell wall. If so, he concluded, it might as well exert an antibacterial effect. In numerous animal experiments, Ehrlich started exploring organic staining compounds. They all contained arsenic even though this limited their therapeutic use. One of the compounds called Salvarsan® reached notoriety as treatment of syphilis. Following up on Ehrlich's work, the German Farbwerke developed sulfonamides that were based on azo groups instead of arsenic. The most important early sulfonamide was Prontosil® [49]. At about the same time, Alexander Fleming described the bacteriostatic effect of a substance originating from a fungi culture [50]. It was not until 10 years after Fleming's observation that structured research led to penicillin. In early antibiotic development, altruism went along with scientific interest and business orientation.

As a result of the mass use of antibiotics, bacteria develop resistance. New antibiotics are needed. Market mechanisms fail to address the need. The return-on investment is low due to the short drug administration time and generic pricing. Politicians have realized the dilemma and propose incentives such as subscription payments, market entry rewards, exclusivity extensions and direct funding [51].

By the end of the twentieth century, the arsenal of chemically synthesized or biologically produced drugs was almost impossible to keep track of. Since the 1990s, even the most extreme forms of arterial hypertension have been treatable. Today, Franklin D. Roosevelt would no longer have to let Stalin talk him into drowsiness when his systolic blood pressure was above 200 mmHg [52]. Randomized controlled trials have shown that normalizing cholesterol levels is not laboratory cosmetics but prolongs life. Anticoagulation prevents strokes in patients with atrial fibrillation, and if an occlusive stroke does occur, acute lysis is offered. A new class of antidiabetics not only corrects glucose but is reno- and cardioprotective. Rheumatoid arthritis is treatable thanks to an array of immune-modulatory biologics. Oncology has made tremendous progress, most recently with the arrival of immune- and CAR-T-cell therapy. The number of fatal cancer cases has fallen significantly. Hepatitis C can be cured. Antiretroviral drugs have changed AIDS from a death sentence to a chronic disease. Drugs are available to treat rare diseases like IPF.

At the same time, drug development suffers drawbacks and disappointments. The negative results of the CAST trial shocked more than just arrhythmia experts [53]. It sparked a rethink, which led to higher demands on benefit/risk assessment during clinical development. The randomized, controlled trial became the ultimate proof of efficacy.

Dementia incidence, particularly that of the Alzheimer's type, is increasing [54]. Basic research has been in full swing for decades. Billions have been spent [55]. However, companies withdraw from Alzheimer's research [56]. Out of hundreds of clinical trials, few drugs with questionable efficacy have emerged [57]. Yet these programs looked so hopeful, animal models had promised so much [58]. The approval of donanemab and lecanemab by the FDA in 2023 and 2024 [59] and that of lecanemab by the EMA in 2024 [60] may spark renewed optimism among deciders in drug development.

The majority of drugs which work in animal models do not do in humans. Translation fails because biology is not understood. Preclinical models are based on receptor pharmacology—monocausal scenarios are transferred into multidimensional interdependencies. Better understanding of human and non-human biology is needed.

Identifying biomarkers has been the talk of the town for decades. Biomarkers indeed revolutionized the diagnostic landscape like, for example, in tumor classification. However, biomarkers as surrogates for efficacy are another story. Biomarkers are epiphenomena that do not close the gap between animals and humans. They support drug profiling on levels of increasing relevance.

A target engagement marker proves that a drug binds to a receptor: for example, if vascular endothelial growth factor decreases after administration of an antibody. Pharmacological principle is demonstrated when binding to the receptor has an indirect effect: for example, if a diuretic causes a drop in serum potassium. Efficacy is likely if the biomarker indicates disease-specific changes: for example, if blood pressure goes down. On the highest level of significance, a biomarker predicts clinically relevant (pain reduction, disability prevention) or hard (heart attack, stroke, mortality) endpoints. The latter will be requested by regulators before accepting a biomarker as surrogate endpoint.

Demonstrating that a drug reduces the risk of serious but rare complications constitutes a challenge. Asthma exacerbations, myocardial infarction or cancer mortality are clinically important—but trials exploring these endpoints require a large sample size. For some indications, innovation is at risk unless validated surrogate biomarkers are found.

Most drugs fail due to lack of efficacy, or they are much weaker in humans than in preclinical models. Animals are another species but more than that. Pharmacological models are established in otherwise healthy animals, whereas patients have concomitant diseases. In animals, the modeled disease develops over a short period of time. In the patient, it may have evolved over decades. Patients have comedication whereas laboratory animals do not. Animal diseases are different: In the short-lived and highly reproductive mice, tumors grow rapidly and react easily to treatment [61]. Last but not least, humans are subject to complex psychological, social, hereditary and environmental, nutritional and behavioral factors that cannot be reflected in animal models.

If a placebo-controlled clinical trial fails, it is tempting to claim that the placebo had an unusually strong effect [62]. Overestimating natural decline is common. At the time the trial is conducted, patients fare better compared to years before. New background treatment, improved care and diagnostic standards render prognosis more favorable than in published data. In addition, experts who publish have a selection bias toward severe cases. Historical data must be critically assessed.

The life of trial participants is not standardized. Accuracy and precision are difficult to achieve. Confounding factors, bias or broad inclusion criteria drive endpoint variability. Data points are lost due to premature withdrawal. Logistics and operational challenges capture the attention of trial teams. As a consequence, measurement variability increases, endangering statistical significance.

Sometimes it is better to start low, with a small, highly responding patient population. Once the drug shows signs of efficacy, the patient population is expanded. This is what happened with alteplase in stroke lysis. The post-stroke time window gradually expanded in sequential clinical trials. The initially short interval (up to 3 hours) would have reached only a fraction of the patients who benefit from lysis [63].

Sponsors may consider termination of development if a similar drug has a safety problem, or lack of efficacy. However, it is usually unknown whether the cause is a class effect. While ximelagatran, the first direct thrombin inhibitor, had to be taken from the market due to hepatotoxicity, dabigatran, with the same mechanism of action, is safe. It was a good decision to not terminate the development of dabigatran when the negative safety data on ximelagatran became known [64].

Patient input is crucial. The first inhaled insulin rapidly disappeared from the market. Sales were lower than expected. The majority of patients preferred injections as compared to the cumbersome inhalation [65]. It is important to know what benefit the patients expect and what they actually experience.

If a hypothesis is overwhelmingly plausible even though a trial was negative, one should not give up too quickly. Results can be false negative. For example, early clinical trials on tiotropium did not show a convincing effect on asthma. Tiotropium was approved for COPD only. However, case reports suggested that also asthma patients benefited from tiotropium. A subsequent clinical trial program, starting with tiotropium in severe [66], then moderate, then mild asthma, provided clear evidence of efficacy in asthma. Today, the number of publications on tiotropium in asthma is almost incalculable [67].

What ultimately counts is the totality of the data. As described above, survival is the most convincing endpoint, but regulatory authorities may accept less strict endpoints if the overall evidence is convincing: if all data point in the same direction, if sensitive analyses support the primary endpoint, if secondary endpoints are in line with the primary, if survival shows a trend and if PROs support efficacy. Developing a drug is an art. Drugs do not disclose their potential freely. Efficacy must be carefully established through in-depth scrutiny of all available data. Drugs must be prevented from being prematurely declared dead.

### 2.5 Quo vadis?

A press release on blockchain technology in clinical research generated millions of clicks [68]. Media and the interested public react with great sensitivity as soon as digitization and life sciences are mentioned together. Indeed, fascinating progress is seen. Artificial hearts function, even if only for a limited period [69]. CAR T-cell therapy heralds the age of individualized medicine, but at tremendous cost [70, 71]. Highly controversially, He Jiankui edited the genes of human embryos [72]. Devices worn as a bracelet can measure blood pressure, monitor respiratory and heart rate, or transmit oxygen saturation [73]. However, quality and data protection issues remain a matter of discussion around wearable technology [74]. The use of artificial intelligence has become standard technology in basic pharmaceutical research. Its breathtaking potential should not let forget limitations [75].

Despite modeling, simulation and virtual biomathematics, animal experiments remain indispensable. The translation of animal data to humans still represents a hurdle. Promising concepts take long from bench to bedside. Oncolytic viruses were genetically modified already at end of the last century [76]. Only a handful of them achieved approval since 2005 [77]. Much has been published on glucose-sensing lenses, but no such device is yet marked. However, for a different purpose a smart lens made it to approval [78, 79]. Things are progressing, but they take longer than hoped for.

In CAR-T cell therapy, an individual's T cells are genetically modified so that they develop receptors against surface antigens of a cancer cell. Following re-infusion, the cells attack the cancer. As they divide and multiply, they retain the receptor. Fourth generation CAR-T cells have been coupled with immune modulators [80]. The idea of collecting a patient's T cells, subjecting them to treatment and then re-infusing them is not new. Extracorporeal photopheresis was used in the 1980ies to treat lymphoma and immunological disorders. After removal, T cells were exposed to 8-methoxypsoralen that binds DNA strands under UVA irradiation. It was hoped that the immune system would react in a vaccination-like fashion when the T cells were re-infused. With today's CAR-T cell therapy, immunological knowledge and genetic engineering have developed a speculative idea into a scientifically sound concept.

Artificial intelligence holds great promise [75]. Artificial intelligence can pull critical information from publicly available databases that support patient recruitment, predict dropouts, analyze video surveillance of medication intake, change scientific to lay language, handle missing data points, generate reports or clean data. Self-learning programs are particularly promising in the field of diagnostics. However, accuracy and precision of AI remain challenging. Human review remains indispensable [75]. Artificial intelligence lacks reliability [81]. Validation of AI is in its early phase. Imaging and pattern analysis are widely used but so far did AI not replace the radiologist [82]. Computer-assisted emotion recognition technology may become useful in psychiatric trials [83], but data protection causes concern. There is no consistent concept yet on how identifiable patient data will be protected and what level of informed consent is required.

The inflationary use of the word disruption may not always stand on the technical grounds set by Christensen [84, 85]. Still, industry leaders believe in it. People with fancy ideas are sought after. Human resources want digital natives, already waiting for the alpha generation [86]. Disruptive leaps are celebrated—preferably in retrospect [87]. Speakers praise paradigm shift and rarely leave the iPhone story unmentioned [88]. Disruptive innovations in the field of medicine are crowned by the Nobel Committee—after a considerable time has passed. Helicobacter was discovered in 1983 and initiated a disruptive reorientation of stomach ulcer therapy. Sixteen years later, the describers received the Nobel Prize [89]. Beta-blockers, antihistamines and a series of drugs like mercaptopurine, trimethoprim, azathioprine, allopurinol, acyclovir or zidovudine likewise were crowned in retrospect [90]). Viewed from a historical distance, these innovations were disruptive.

In the daily work of researchers, incremental changes develop into disruptive innovations [91]. Tenacity and determination are essential. Software as Medical Device (SaMD), for example, evolves step by step [92]. Transitions between incremental and breakthrough innovations are fluid. Those looking for breakthrough innovation must not shy away from hard work. At the same time, the minds must remain open. Paul Ehrlich came up with the brilliant idea of using dyes against bacteria but left the development of sulfonamides to others [93, 94]. Alexander Fleming noticed the bacteriostatic effects of penicillin but did not succeed in isolating a drug [95].

Disruptive concepts grow on the grounds of curiosity, intellectual exchange and openness. Cooperation, assertiveness, flashes of inspiration and the prospect of economic success might be a good mix from which innovation and progress evolve. Not to forget serendipity—good luck and the art of grabbing the chance. However, as science deciphers the language of biology, new risks pop up. A recent example of concern is the creation of mirror life—microbes that are resistant to all available treatment [96]. Global consensus will be crucial to make sure that the scientific and technological progress serves mankind.

### 2.6 Drug development in minors

Around 30% of drugs used in children's hospitals are administered off-label, that is, without specific approval for the age group and thus without having been clinically tested [97]. Around 40% of all children experience side effects during inpatient treatment [98]. Two thirds of the side effects relate to drugs administered off-label [99]. Adverse drug reactions due to dosing errors are also common in children [100]. The benefit-risk evidence of many drugs used in minors is unclear [101].

A child is not a small adult. Both pharmacokinetics and pharmacodynamics can largely differ between minors and adults. Drug effects in adults cannot be extrapolated to adolescents, children or newborns by simply adjusting the dose. The organism is under constant development from birth to adulthood. The gastrointestinal tract and kidneys mature during the first year of life and the lungs until the end of the second year. The development of the central nervous system and the sexual organs is not completed until adolescence. The skeleton does not even reach its final shape and size until the age of 25. The immune system, liver and gall bladder undergo postnatal maturation. The hepatic detoxification capacity is built up in the first year of life and continues to develop afterward [102]. Many metabolic functions that are of critical importance for drugs, for example, enzymes of the cytochrome P450 system, change throughout childhood and adolescence [103]. The skin of newborns is thin, allowing drugs to be easily absorbed. In contrast, drug absorption following intramuscular injection is reduced in newborns. When inhaled, drug absorption in minors is higher than in adults. The plasma protein-binding capacity of newborns is low due to the low protein content, which results from relatively more body water [102]. In conclusion: clinical trials in minors are urgently needed. However, there is an ethical dilemma.

In 1796, Edward Jenner injected his gardener's 8-year-old son with secretions from a cowpox pustule. After a few weeks and a mild cowpox infection, he re-injected the child with secretions from a human smallpox pustule [104]. The boy survived smallpox. In the nineteenth century, clinical trials with children were rarely challenged. A century later, Albrecht Neisser infected healthy young girls with syphilis for research purposes. The case became a scandal, and Neisser received a small fine [105]. The first guidance on human medical research followed, including the request for written informed consent [106]. Around 30 years later, experimental vaccination caused fatal side effects in children [107]. Guidelines on clinical research were issued again. Under the National Socialist dictatorship, the German medical profession threw ethical principles overboard. Research became murder, including that of children. The Nuremberg Code of 1947 prohibited clinical trials in minors [108]. In 1964, however, the World Medical Association relativized the norm [109]. Today, minors can be legally included in clinical trials in most countries.

The EU's Clinical Trial Regulation 536/2014 sets rules for the conduct of clinical trials in minors [110], with detail provided by the EU Pediatric Regulation

1901/2006 [111, 112]. A Pediatric Investigational Plan (PIP) must be written for all clinical development programs. It is requested even if the development for adults is abandoned. The PIP has to describe all clinical trials to be conducted in adolescents and children, and possibly also in infants and newborns. The PIP is developed in discussion with the Pediatric Committee (PDCO) of the EMA [112].

The PIP trials are conducted during or after Phase 3 of the adult clinical development. However, there is no mandatory standard. If the disease occurs only in children, waiting for adult data may not be considered necessary. If the medical need is not urgent, more time may be allowed. It will be wise to begin the pediatric trial program with adolescents, and then go down in age from children to infants as adequate. The EMA offers PIP deferral if it is justified to complete adult studies first. The PIP can be waived only if the drug is not expected to be safe or effective in children, or if the drug, by its mechanism, is restricted to adult disease. All age groups have to be taken into consideration.

In line with a stick-and-carrot principle, regulatory authorities offer incentives. The EU grants an extension of patent protection by 6 months if all parts of the PIP have been completed as agreed. Technically, it is an extension of the Supplementary Protection Certificate (SPC) on intellectual property rights [113]. If the PIP is not followed, the EMA threatens to blame and shame the company by publishing its name. A fine can be imposed. The EMA even reserves the right to refuse adult approval of the drug concerned [112].

It is often challenging to conduct trials which fulfill PDCO's expectation. The PDCO, based on scientific rationale, may require study designs that cannot be approved due to ethical concerns or are considered technically impossible. In the years since the PIP was introduced, however, a great deal of understanding and expertise has grown. The early involvement of patient organizations and children's networks has proven particularly helpful. However, sometimes, despite careful planning it is impossible to recruit the agreed sample size for a pediatric clinical trial.

Toxicological, pharmacological and pharmacokinetic studies on juvenile animals are prerequisites for pediatric clinical trials. Respective guidelines were published by the EMA in 2008 [114] and by the US FDA in 2006 [115]. Specific formulations may be needed for children. The drug's size or volume should be as small as possible. The taste should not be repulsive, but also not too tasty. Excipients must be safe for children [116].

Before a trial starts, information brochures must be developed for all age groups. The information session requires patience by the minor, parents and the pediatrician who explains the trial. In most countries, both parents must be present and consent. The child or adolescent must give assent, as a replacement for legal consent. An explicit refusal by the minor must be respected. No incentives are allowed. The clinical trial must relate to a medical condition from which the minor suffers. Medical benefit should be expected from trial participation; if not, the trial must benefit the population represented by the minor. Risk and burden caused by trial participation must be minimal. If an adolescent turns 18 during an ongoing trial, legal consent must be obtained [117].

**Figure 1** presents a PIP example. By the time the PIP was designed, safety data from adults were available. The PIP consisted of a total of seven clinical trials in the age groups 0–5 years, 6–11 years and 12–17 years. The program lasted for 4 years. Between 100 and 500 children and adolescents were included in each of the individual clinical trials.

Following the Pediatric Regulation, which has been in force in Europe since 2006, the number and proportion of pediatric clinical trials increased noticeably, although

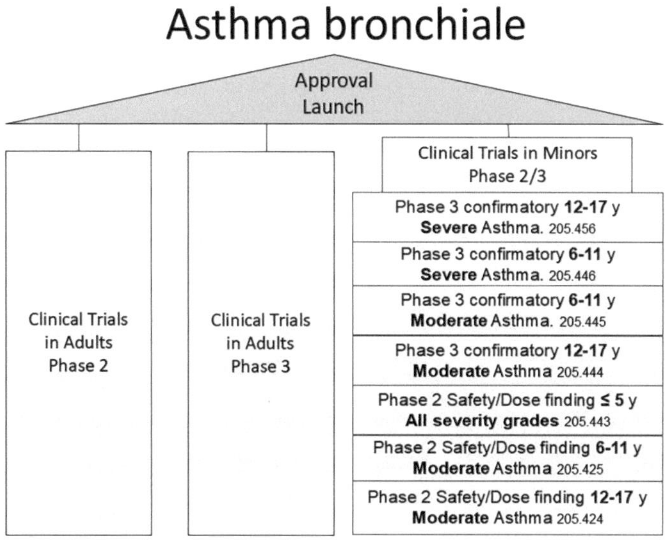


**Figure 1.**
*Pediatric clinical development of tiotropium in asthma. For trial descriptions, see ClinTrialsGov [118]. Source: Author.*

not as much as hoped for. By the end of 2016, 131 PIPs had been completed [119]. Public and published opinions are gradually recognizing the need for clinical trials in minors. New concepts of how to best manage clinical trials in minors are adopted and implemented. Innovative trial designs consider the specific challenges while fostering scientifically valid results.

## 3. Conclusion

Drug development is ethically challenging. Science-based research creates knowledge that slowly but steadily replaces trial and error. Science can run out of control, and it can be misused. Ethics must keep pace with natural science.

Focus on medical need can resolve the antagonism between business and altruism. As long as the search for profit does not get out of hand, the road to success remains open.

The joint undertaking of multiple contributors, including the patients who participate in clinical trials, is rewarded with therapeutic progress and return-on investment.

Success in developing a drug can never be guaranteed, but much can be done to increase its likelihood. The large room to be filled with knowledge and understanding is what makes drug development so fascinating.

The global innovation machine is humming. Science is confident that 1 day even the most challenging diseases can be treated. The chance is there if mankind works together, beats swords into plowshares and contains the risks associated with technological progress.

## Conflict of interest

The author is a retired employee of Boehringer Ingelheim.

## Author details

Matthias Klüglich
Internist, Clinical Pharmacologist, Biberach, Germany

*Address all correspondence to: matthias.klueglich@posteo.de

## References

[1] National Geographic. The Future of Medicine [Internet]. Washington, USA: National Geographic Partners, LLC; 2019. Available from: https://www.nationalgeographic.com/magazine/issue/january-2019 [Accessed: January 21, 2025]

[2] Pew Research Center, Kennedy B, Tyson A. American's Trust in Scientists, Positive Views of Science Continue to Decline [Internet]. Washington, USA: Pew Research Center; 2023. Available from: https://www.pewresearch.org/science/2023/11/14/americans-trust-in-scientists-positive-views-of-science-continue-to-decline/ [Accessed: January 21, 2025]

[3] Vosoughi S, Roy D, Aral S. The spread of true and false news online. Science. 2018;**359**:1146-1151. DOI: 10.1126/science.aap9559

[4] Weindling P, von Villiez A, Loewenau A, Farron N. The victims of unethical human experiments and coerced research under National Socialism. Endeavour. 2015;**40**(1):1-6. DOI: 10.1016/j.endeavour.2015.10.005

[5] ICH. Guideline for Good Clinical Practice E6(R2) [Internet]. Amsterdam, The Netherlands: European Medicines Agency; 2016. Available from: https://www.ich.org/page/efficacy-guidelines [Accessed: January 21, 2025]

[6] Jonklaas S. Optimal thyroid hormone replacement. Endocrine Reviews. 2022;**43**(2):366-404. DOI: 10.1210/endrev/bnab031

[7] Bynum W. Nature's helping hand. Nature. 2001;**414**:21. DOI: 10.1038/35102123

[8] Lagay F. The legacy of humoral medicine. Virtual Mentor. 2002;**4**(7):206-208. DOI: 10.1001/virtualmentor.2002.4.7.mhst1-0207

[9] Pearce J. The doctrine of signatures. European Neurology. 2008;**60**(1):51-52. DOI: 10.1159/000131714

[10] Relton C, Cooper K, Viksveen P, Fibert P, Thomas K. Prevalence of homeopathy use by the general population worldwide: A systematic review. Homeopathy. 2017;**106**:69-78. DOI: 10.1016/j.homp.2017.03.002

[11] Mackenbach JP. The origins of human disease: A short story on "where diseases come from". Journal of Epidemiology and Community Health. 2006;**60**:81-86. DOI: 10.1136/jech.2005.038661

[12] Bhikha R, Glynn J. The theory of humours revisited. International Journal of Development Research. 2017;**7**(9):15029-15034. DOI: 10.37118/ijdr

[13] Diamond A. That Signature Look: An Introduction to the Doctrine of Signatures [Internet]. Lyme, USA: Northern Woodlands; 2014. Available from: https://northernwoodlands.org/articles/article/doctrine-signatures [Accessed: January 21, 2025]

[14] Mukerji N, Ernst E. Why homoeopathy is pseudoscience. Synthese. 2022;**200**(394):1-29. DOI: 10.1007/s11229-022-03882-w

[15] Hafliðadóttir SH, Juhl CB, Nielsen SM, Henriksen M, Harris IA, Bliddal H, et al. Placebo response and effect in randomized clinical trials: Meta-research with focus on contextual effects.

Trials. 2021;**22**(493):1-15. DOI: 10.1186/s13063-021-05454-8

[16] Decety J, Fotopoulou A. Why empathy has a beneficial impact on others in medicine: Unifying theories. Behavioral Neuroscience. 2015;**8**(457):1-11. DOI: 10.3389/fnbeh.2014.00457

[17] Wikipedia. Death of Wolfgang Amadeus Mozart. 2025. Available from: https://en.wikipedia.org/wiki/Death_of_Wolfgang_Amadeus_Mozart#Theories_involving_disease [Accessed: January 21, 2025]

[18] University of Zurich. The Zurich Paracelsus Project. Winterthur, Switzerland: Urs Leo Gantenbein; 2024. Available from: https://www.paracelsus.uzh.ch/paracelsus.html [Accessed: February 14, 2025]

[19] Valtonen J, Ilmarinen V-J, Lönnqvist J-E. Political orientation predicts the use of conventional and complementary/alternative medicine: A survey study of 19 European countries. Social Science & Medicine. 2023;**331**(116089):1-10. DOI: 10.1016/j.socscimed.2023.116089

[20] Lanigan T, Kopera H, Saunders T. Principles of genetic engineering. Genes. 2020;**11**(291):1-21. DOI: 10.3390/genes11030291

[21] Food and Drug Administration. 100 Years of Insulin. Maryland, USA: U.S. Food and Drug Administration; 2022. Available from: https://www.fda.gov/about-fda/fda-history-exhibits/100-years-insulin# [Accessed: January 21, 2025]

[22] Malavija A, Mehra N. A fascinating story of the discovery & development of biologicals for use in clinical medicine. The Indian Journal of Medical Research. 2018;**148**:263-278. DOI: 10.4103/ijmr.IJMR_1471_18

[23] Dumont J, Euwart D, Mei B, Estes S, Kshirsagar R. Human cell lines for biopharmaceutical manufacturing: History, status, and future perspective. Critical Reviews in Biotechnology. 2016;**36**(6):1110-1122. DOI: 10.3109/07388551.2015.1084266

[24] Bloom JD, Chan YA, Baric RS, Bjorkman PJ, Cobey S, Deverman BE, et al. Investigate the origins of COVID-19. Science. 2021;**372**(6543):694. DOI: 10.1126/science.abj0016

[25] World Health Organisation. Biological Weapons. Geneva, Switzerland: World Health Organisation; 2025. Available from: https://www.who.int/health-topics/biological-weapons#tab=tab_1 [Accessed: January 21, 2025]

[26] Roslund H. Factfulness: Ten Reasons we're Wrong about the World. English ed. USA: MacMillan Publishers; 2018. 352 p. ISBN 9781473637474.

[27] Willigers B, Jones B, Bratvold R. The net-present-value paradox: Criticized by many, applied by all. Economics & Management. 2017;**9**(4):1-13. DOI: 10.2118/187937-PA

[28] European Medicines Agency. Paediatric Committee (PDCO). Amsterdam, The Netherlands: European Medicines Agency; 2025. Available from: https://www.ema.europa.eu/en/committees/paediatric-committee-pdco [Accessed: January 21, 2025]

[29] Thomsen MD. Global pediatric drug development. Current Therapeutic Research. 2019;**90**:135-142. DOI: 10.1016/j.curtheres.2019.02.001

[30] European Medicines Agency. Orphan Designation: Overview. Amsterdam, The Netherlands: European Medicines Agency; 2025. Available

from: https://www.ema.europa.eu/en/human-regulatory-overview/orphan-designation-overview [Accessed: January 21, 2025]

[31] Food and Drug Administration. Orphan Drug Act – Relevant Excerpts. 2025. Available from: https://www.fda.gov/industry/designating-orphan-product-drugs-and-biological-products/orphan-drug-act-relevant-excerpts [Accessed: January 21, 2025]

[32] European Medicines Agency. Orphan incentives. 2025. Available from: https://www.ema.europa.eu/en/human-regulatory-overview/research-development/orphan-designation-research-development/orphan-incentives [Accessed: January 21, 2025]

[33] Gates B, Gates M. Imagine a World Built on Generosity. Washington, USA: Gates Foundation; 2025. Available from: https://www.gatesfoundation.org/ [Accessed: January 21, 2025]

[34] Clinton Health Access Initiative (CHAI). 2025. Available from: https://www.clintonhealthaccess.org/ [Accessed: January 21, 2025]

[35] Dramé A. Insights from Cuba's public health achievements: Implications for African countries. Journal of Public Health and Epidemiology. 2024;**16**(2):41-50. DOI: 10.5897/JPHE2024.1486

[36] Minja N, Nakagaayi N, Aliku T, Zhang W, Ssinabulya I, Nabaale J, et al. Cardiovascular diseases in Africa in the twenty-first century: Gaps and priorities going forward. Frontiers in Cardiovascular Medicine. 2022;**9**(1008335):1-20. DOI: 10.3389/fcvm.2022.1008335

[37] Chhatwal J, He T, Hur C, Lopez-Olivo MA. Direct-acting antiviral agents for patients with hepatitis C virus genotype 1 infection are cost-saving. Clinical Gastroenterology and Hepatology. 2017;**15**:827-837. DOI: 10.1016/j.cgh.2016.09.015

[38] Mireku A. Jardiance and Ofev propel Boehringer's human pharma sales. Pharmaceutical Technology. 2024. Available from: https://www.pharmaceutical-technology.com/news/jardiance-and-ofev-propel-boehringers-human-pharma-sales/?cf-view [Accessed: January 21, 2025]

[39] Bible KJ. Matthew 6:33. 2025. Available from: https://thekingsbible.com/Bible/40/6 [Accessed: January 21, 2025]

[40] Harris R. ACT made simple. 2nd ed. Oakland, California, US: New Harbinger Publications Inc.; 2019. 374 p. ISBN 9781684033010

[41] Murphy A, Bere N, Vamvakas S, Mavris M. The added value of patient engagement in early dialogue at EMA: Scientific advice as a case study. Frontiers of Medicine. 2022;**8**:811855. DOI: 10.3389/fmed.2021.811855

[42] Mercieca-Bebber R, King M, Calvert M, Stockler M, Friedlander M. The importance of patient-reported outcomes in clinical trials and strategies for future optimization. Patient Related Outcome Measure. 2018;**9**:353-367. DOI: 10.2147/PROM.S156279

[43] Compass International Inc. The Global Construction Newsletter. 2023. Available from: https://compassinternational.net/order-magnitude-road-highway-costs/#:~:text=USA%20%246.46%20million%20per%20mile,USA%20%24%206.75%20million%20per%20mile [Accessed: January 21, 2025]

[44] Reuters SD. U.S. Judge Approves $14.7 Billion Deal in VW Diesel Scandal.

Toronto, Canada: Reuters; 2016. Available from: https://www.reuters.com/article/us-volkswagen-emissions-idUSKCN12P22F/ [Accessed: January 21, 2025]

[45] Kepplinger E. FDA's expedited approval mechanisms for new drug products. Biotechnology Law Report. 2015;**34**(1):15-37. DOI: 10.1089/blr.2015.9999

[46] International Council for Harmonization of Technical Requirements for Pharmaceuticals for Human Use (ICH). Guideline for Good Clinical Practice E6(R2). 2016. Available from: https://database.ich.org/sites/default/files/E6_R2_Addendum.pdf [Accessed: January 21, 2025]

[47] Rennane S, Baker L, Mulcahy A. Estimating the cost of industry Investment in Drug Research and Development: A review of methods and results. The Journal of Health Care Organization, Provision, and Financing. 2021;**58**:1-11. DOI: 10.1177/00469580211059731

[48] Sertkaya A, Beleche T, Jessup A, Sommers B. Costs of drug development and Research and Development intensity in the US 2000-2018. Jama Network Open. 2024;**7**(6):1-13. DOI: 10.1001/jamanetworkopen.2024.15445

[49] The Nobel Prize Organisation, Domagk G. Further Progress in Chemotherapy of Bacterial Infections. Stockholm, Sweden: Nobel Prize Outreach 2025; 1947. Available from: https://www.nobelprize.org/uploads/2018/06/domagk-lecture.pdf [Accessed: January 21, 2025]

[50] The Nobel Prize Organisation, Fleming A. Penicillin. Stockholm, Sweden: Nobel Prize Outreach 2025; 1945. Available from: https://www.nobelprize.org/uploads/2018/06/fleming-lecture.pdf [Accessed: January 21, 2025]

[51] Anderson M, Panteli D, van Kessel R, Ljungqvist G, Colombo F, Mossialos E. Challenges and opportunities for incentivising antibiotic research and development in Europe. The Lancet. 2023;**33**(100705):1-12. DOI: 10.1016/j.lanepe.2023.100705

[52] Messerli FH. This day 50 years ago. New England Journal of Medicine. 1995;**332**(15):1038-1039. DOI: 10.1056/NEJM199504133321518

[53] Echt DS, Liebson PR, Mitchell BL, Peters RW, Obias-Manno D, Barker AH, et al. Richardson: Mortality and morbidity in patients receiving Encainide, Flecainide, or placebo — The cardiac arrhythmia suppression trial. New England Journal of Medicine. 1991;**324**(12):781-788. DOI: 10.1056/NEJM199103213241201

[54] Li X, Feng X, Sun X, Hou N, Han F, Liu Y. Global, regional and national burden of Alzheimer's disease and other dementias, 1990-2019. Frontiers in Aging Neuroscience. 2022;**14**(937486):1-17. DOI: 10.3389/fnagi.2022.937486

[55] Cummings J, Goldmann D, Simmons-Stern N, Ponton E. The costs of developing treatments for Alzheimer's disease: A retrospective exploration. Alzheimers and Dementia. 2021;**18**:469-477. DOI: 10.1002/alz.12450

[56] British Broadcasting Company BBC. Pharma Giant Pfizer Pulls out of Research into Alzheimer's. London, UK: British Broadcasting Corporation; 2018. Available from: https://www.bbc.com/news/health-42633871 [Accessed: January 21, 2025]

[57] Medical News Today, Shukla D. Alzheimers: Are Newly Approved Drugs Making a Real-Life Difference? London, UK: Healthline Media; 2024. Available from: https://www.medicalnewstoday.com/articles/alzheimers-are-newly-approved-drugs-making-a-real-life-difference [Accessed: January 21, 2025]

[58] Franco R, Cedazo-Minguez A. Successful therapies for Alzheimer's disease: Why so many in animal models and none in humans? Frontiers in Pharmacology. 2014;**5**(146):1-13. DOI: 10.3389/fphar.2014.00146

[59] Food and Drug Administration FDA. FDA Approves Treatment for Adults with Alzheimer's Disease. Maryland, USA: U.S. Food and Drug Administration; 2024. Available from: https://www.fda.gov/drugs/news-events-human-drugs/fda-approves-treatment-adults-alzheimers-disease [Accessed: January 21, 2025]

[60] European Medicines Agency EMA. Leqembi Recommended for Treatment of Early Alzheimer's Disease. Amsterdam, The Netherlands: European Medicines Agency; 2024. Available from: https://www.ema.europa.eu/en/news/leqembi-recommended-treatment-early-alzheimers-disease [Accessed: January 21, 2025]

[61] Dujon A, Boutry J, Tissot S, Lemaitre JF, Boddy A, Gerard AL, et al. Cancer susceptibility as a cost of reproduction and contributor to life history evolution. Frontiers in Ecology and Evolution. 2022;**10**(861103):1-18. DOI: 10.3389/fevo.2022.861103

[62] Kaptchuk T, Miller F. Placebo effects in medicine. New England Journal of Medicine. 2015;**373**(1):8-9. DOI: 10.1056/NEJMp1504023

[63] Ma H, Campbell BVC, Parsons MW, Churilov L, Levi CR, Hsu C, et al. Thrombolysis guided by perfusion imaging up to 9 hours. New England Journal of Medicine. 2019;**380**(19):1795-1803. DOI: 10.1056/NEJMoa1813046

[64] Keisu M, Anderson T. The case of ximelagatran. Handbook of Experimental Pharmacology. 2010;**196**(196):407-418. DOI: 10.1007/978-3-642-00663-0_13

[65] Oleck J, Kassam S, Goldman J. Why was inhaled insulin a failure in the market? Pharmacy and Therapeutics. 2016;**29**(3):180-184. DOI: 10.2337/diaspect.29.3.180

[66] Kerstjens HA, Disse B, Schröder-Babo W, Bantje T, Gahlemann M, Sigmund R, et al. Tiotropium improves lung function in patients with severe uncontrolled asthma: A randomized controlled trial. The Journal of Allergy and Clinical Immunology. 2011;**128**(2):308-314. DOI: 10.1016/j.jaci.2011.04.039

[67] Mansfield L, Bernstein J. Tiotropium in asthma: From bench to bedside. Respiratory Medicine. 2019;**154**:47-55. DOI: 10.1016/j.rmed.2019.06.008

[68] Boehringer Ingelheim Canada Ltd, McClelland S, Boehringer Ingelheim (Canada) Ltd. IBM Canada Announce First of its Kind Collaboration to Integrate Blockchain Technology into Clinical Trials. Ontario, Canada: Boehringer Ingelheim; 2019. Available from: https://www.boehringer-ingelheim.com/ca/boehringer-ingelheim-canada-ltd-and-ibm-canada-announce-first-its-kind-collaboration-integrate#:~:text=and%20IBM%20Canada%20aim%20to,patient%20safety%20at%20reduced%20cost [Accessed: January 21, 2025]

[69] Duke Health, McCollum J. Duke Implants Second-in-Human Total

Artificial Heart. North Carolina, USA: Duke University Health System; 2024. Available from: https://physicians.dukehealth.org/articles/duke-implants-second-human-total-artificial-heart [Accessed: January 21, 2025]

[70] Wikipedia. CAR T Cell. 2024. Available from: https://en.wikipedia.org/wiki/CAR_T_cell [Accessed: January 21, 2025]

[71] Scheffer E, Kelkar A, Russler-Germain D, Tessema F, Raymakers A, Feldman W, et al. High Cost of Chimeric Antigen Receptor T-Cells: Challenges and Solutions2023. pp. 1-11. DOI: 10.1200/EDBK_397912

[72] Wikipedia. He Jiankui genome editing incident. 2024. Available from: https://en.wikipedia.org/wiki/He_Jiankui_genome_editing_incident [Accessed: January 21, 2025]

[73] Surantha N, Atmaja P, Wicaksono M. A review of wearable internet-of-things device for healthcare. Procedia Computer Science. 2021;**179**:936-943. DOI: 10.1016/j.procs.2021.01.083

[74] Canali S, Schiaffonati V, Aliverti A. Challenges and recommendations for wearable devices in digital health: Data quality, interoperability, health equity, fairness. PLOS Digital Health. 2022;**1**(10):e0000104. DOI: 10.1371/journal.pdig.0000104

[75] Hutson M. Cutting to the chase. Nature. 2024;**627**:S2-S5. DOI: 10.1038/d41586-024-00753-x

[76] Kelly E, Russel S. History of oncolytic viruses: Genesis to genetic engineering. Molecular Therapy. 2007;**15**(4):651-659. DOI: 10.1038/mt.sj.6300108

[77] Wikipedia. Oncolytic Virus. California, USA: Wikipedia Foundation Inc.; 2024. Available from: https://en.wikipedia.org/wiki/Oncolytic_virus [Accessed: January 21, 2025]

[78] Shetty K, Desai D, Patel H, Shah D, Willcox M, Maulvi F. Contact lens as an emerging platform for non-invasive bio-sensing: A review. Sensors and Actuators: A. Physical. 2024;**376**:115-617. DOI: 10.1016/j.sna.2024.115617

[79] Toris C, Gagrani M, Ghate D. Current methods and new approaches to assess. Expert Review of Ophthalmology. 2021:1-21. DOI: 10.1080/17469899.2021.1902308

[80] Huang R, Li X, He Y, Zhu W, Gao L, Liu Y, et al. Recent advances in CAR-T cell engineering. Journal of Hematology and Oncology. 2020;**13**(88):1-19. DOI: 10.1186/s13045-020-00910-5

[81] Ludwig-Maximilians-Universität München. Kutyniok G. 2024. How can reliability of artificial intelligence be ensured. Available from: https://www.ai.math.uni-muenchen.de/publications/survey/reliability1.pdf [Accessed: January 21, 2025]

[82] Cacciamani G, Sanford D, Chu T, Kaneko M, De Castro AA, Duddalwar V, et al. Is artificial intelligence replacing our radiology stars? Not yet! European Urology Open Science. 2023;**48**:14-16. DOI: 10.1016/j.euros.2022.09.024

[83] Guo R, Guo H, Wang L, Chen M, Yang D, Li B. Development and application of emotion recognition technology — A systematic literature review. British Medical Journal Psychology. 2024;**12**(95):1-15. DOI: 10.1186/s40359-024-01581-4

[84] Christensen C, McDonald R, Altman E, Palmer J. Disruptive

innovation: An intellectual history and directions for future research. Journal of Management Studies. 2018;**55**(7):1043-1078. DOI: 10.1111/joms.12349

[85] Wonkhe, Miller C. Let's Stop Talking about Disruptive Research. London, UK: Wonkhe Ltd.; 2024. Available from: https://wonkhe.com/blogs/lets-stop-talking-about-disruptive-research/ [Accessed: January 21, 2025]

[86] TriNet. Generational Differences in the Workplace: Boomers, Gen X, Gen Y, and Gen Z Explained. California, USA: TriNet Group Inc.; 2024. Available from: https://www.trinet.com/insights/generations-in-the-workplace-boomers-gen-x-gen-y-and-gen-z-explained [Accessed: January 21, 2025]

[87] Institute for Management Development IMD. What is disruptive innovation? 10 real-world examples. 2025. Available from: https://www.imd.org/blog/innovation/what-is-disruptive-innovation/ [Accessed: January 21, 2025]

[88] Christensen CM, Raynor ME, McDonald R. Harvard Business Review. What is Disruptive Innovation? Massachusetts, USA: Harvard Business School Publishing; 2015. Available from: https://hbr.org/2015/12/what-is-disruptive-innovation [Accessed: January 21, 2025]

[89] Marshall B, Adams P. Helicobacter pylori: A Nobel pursuit? Canadian Journal of Gastroenterology. 2008;**22**(11):895-896. DOI: 10.1155/2008/459810

[90] Nobel Prize. All Nobel Prizes. Stockholm, Sweden: Nobel Prize Outreach 2025; 2024. Available from: https://www.nobelprize.org/prizes/lists/all-nobel-prizes/ [Accessed: January 21, 2025]

[91] Zhang X. Incremental innovation: Long-term impetus for design business creativity. Sustainability. 2022;**14**:1-24, 14697. DOI: 10.3390/su142214697

[92] Yu J, Zhang J, Sengoku S. Innovation process and industrial system of US Food and Drug Administration–approved software as a medical device: Review and content analysis. Journal of Medical Internet Research. 2023;**25**:e47505. DOI: 10.2196/47505

[93] Bosch F, Rosich L. The contributions of Paul Ehrlich to pharmacology: A tribute on the occasion of the centenary of his nobel prize. Pharmacology. 2008;**82**:171-179. DOI: 10.1159/000149583

[94] Morrant J. Never say dye. British Columbia Medical Journal. 2012;**54**(2):68-69. Available from: https://bcmj.org/newsnotes/special-feature-never-say-dye [Accessed: January 21, 2025]

[95] Gaynes R. The discovery of penicillin—New insights after more than 75 years of clinical use. Emerging Infectious Diseases. 2017;**23**(5):849-853. DOI: 10.3201/eid2305.161556

[96] Adamala K, Adashe G, Belkaid Y, Matias de Bittencourt D, Cai Y, Chang MW, et al. Confronting risks of mirror life. Science. 2024;**386**(6728):1351-1353. DOI: 10.1126/science.ads9158

[97] Knopf H, Wolf IK, Sarganas G, Zhuang W, Rascher W, Neubert A. Off-label medicine use in children and adolescents: Results of a population-based study in Germany. BMC Public Health. 2013;**13**(631):1-12. DOI: 10.1186/1471-2458-13-631

[98] Aagaard L, Hansen E. Information about adverse drug reactions reported in children: A qualitative review

of empirical studies. BMC Clinical Pharmacology. 2010;**70**(4):481-491. DOI: 10.1111/j.1365-2125.2010.03682.x

[99] Saiyed M, Lalwani T, Rana D. Is off-label use a risk factor for adverse drug reactions in pediatric patients? A prospective study in an Indian tertiary care hospital. The International Journal of Risk & Safety in Medicine. 2015;**27**(1):45-53. DOI: 10.3233/jrs-150642

[100] Wimmer S, Neubert A, Rascher W. The safety of drug therapy in children. Deutsches Ärzteblatt International. 2015;**112**(46):781-187. DOI: 10.3238/arztebl.2015.0781

[101] Ito S. Drugs for children. Clinical Pharmacology and Therapeutics. 2017;**101**(6):704-706. DOI: 10.1002/cpt.675

[102] Elzagallaai A, Greff M, Rieder M. Adverse drug reactions in children: The double-edged sword of therapeutics. Clinical Pharmacology & Therapeuticsz. 2017;**101**(6):725-735. DOI: 10.1002/cpt.677

[103] Kearns G, Abdel-Rahman S, Alander S, Blowey D, Leeder J, Kauffman R. Developmental pharmacology - drug disposition, action and therapy in infants and children. New England Journal of Medicine. 2003;**349**(12):1157-1167. DOI: 10.1056/NEJMra035092

[104] Vaishali P, Boopathy N. Edward Jenner: The Pioneer of vaccination and his enduring legacy in modern medicine. Cureus. 2024;**16**(9):e68805. DOI: 10.7759/cureus.68805

[105] Krischel MF. The genesis of informed consent in the context of medical research ethics 1900-1931. Urologie. 2023;**62**(3):261-270. DOI: 10.1007/s00120-023-02042-3

[106] Vollmann J, Winau R. The Prussian regulation of 1900: Early ethical standards for human experimentation in Germany. IRB: Ethics & Human Research. 1996;**18**(4):9-11. DOI: 10.2307/3564006

[107] Donald P, Kaufmann S, Thee S, Mandalakas A, Lange C. Pathogenesis of tuberculosis: The 1930 Lübeck disaster revisited. European Respiratory Review. 2022;**31**:1-13, 220046. DOI: 10.1183/16000617.0046-2022

[108] Wikipedia. Nuremberg code. 2024. Available from: https://en.wikipedia.org/wiki/Nuremberg_Code [Accessed: January 21, 2025]

[109] World Medical Association. Declaration of Helsinki. 2024. Available from: https://www.wma.net/policies-post/wma-declaration-of-helsinki/ [Accessed: January 21, 2025]

[110] European Union. Eur Lex. Regulation (EU) No 536/2014 of the European Parliament and of the Council of 16 April 2014 on clinical trials on medicinal products for human use. Amsterdam, The Netherlands: European Medicines Agency; 2014. Available from: https://eur-lex.europa.eu/eli/reg/2014/536/2022-12-05 [Accessed: January 21, 2025]

[111] European Medicines Agency. Paediatric Regulation. 2007. Available from: https://www.ema.europa.eu/en/human-regulatory-overview/paediatric-medicines-overview/paediatric-regulation [Accessed: January 21, 2025]

[112] European Union. Eur Lex. Regulation (EC) No 1901/2006 of the European Parliament and of the Council of 12 December 2006 on medicinal products for paediatric use. 2006. Available from: https://eur-lex.europa.eu/legal-content/EN/TXT/?uri=CELE

X:32006R1901&qid=1621344437946 [Accessed: January 21, 2025]

[113] European Commission. Supplementary Protection Certificates for Pharmaceutical and Plant Protection Products. Luxembourg, Luxembourg: European Commission; 2024. Available from: https://single-market-economy.ec.europa.eu/industry/strategy/intellectual-property/patent-protection-eu/supplementary-protection-certificates-pharmaceutical-and-plant-protection-products_en [Accessed: January 21, 2025]

[114] European Medicines Agency. Guideline on the Need for Non-clinical Testing in Juvenile Animals of Pharmaceuticals for Paediatric Indications. Committee for Human Medicinal Products; 2008. Available from: https://www.ema.europa.eu/en/documents/scientific-guideline/guideline-need-non-clinical-testing-juvenile-animals-pharmaceuticals-paediatric-indications_en.pdf [Accessed: January 21, 2025]

[115] Food and Drug Administration. Guidance for Industry Nonclinical Safety Evaluation of Pediatric Drug Products. Maryland, USA: U.S. Food and Drug Administration; 2006. Available from: https://www.fda.gov/media/119658/download [Accessed: January 21, 2025]

[116] European Medicines Agency. Committee for Human Medicinal Products. Reflection Paper: Formulations of Choice for the Paediatric Population. Amsterdam, The Netherlands: European Medicines Agency; 2006. Available from: https://www.ema.europa.eu/en/documents/scientific-guideline/reflection-paper-formulations-choice-paediatric-population_en.pdf [Accessed: January 21, 2025]

[117] Expert group on clinical trials for the implementation of Regulation (EU) No 536/2014 on clinical trials on medicinal products for human use. Ethical considerations for clinical trials on medicinal products conducted with minors. 2017. Available from: https://health.ec.europa.eu/system/files/2018-02/2017_09_18_ethical_consid_ct_with_minors_0.pdf [Accessed: January 21, 2025]

[118] National Library of Medicine. ClinicalTrials.gov. 2024. Available from: https://clinicaltrials.gov/ [Accessed: January 21, 2025]

[119] European Commission. State of Paediatric Medicines in the EU. Luxembourg, Luxembourg: European Commission; 2017. Available from: https://health.ec.europa.eu/document/download/cbb2bd84-4770-4166-b988-d9097e8d6bb3_en [Accessed: January 21, 2025]

Section 3

# Death and Dying

Chapter 8

# Medical Homicide and Perverse Incentives in Global Perspective

*Kirk C. Allison*


## Abstract

Global pertains to a whole as well as geography. The nexus between intentional lethality and medicine is expanding globally. In Latin etymology *homo + cidium* concerns human death and agency (self or other) under intent (responsibility) and efficient effect. 'Medical' involves a domain of ends, means, agents, and roles, tracing through Latin *medicus* (physician, ...) and protoindoeuropean root **med-*, indicating appropriate measures. Means involve technical, institutional and philosophical mediations: formularies (φάρμακον ... θανάσιμον, lethal drug), procedures (injection, explantation), hospitals, state-political appropriations (medicalized execution; executee organs), (re)definitions to reify or territorialize lethality in(to) a medical domain. Ends involve the 'to or for what' of an act, often with intersecting layers of intent and utility (personal, medical, economic, state-political) and private and public concern. At the nexus, medical or medicalized actors include patients, physicians, nurses, technologists, pharmacists, bioethicists, professional associations, but also corporations, legislators, courts, bureaucracies, functionaries and instruments of state power. Incentives elicit specific behaviors or outcomes. 'Perverse incentives' may be structurally ironic or malign, with intersections recently spanning from organ to public housing demand. This chapter explores contexts involving medicine, lethality, and incentives, intramural and external, and affected populations, including in China, Europe, and North America: a nexus changing medicine and much else.


**Keywords:** medical homicide, euthanasia, assisted suicide, autonomy, perverse incentives, bureaucracy, definition of death, determination of death, vulnerable populations, transplantation, North America, Europe, China

## 1. Introduction

Global pertains to a whole as well as geography. The nexus between intentional lethality and medicine is expanding globally ranging from assisted suicide and euthanasia to organ harvesting under both totalitarian and liberal democratic contexts. Historically and presently there has been an intersection between state and medical actors concerning execution. Increasingly medical lethality is becoming a backstop solution to social, including governmental, failures. In the English speaking world since Blackstone, and before, matters such as homicide and suicide and have been recognized understood as matters of public concern also involving public wrongs or harms, not solely matters of private agency or conscience.

In Latin etymology *homo* + *cidium* concerns human death by human agency (self or other) causally involved [1]; in legal and moral contexts homicide implies intent or responsibility. *Medical homicide* adds specific context and color of action through late Latin genitive *medicalis* "of a physician" (a *medicus*), one not acting in a personal, private or other capacity. Notably the Protoindoeuropean root **med-* indicates to "take appropriate measures" [2]. Appropriate has content in relationship to a particular end (*telos*) and context. One is a *medicus* only when acting under this description but not if acting merely 'under color of ...'. Medical actors include physicians, nurses, technologists, pharmacists, bioethicists, even professional associations.

Means of medicalized homicide could include a formulary (a φάρμακον ... θανάσιμον, lethal drug, in Hippocratic language), procedure (explantation), appropriation (medicalized execution), or definition. Ends concern the 'to or for what' of an act and can accommodate multiple layers of intent. This includes the intersections of private and public acts, laws and institutions. At the nexus, medical or medicalized actors include patients, physicians, nurses, technologists, pharmacists, bioethicists, professional associations, but also corporations, legislators, courts, bureaucracies, functionaries and instruments of state power. Incentives elicit specific behaviors or outcomes. 'Perverse incentives' may be structurally ironic or malign. Intersections recently span from organ to public housing demand. This chapter probes contexts involving medicine, lethality, and incentives, intramural and external, and affected populations, including in China, Europe, and North America: a nexus changing medicine and much else. The intersection of lethality and medicine is at a cost.

## 2. Of public or private concern: Homicide, suicide, medical lethality

### 2.1 Blackstone on private and public wrongs: Homicide

Introducing the *Commentaries on the Laws of England* (1765–1769), Blackstone states "LAW, in its moft general and comprehenfive fense signifies a rule of action"; concerning "human action or conduct", a precept regulating behavior. This, per Blackstone, spans natural law, revelation, and conventional law, often converging. Natural law is general, aligning with pursuit of human happiness under agencies of reason and free will, while "[a] being, independent of any other, has no rule to purfue, but fuch as he prefcribes to himfelf. Blackstone quotes Justinian on intents of law socially: to live honesty, hurt no one, and render to each what is due. A rejection of arbitrary autonomy also judges conventional law under natural law (which he also calls ethics), "binding over all the globe," with a claim that "no human laws are of any validity, if contrary to this" [3].

*Book the Fourth, Of Public Wrongs* addresses Homicide ("the killing of any human creature", IV.14.17); the first three books concerned *Of Rights of Persons*; *Of Rights of Things*; and *Of Private Wrongs*: of the latter, "firft, private wrongs, which, being an infringement merely of particular rights, concern individuals only, and are called civil injuries; and fecondly, public wrongs, which, being a breach of general and public rights, affect the whole community, and are called crimes and mifdemefnors" (I.1.118). Civil actions are brought by individuals in private capacity regarding private wrong whereas public wrongs are "a matter of univerfal concern" prosecuted *in stead* by the crown "in whom centers the majefty of the whole community" (IV.1.2), not as *pars pro toto* but rather *pars qua totum*, as each in the community has substantial interest, not mere bystander curiosity. Hence public wrongs "are of a much more extenfive consequence, violating the laws of nature, moral and political rules of right; almost always breaching public peace;" and "in tendency they threaten and endanger the fubverfion of all civil fociety" (IV.14.176–177).

Homicide, states Blackstone, is in all cases a matter of universal concern but "is of three kinds; juftifiable, excufable, and felonious", the latter being "the higheft crime againft the law of nature" (IV.14.177–178).

### 2.2 Blackstone on private and public wrongs: Suicide

Both homicide and suicide are considered a matter of public concern, either possible species of murder as an intentional killing of an innocent: in suicide one person holds divided moral status as victim (innocent) and actor (culpable).

Blackstone broaches suicide as "SELF-MURDER, the pretended heroifm, but real cowardice, of the Stoic philofophers, who deftroyed themfelves to avoid thofe ills which they had not the fortitude to endure, though the attempting it feems to be countenanced by the civil law, yet was punifhed by the Athenian law" (IV.14.189) –indirectly citing Arrius Menander (*Military Law*, book 3) on soldiers: "Si quis impatientia doloris, aut taedio vitae, aut morbo, aut furore, aut pudore, mori maluit, non animadvertatur in eum" ("If any one, under the pressure of grief, weariness of life, disease, madness, or shame, prefers death, his conduct shall not be considered to the prejudice of his character" [4]), neither validating nor valorizing the attempt. Save for military desertion, Roman and Greek law did not consider suicide a punishable act [5].

Blackstone states suicide constituted a reflexive double offense (spiritual/political), a "peculiar species of felony, a felony committed on onefelf" (*felo de se*) with sanctions limited to reputation and property (forfeited to the crown); others historically included denial of consecrated burial or desecration (being subjected to dissection for medical training was reserved for executees) [6]. An inquest judgment of *non compos mentis* (widely already by the 17th C) freed a deceased and survivors from formal and material penalty [7]. Were one's death was assisted by another, English and Scots law assigned responsibility to the proxy: "he who desires and persuades another man to kill him, is not a felo de se; his assent being void in law, and the person killing him a murderer. Kelw. 136" [8]. Responsibility to reject the request lay with the fulfiller.

Decriminalization of suicide appears as extension of self-sovereignty. In modernity an axiological shift regarding suicide traverses negative legal sanction, to decriminalization, to destigmatization within psycho-therapeutic language (suicide now 'attempted' and 'completed' not 'committed'), to medical-institutionalization ('assisted'). Voluntary stopping of eating and drinking assumes responsibility for one's own death in both decision and instrument, free also to reverse course [9, 10]. Not imposing on medicine an expectation to provide an efficient lethal means avoids a conundrum: which suicides to prevent or abet [11, 12]. As John Kelly of Not Dead Yet noted, were suicide assistance a general right, it ceases to be *medical* [13].

Still, suicide is a social act, not merely individual. So-called *Werther effects* arose in the wake of Goethe's epistolary novel *Die Leiden des jungen Werthers* of 1774 (*The Sorrows of Young Werther*), whose preface offers the book as friend and comfort to those suffering similar sorrows [14]. An 18th C *Werther* contagion including emulation in style and action. Involving celebrities ('influencers') Lutter et al. found suicide is socially more impactful than death by unexpected accident; additional suicides follow as wake or imitation more so than following accident (anomie) [15] although both abruptly rupture relationships (direct, mediated, imaginal). Accidents are not considered communication or statement.

Valorizing coverage of assisted suicide has led to calls for communicative probity [16]; intensive media coverage of 'suicide tourism' increased the same [17]. In the US in 2014 Brittany Maynard publicly shared progression of her glioblastoma in social media and publicly pursued and advocated for expansion of access to assisted suicide also with an advocacy organization. She received quasi-official iconic status in *People Magazine* on 24 October 2014: a cover story under the rubric 'Celebrity'. Framed exclusively in terms of first-person autonomy, her advocacy and media prominence inspired attempted imitation even absent a terminal diagnosis [18]. Such deaths transcend private acts in public secondary impacts.

### 2.3 Medicalized state homicide: The physician as expert and executioner

Consistent with Hippocratic proscriptions, physicians have often rejected instrumental involvement in executions invoking integrity of profession beyond private integrity or conscience. Sikora and Fleishman state "[t]he redefinition of the relationship between doctors and their patients represented by physician involvement in capital punishment is inconsistent with the integrity of medicine as a profession" [19]. Latin *integritas* indicates "'soundness, wholeness, completeness' figuratively 'purity, correctness, blamelessness' from *integer* 'whole'" [20]. Integrity, integer, and integral all indicate something untouched (*in* ~ not, *tangere* and PIE root **tag* ~ touch, handle) [21]. Antonym of integer is fraction (Latin *frangere* "to break (something) in pieces, shatter, fracture," via Proto-Italic **frang-* nasalized from PIE root **bhreg-* "to break") [22]. One should ask: What is the integer of medicine? What remains after fracturing?

#### *2.3.1 L'Humanité and lethal efficiency in the name of public good*

Innovating means of execution historically has not been completely foreign to those bearing the title physician, most famously 6 articles introduced in France's Assembly on 10 October 1789 by member Dr. Joseph-Ignace Guillotin. A lawyer's son, previously tonsured, Dr. Guillotin was *docteur-régent* of the Paris Faculty of Medicine in anatomy, physiology, and pathology. The legislator-physician offered a comprehensive prescription to the body politic: Article 1 required identical penalties for identical offenses regardless of rank or station. Article 2 required one mode of capital punishment whatever the crime (without torture) by decapitation via "a simple mechanism." Articles 3, 4 and 5 prohibited defaming or disadvantaging immediate family, punishing relatives, and property confiscation. Article 6 returned the body of the executed to the family on request for normal burial, "and no reference shall be made on the register to the nature of the death" – a privacy measure [23].

The proposal received acclaim in *Le Journal de Paris*; *La Gazette de Paris*; and *Le Moniteur* 1, 3, and 17 days after its 1 December 1789 second reading. Although Article 2, standardizing and democratizing execution, never passed, decapitation was approved as method on 3 June 1791, codified in September, with technological principle stipulated on March 1792.

Despite eponymous fame, the instrument was designed by Dr. Antoine Louis, secretary of the *Académie Chirurgical* whose March 1792 treatise for the Legislative Committee detailed legal requirements, execution botches, cutting mechanics, and human anatomy. The Committee's encomium: "the reflections born of your humanity and your profound anatomical knowledge have been adopted by the Committee [....] You thus have the merit of having benefited humanity even when the law's blade strikes the head of the guilty" [23].

Clinical trials followed construction in April 1792. Chief surgeon Dr. Cullerier provided corpses from Bicêtre prison/hospital/geronton near Paris. Among attending in one account were *médecins* Louis, Cullerier, Cabanis, Philippe Pinel, and Guillotin. The trials were an anatomical success (45–47). On inspection, the professional *bourreau* (executioner) Charles-Henri Sanson expressed an inkling of moral hazard: "a fine machine – so long as its facility is not abused" [23]. The first *homme vivant* was dispatched on 25 April 1792 at Place de Grève where members of the legislature followed in due time. Post technical input by *médecins*, operation was left to other professionals (often generational): the *bourreau*, at a distance from medicine.

Claims that consciousness was immediately extinguished by such a mechanism was rejected by Dr. Pierre Guatier already in 1776. Despite humanitarian trappings, in 1795 German anatomist S. T. Sommering, given consciousness in brain, decried "the barbarous horrors of this butchery," calling it a "cruel and painful type of execution" [23]. Others (Wedekind, Le Pelletier, Sedillot) offered rebuttal. In1905, a Dr. Beurieux, seconds after a privatized execution, reported prisoner eyes opening twice with focus in response to his name, similarly reported by Drs. Piedlievre and Fournier in 1956.

### *2.3.2 L'Humanité and lethal efficiency: Medicalized capital punishment presently*

An active role for physicians in execution has been debated and proposed in the US given technical competences as in the day of Drs. Guillotine and Louis, especially when carried out with medical trappings: IV bags, tubing, needles, formulary, discussions on what *pharmakon* mix is *safe and effective* (physically painless death defined as success and survival judged technical and legal failure). To an instrumental mind who better than a physician or other certified person to efficiently access a vein sufficient for physiological efficiency and lethal outcome? Multiple sides of the semantics of *pharmakon* (φάρμακον) are in play simultaneously for the body politic: [24] a drug (healing or noxious), remedy (for injustice), enchanted potion (putting to 'sleep', restoring moral order, preceded by recitation of the Warrant of Execution), a poison (killing the body), and lye (cleansing society).

Revealing are the ethical tone and technical requirements of an 18 February 2025 letter and directive from the Secretary of the Florida Department of Corrections to Governor Ron Desantis titled "Execution by Lethal Injection Procedures" [25]. The letter's moral-ethical tone is similar to other medicalized contexts: "the procedure has been reviewed and is compatible with evolving standards of decency that mark the progress of a maturing society, the concepts of the dignity of man, and advances in science, research, pharmacology, and technology [....] The foremost objective of the lethal injection process is a humane and dignified death" while "emotions of all those involved must be addressed."

The document details credentialling and technical requirements. The execution team comprises medically certified or licensed actors. The "executioner's sole function is to inject the chemicals into the IV access port by physically pushing the chemicals from the syringe." Secretary and warden ensure "necessary licensure and certification" for specific functions: For "achieving and monitoring peripheral venous access" a certified phlebotomist; certified paramedic or EMT; licensed LPN, RN, APRN;

physician or physician's assistant. For "attaching the leads to the heart monitors and observing the monitors" similar minus phlebotomists. For "purchasing, maintaining and mixing the lethal chemicals" a licensed physician or licensed pharmacist. Identities are statutorily confidential (shielded from public and credentialing body scrutiny).

Preparation is dense in medical, technical detail: Etomidate injection (to render unconscious): 4 syringes x (60 cc, 2 mg/ml, 100 mg); Rocuronium bromide (neuromuscular blocking agent): 4 syringes x (60 cc, 500 mg); Potassium acetate (to produce electrolytic lethal cardiac hyperkalemia): 4 syringes (60 cc, 120 mEq); Saline solution (flushing): 4 syringes x (20 cc, 20 ml); aseptic technique with 2 standard intravenous (IV) infusion sets. The warden "will explain the lethal injection preparation procedure to the inmate and ensure the provision of any medical assistance or care deemed appropriate" and offer noncompulsory "intramuscualar injections of hydroxyzine, in appropriate dosages relative to weight, to ease anxiety."

The executioner at each stage will "push the entire contents of that syringe into the IV port at a rate that meets the injection resistance of the cannula": 2x 100 mg etomidate; 20 ml saline; check unconsciousness (if conscious, use secondary infusion site or establish another with or without surgical venous cut-down; repeat sequence); 2 x 500 mg rocurionium bromide; 20 ml saline; 2x 120 mEq potassium acetate. If heart monitor returns a flat line during or following administration, "a physician will examine the inmate to determine whether there is complete cessation of respiration and heartbeat" to certify death.

Of all disciplines, anesthesiology understands what would be pharmacologically efficient to kill a person, given relevant factors. Given possible *pharmakon* combinations, botched executions, under banner of reducing suffering some physicians offer themselves (or others similarly situated) [26]. Indeed in 1977 an anesthesiologist first suggested the protocol of sodium thiopental, to render unconscious; pancuronium bromide, to paralyze muscles; followed by potassium chloride to stop the heart ('treating' simultaneously the condemned and body politic under color of medicine).

Pancomioum bromide (Pavulon™) is a nexus of confluences and contradictions, blocking muscle activation (not sensation), used in US execution protocols and euthanasia protocols in Belgium and Netherlands, plus in simple murder [27]. Presently under UK export control, it is banned for the US under "torture and capital punishment goods" but not for lethal use in Belgium or Netherlands [28]. Supply bottlenecks for lethal *pharmakoi* in the US have resulted in reversions to nonmedicalized methods [29].

The AMA's *Code of Medical Ethics Opinion 9.7.3 Capital Punishment* [30] provides a rationale parallel to its opposition to lethal actions in clinical contexts, distinguishing individual and professional *personae*: "An individual's opinion on capital punishment is the personal moral decision of the individual. However, as a member of a profession dedicated to preserving life when there is hope of doing so, a physician must not participate in a legally authorized execution". Physician participation includes directly causing death; assisting, supervising, or contributing to another's ability to directly cause death; or aiding automating execution. All instrumental functions described in Florida's process are proscribed plus determining prisoner competency for execution; treating an incompetent prisoner to regain competency for execution; attending or observing *as* a physician. Not proscribed is relieving acute suffering (tranquilizers) if requested by prisoner. One may certify but not declare death. Participation is framed as medical betrayal. It also holds prisoner organs may be harvested only if a donation decision was pre-conviction;

harvesting after declared dead outside the execution chamber, no advising or modifying of execution method to yield better quality organs.

In 1981 the World Medical Association passed a *Resolution on Physician Participation in Capital Punishment* (revised 2000, 2008; merged into the *WMA Resolution on Prohibition of Physician Participation in Capital Punishment* in 2018) [31]. Centrally: "There is universal agreement that physicians must not participate in executions because such participation is incompatible with the physician's role as healer." The WMA urges physicians to lobby governments against involvement. In parallel is the 2019 *WMA Declaration on Euthanasia and Physician-Assisted Suicide* proscribing both and reserving a right not to make referrals for such [32].

Intentionally lethal acts under color of medicine in countries prohibiting judicial executions reject medical homicide only as punishment. Once lethality is on the menu, acting as de facto executioner is not so easily avoided. Belgium has no death penalty, however on 28 February 2023, Genevieve Lhermitte, guilty of first-degree murder, was killed at her own request on the 16th anniversary of murdering her son and four daughters ages 3–13. A psychologist characterized the timing as a "symbolic gesture in respect for her children" [33] – a de facto self-execution with medical collaboration.

Systems of medical homicide can hold effective veto against justice for victims of crime. In Spain on 14 December 2021, a fired security guard shot 3 former colleagues and a police officer before sustaining paraplegic injuries [34]. Medical homicide was legalized after in Spain in March 2022. Before trial, the gunman was granted medical death claiming "unbearable pain" and under the rubric of not violating the shooter's dignity and rights but depriving his victims their day in court and facing his own remorseless responsibility with any concept of punitive justice eliminated [35].

Prisoner medically assisted deaths in Canada are rising with slightly under one third approved vs. 81% outside [36]. Canada's Office of the Correctional Investigator expressed concern that such were exempted from standard investigation oversight. Correctional Services of Canada indicated circa 75% of incarcerated have a mental health diagnosis. Prisoners floated medicalized de facto execution on request to replace long sentences, noting economic efficiency for government and 'society' [37].

## 3. Medical homicide: A PubMed query

Homicide as term and topic appears increasingly over time in medical literature, exponentially after 1950. A PubMed query of 'homicide' through 2024 returned 28,793 results [38]. The first is in the 1832 *Edinburgh Medical Surgical Journal* concerning exculpation due to insanity [39]. Save 2 in 1838 by one author, there are no more than 1 yearly through 1944. 1945 yielded 13 with 8 having psychological/psychiatric dimensions. Counts expand thereafter: 9–92 (1945–1967), 117–265 (1968–1983), 307–517 (1984–1991), and 601–822 (1992–2024) (**Figure 1**) [40].

A sentinel event spanning 1972–1973 corresponds to a single year gap-up from 130 to 223 items: the 22 January 1973 US Supreme Court abortion decisions *Roe v. Wade* and *Doe v Bolton*. Might expansion of antenatal medical lethality increase consideration of postnatal medical lethality, at least in discussion?

A natural experiment query on 'homicide' a year prior and post (22 Jan 1972–2021 Jan 1973/22 Jan 1973–2021 Jan 1974, inclusive) returned 137 and 238 results respectively. Partitioning using medical subject heading (MeSH) terms ([induced] Abortion, [human] Euthanasia/PAS, Both, or Other homicide) yielded percentages

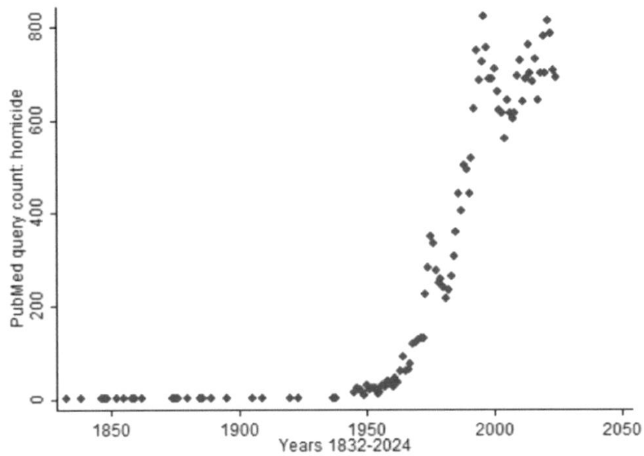


**Figure 1.**
*PubMed query "homicide".*

before and after: Abortion (6.6, 7.6%), [human] Euthanasia/PAS (17.5, 31.9%), Both (3.6, 4.6%), and Other homicide (71.5, 55.9%). Abortion and Both remained within 1% while Euthanasia/PAS articles increased +14.4% proportionally and Other homicide articles decreased −15.6% - across the 4 categories (Chi-Square 10.56, df 3, p = 0.0144) consistent with the thesis of judicial decisions energizing post-natal lethality discussions.

A search of 'medical homicide' returned only 7 results: 5 on forensic investigation (3 in 1946) [41] and 2 (1991) concerning medical actors, one re extreme negligence while not intending the death [42]. Nonintentional dosing error was often certified as accident, but if "the physician intentionally injected the patient to cause death it would be certified as homicide" given *actus reus* (having caused a death) and *mens rea* (intention). However, "[i]f a patient administers (by his/her own hand) a lethal dose of medication with intent to cause death, the manner is suicide" while"[i]f that same person allows another person knowingly to administer the lethal cocktail, the manner is homicide (death at hand of another)". Were the other qua physician or nurse then medical homicide. The second 1991 article argued for "necessity to palliate pain and suffering as a defense to medical homicide," legally considered positing a medical-ethical-legal obligation to respect patient autonomy instrumentally to *maximally* relieve pain and suffering at end of life, including causing death with intent: "[i]t is the proximate action that is the responsible one, not any precedent causes" [43].

## 4. What's in a name?

### 4.1 Suicide and euthanasia

Attempts to banish 'suicide' regarding physician assisted suicide in the US or elsewhere, in concept, nomenclature, and culture, including statutory or regulatory prohibitions, ignore the clear etymological sense of the word.

On 30 October 2017 the American Association of Suicidology (AAS) Board adopted the statement "'Suicide' is not the same as 'Physician Aid in Dying'", drafted primarily by proponents to conceptually distinguish the latter and distance it from the american association of suicidology (AAS) sphere of concern [44, 45]. The statement, retired on 24 February 2023, offered 15 possible differences and an encomium to psychological screening safeguards that in truth, save in Hawai'i, are rarely engaged in US context (e.g. Oregon's < 3% screening referral [46]; a prechecked screening report form finding competence [47]; and depression-consistent indicators reported as 'concerns' by attending physicians only post mortem [48]). The Executive Summary's policy-political conclusion: "legal physician assisted deaths should not be considered to be cases of suicide and are therefore a matter outside the central focus of the AAS" with implications for research, monitoring, and (non)intervention. It closes proposing a quasi *Sprachverbot*: "we believe that the term 'physician-assisted *suicide*' in itself constitutes a critical reason why these distinct death categories are so often conflated, and should be deleted from use." Ironically an overlapping 3-year AMA process concluded "ethical deliberation and debate is best served by using plainly descriptive language", specifically "'physician assisted suicide' describes the practice with the greatest precision" and "[m]ost importantly, it clearly distinguishes the practice from euthanasia" [49].

On 10 June 2019 the AMA House of Delegates voted 360–190 (65%) confirming the above language and 71% reaffirmed *AMA Code of Ethics* Opinion 5.7 Physician Assisted Suicide stating "Physician-assisted suicide is fundamentally incompatible with the physician's role as healer, […]" [50]. An introductory statement accompanying Opinion 5.7 provided proponents less than half a loaf, but inaccurately stating "Opinion 1.1.7 ["Physician Exercise of Conscience"] articulates the thoughtful moral basis for those who support assisted suicide" while Opinion 1.1.7 mentions only to "honor patients' informed decisions to refuse life-sustaining treatment" [51].

Opinion 5.8 on Euthanasia amplified presciently: "Euthanasia is fundamentally incompatible with the physician's role as healer, would be difficult or impossible to control, and would pose serious societal risks. Euthanasia could readily be extended to incompetent patients and other vulnerable populations. The involvement of physicians in euthanasia heightens the significance of its ethical prohibition. The physician who performs euthanasia assumes unique responsibility for the act of ending the patient's life" [52]. The semantic circle is impoverished: Since mid-seventeenth century 'euthanasia' indicated a 'gentle, easy death' (Greek *eu-* (good) *thanatos* (death)); 'legally sanctioned mercy killing' is found circa 1869 [53].

John Dolan asks whether *physician* assisted suicide is *possible* noting in extremis 'better off dead' need not entail 'better off killed' [54]. Introduction of lethal intent – *healing by killing* - inverts fundamental intuitions: survival as failure (*mal*practice). Dolan notes Pieter Admiraal's practice of removing his white coat before performing a lethal act, reflecting a sense of a constitutive rule being set aside: a Hippocratic confession of sorts as the Oath rejected lethal interventions: "I will use treatment to help the sick according to my ability and judgment, but never with a view to injury and wrong-doing. Neither will I administer a lethal φάρμακον to anybody [οὐδενὶ *not to one*] when asked to do so, nor will I suggest such a course" [55]. οὐδενὶ is unrestricted, not merely refusing participating in political assassination plots as has been suggested [56]. Directly follows: ἁγνῶς δὲ καὶ ὁσίως διατηρήσω βίον τὸν ἐμὸν καὶ τέχνην τὴν ἐμήν, with purity and holiness to conduct one's life and art. Admiraal's undonning raises a question: if not acting as physician (having taken off the white coat), then acting as …? [54] A different practice, once legally legitimized, regularization and institutionalization follow [57].

## 4.2 Death certification, bureaucracies, and legal fictions

Legal performatives are modern magic: 'for the purpose of' within the Definitions section of a statute, one can establish a round square or refer a signifier to its prior opposite. J.L. Austin notes: "Of all people, jurists should be best aware of the true state of affairs [....]. Yet they will succumb to their own timorous fiction, that a statement of 'the law' is a statement of fact" [58]. Health practitioners are also not immune.

The US Centers for Disease Control *Physician's Handbook for the Medical Certification of Death* (revised 2003) Cause of Death section follows World Health Association recommendations [59]. On the *US Standard Certificate of Death* Box 32 Cause of Death, Part I, line (a.) is "IMMEDIATE CAUSE (final disease or condition resulting in death)". A lethal *pharmakon* would be the proximate efficient cause of death. Subsequent causal chain entries end with the *underlying cause of death* ("Enter the UNDERLYING CAUSE (disease or injury that initiating events resulting in death) LAST"). Liver cancer could qualify. Part II allows additional context ("Enter other significant conditions contributing to death but not resulting in the underlying cause given in PART I"). Box 37 partitions Manner of death into natural, accident, homicide, suicide, pending investigation, and undetermined. It intersects the final cause of a process where present: for what or to what motivates the efficient action? Manner is first a descriptive classification not an assessment of legal responsibility (for example homicide may be justified or culpable) [60]. In this context Aristotelean causality is helpful (material, efficient, formal, and final).

### *4.2.1 Oregon's suggestion*

Oregon was first in the world in positively legalizing assisted suicide after referendum, coming into effect in 1998, with Washington State following. Oregon's performative declaration in ORS 127.880 became adopted as canonical form in other state statutes, specifically "Actions taken in accordance with ORS 127.800–127.897 shall not, for any purpose, constitute suicide, assisted suicide, mercy killing or homicide, under the law"- Austin's timorous fiction. Lacking explicit statutory language [61], the Oregon Health Authority Center for Health Statistics "recommends that physicians record the underlying terminal disease as the cause of death and mark the manner of death 'natural' for patients who die under Oregon's Death with Dignity Act (DWDA)" [62], i.e. to falsify the physiological causal chain and manner of death, where voluntary lethal ingestion would be accurate. Their rational: "to balance the confidentiality of patients and their families, while ensuring that we have complete information for statistical purposes" (sans individual data vectors), while asking physicians to impale their integrity. Given the voluntary nature of the action, why this category deserves more privacy than general suicide or succumbing to alcohol poisoning, is not explained.

### *4.2.2 A Washington coercion*

Washington State's 4 November 2008 Initiative Measure I-1000 (*The Washington Death with Dignity Act* (RCW 70.245, 2008)) codified Oregon's cause of death 'recommendation' as explicit requirement. A one-page *Instructions for Physicians and Other Medical Certifiers for Death Certificates: Compliance with the Death with Dignity Act* [63] quotes then RCW 70.245's contrafactual imperative: "... the patient's death certificate ... shall list the underlying terminal disease as the cause of death" followed by canonical language derived from Oregon: "Actions taken in accordance with this chapter do not, for any purpose, constitute suicide, assisted suicide, mercy killing, or homicide, under the law." Moral distress is served up again to the physician with integrity, a commitment to facts (*factus est* – what was done): "you must comply with the strict requirements of the law when completing the death record" - also contrary to CDC requirements. Additionally: "the manner of death must be marked as 'Natural'" although a lethal pharmakon intentionally administered to effect death is quite unnatural even when permissible homicide.

Prior to the vote, Washington State Medical Association president, Brian P. Wicks, stated "[t]o my knowledge, there's no other situation in medicine in which the death certificate is deliberately falsified and in which this falsification is mandated by law" [64].

Bordering on parody, the instruction continues: "the cause of death section may not contain any language that indicates that the Death with Dignity Act was used", not Suicide, Assisted suicide, Physician-assisted suicide, Death with Dignity, I-1000, Mercy killing, Euthanasia, Secobarbital/Seconal, Pentoobarbital/Nembutal, even when used. Should the actual drug(s) be mentioned, the Washington State Registrar will reject until the certifier conforms to the falsification requirements.

In truth, both registrar and certifier are in a double bind, double farce: Per RCW 70.58.030, the State Registrar of Vital Statistics "shall prepare and issue such detailed instruction as may be required to secure the uniform observance of its provision and the maintenance of a perfect system of registration" – here perfect cover up.

The third party in the double bind or limbo is the funeral director. Until trace references to any of the above are eliminated from the death certificate, a permit for disposition of the body will not be issued.

Nonetheless, RCW 70.58A.590 (2) states "Every person who willfully furnishes false information or who makes any false statement to establish a vital record or obtain a certification required by this chapter is guilty of a gross misdemeanor" [65]. The contradiction is cause for moral distress, a corruptive effect and precedent for future falsifications considered socially desirable.

Montana's Supreme Court decision *Baxter v State* (2009) granted physician immunity from prosecution (decriminalization) without refined institutionalization. A law review article on Montana calls falsification of death certificates a 'best practice' and describes a coroner who accurately identified the actual efficient cause of death and manner "ignorant" [66]. In Switzerland assisted suicide is indicated and death registered as non-natural; in the Netherlands as unnatural with assisted suicide, euthanasia or other indicated [67] and under articles 293 and 294 of the Dutch Criminal Code, referred to prosecutor. Advantages in accuracy are legal, research, and oversight transparency [68].

## 5. Medical homicide, transplantation, and perverse incentives

Incentives are second order structures that increase likelihood of a specific behavior or outcome. In context what motivates sufficiently is not the outcome alone but an ancillary factor. The etymology of *incentive* contains musical overtones of setting a tune (PIE roots *en and *kan, to sing, as in enchant). By the 15th C an incentive "moves the mind or stirs the passion" (effecting through thought or affect); *incentivum* in the 16th C via *incentivus is* related to inciting. The economic sense, not the dynamic, emerged much later, in 1943 war economy jargon) [69]. Incentives are often offered to overcome obstacles, disutilities, or indifference (e.g. payments to participate in inconvenient, painful, or higher risk medical research or to obtain biologics - payment-for-plasma versus blood *donation*).

'Perverse incentives' may be imprudent or malign. In economic and policy parlance *perverse incentives* cause the opposite of an intended goal. An axiologically perverse incentive promotes an ill goal or means, possibly effectively; if malign such is never prudent even if efficient. In the realm of medical lethality, a University of Oxford blog titled *Practical Ethics* offered a 2008 entry "Euthanasia and perverse incentives" arguing England *not* establishing 'euthanasia' might motivate a person to travel to Switzerland to end their life sooner than would be the case otherwise [70]. Two propositions may hold simultaneously: Achieving the goal of not changing the nature of medicine as a social-ethical practice yet not preventing self-killing elsewhere.

Incentives also inform commercial payors (insurance). Denials of beneficial treatment with offered coverage of a lethal alternative have been reported anecdotally [71] including after change in lethal option availability [72]. In British Columbia in 2023, a powerpoint on lethal options accompanied information on pension packages sent to healthy retirees by Fraser Health Care, the province's largest provider. The messenger, not simply the message, raises conflict of interest concerns [73]. Another context, intersections of medical homicide with demand for transplantable organs/tissues, is ripe for perverse incentives.

### 5.1 Medical homicide and transplantation under totalitarianism: China

On 6 November 2006 The Transplantation Society, the leading international association for transplantation, published a circular "To TTS Members" on member interaction with China given then Vice Minister of Health and liver transplant surgeon Huang Jiefu's admission that over 90% of transplant organs were sourced from executees [74–76]. Of the prior year's 11,000+ transplants, "[a]lmost all organs are likely to have been obtained from executed prisoners" resulting "in rampant commercialism and transplant tourism." Simultaneously the China International Transplantation Network Assistance Center already boasted "Viscera providers can be found immediately!" intersecting with interests of patients willing to look the other way to reduce wait times from years to a few months, weeks, or even days. The Center's enthusiastic description mirrored a vertically integrated state-medical structure. "The Supreme Demotic Court, Supreme Demotic Law-officer, Police, Judiciary, Department of Health and Civil Administration have enacted a law together to make sure that organ donations are supported by the government. This is unique in the world" [77]. A lucrative international market operating hand in hand with political repression.

HLA matches on short notice would not be possible without a ready-lobster-in-the-tank population of organ sources. Numbers and sites increased exponentially. Evidence mounted of organ sourcing not only from judicial executees but also from prisoners of conscience, chiefly from hundreds of thousands of incarcerated Falun Gong practitioners after the crackdown launched by Jiang Zemin in June 1999. As an indigenous synthesis of Qi Gong, Taoism and Buddhism, FG offered an alternative center of meaning and life practice opposite the Chinese Communist Party (also drawing its members), with practitioners exceeding the CCP, making it a target [78].

Despite the executee pipeline, the TTS pursued ongoing engagement: accept new members if agreeing to TTS policies; reject presentations based on prisoner organ data or tissue; accept attendees from China "to promote dialogue and education"; allow TTS members to conduct research in China *not* directly involving organs or tissues from executees; lecture and share expertise in China as "an excellent opportunity for dialogue" but "ensuring, as far as possible, that such participation" nudges Chinese programs toward TTS standards "and does not promote … transplantation of organs from executed prisoners"; and, astonishingly, "accept clinical or pre-clinical trainees" from China "to educate such trainees in appropriate and effective alternatives" while ensuring "as far as possible" they *intended* to conduct their clinical career compliant with TTS standards. Lectures, expertise and training surgeons only expanded capacity and efficiency in exploiting prisoner organs, despite promises.

Each TTS webpage carried logos of four sponsoring pharmaceutical companies involved in ongoing transplant antirejection drug research in China (large volumes of patients given execution transplantation available for pharmaceutical development – proximate material cooperation with evil) [79]. The 2008 Declaration of Istanbul on "Organ trafficking and transplant tourism and commercialism" with notable TTS participation mentioned tourism to Pakistan not mentioning China as chief violator [80].

In 2009 Swiss pharmaceutical company Roche was queried through its Roche Group Compliance Officer on its procedures to ensure clinical trials were not populated by prisoner organs. The reply letter dated 4 November 2009 offered bioethical camouflage: "… Roche ist in keiner Art und Weise für die Bescahffung von Organen zuständig [….]. Anonymität und Vertraulichkeit der höchstpersönlichen Spenderdaten sind rechtlich geschützt. Roche hat keinen Anspruch zu erfahren, woher oder von welchen Spendern die transplantierten Organen stammen" [81]. "Roche is in no manner or way responsible for the procurement of organs [….]. Anonymity and privacy of the most highly personal donor data are legally protected. Roche has no right to learn from where or from which donors the transplanted organs originate."

TTS led collaborations joined WHO toward developing the China Organ Transplant Response System (COTRS), to allocate all organs after September 1, 2013. COTRS, hidden from external inspection, would increase distributional efficiency from whatever sourcing system obtained. China claimed to cease using prisoner organs on January 1, 2015 [82]. China's *Global Times* reported in July 2017 a quadrafecta: a letter signed by officials from the World Health Organization, Vatican's Pontifical Academy of Sciences, The Transplantation Society, and the Declaration of Istanbul Custodian Group praising progress in China's transplantation system [83]. Thereafter the China Red Cross/COTRS reported data defying patterns of a voluntary system, while exceeding expansion of any known voluntary system mimicking a quadratic formula unseen across 50 country systems [84].

Before the persecution of Falun Gong (biotyped after arrest), among the earliest victims of forced organ harvesting were Uighurs in the 1990s [85]. The Uighur population has also been biotyped during ongoing suppression. In Kashgar Airport in Xinjiang Province an express lane marked "Special Passenger" and "Human Organ Export Channel" was first photographed in 2017 scripted in Chinese/Arabic [86] and later Chinese/English [87]. A European Parliament joint resolution on 5 May 2022 cited past and ongoing medical atrocities, urging members "to raise the issue of forced organ harvesting in its engagement with third countries, especially with its partners in the Gulf region, where Chinese transplant centres have advertised 'halal organs' from Uyghurs and Muslim minorities in China" [88]. Where medical homicide is not *haram* a *halal* organ is simply value added. An independent tribunal led by a former prosecutor of the International Criminal Court confirmed evidence of massive forced organ harvesting beginning with Falun Gong practitioners [89].

The International Society for Heart and Lung Transplantation Statement on Transplant Ethics of December 2022 admonishes: "Members of the ISHLT should also refrain from knowingly teaching visiting physicians the art and science of heart and lung transplantation if it cannot be ascertained and guaranteed that those to be trained will not use their newly acquired knowledge for transplants based on organs from executed prisoners or any other transplant related crime" [90].

Finer transgressions in recent Chinese medical literature include touting brain deaths that could not have been a case or ascertained [91]; others clearly breached the 'dead donor rule' in execution through organ procurement [92].

International discrepancies among brain death criteria and determination practices exist [93]. A study by Ding et al. compared (ironically) a more [94] stringent Chinese multi-test protocol (2009/2013) on 37 neurology unit patients [95] compared to American Academy of Neurology 2010 criteria on those same patients [96]. Under US criteria 33 patients (89.2%) qualified as brain dead without ancillary tests while only 9 (24.3%) qualified under the Chinese protocol. Ding et al. note a perverse incentive to reduce rigor in the Chinese ICU: "The BD diagnosis will be difficult to finish in time when organ donations increase in the future" [94] – a social rather than scientific decision. An incentive also in the US to *not* adopt more thorough practices: stricter criteria could reduce number or rate of available organs.

A need for more rigorous practice within current protocols is clearly indicated by occasional *declared-brain-dead-but-responsive-just-before-organ-harvesting* cases reported in medical and mass media - close calls with significant patient recovery - shoddy and shocking [97]. Where changing the definition of death for a social purpose, the crucial element is not a more rigorous insight into physiology. Glazier and Capron note a contradiction between normothermic regional perfusion (NRP) and circulatory death definitions. Changing definitions solely to maximize transplantation could undermine public trust [98].

## 5.2 Medical homicide and transplantation in liberal democracies

If trust is at risk by introducing intentionally lethal actions and actors into the medical space, the specter of a different enterprise arises at intersection of medical homicide and transplantation also in liberal democracies. Having created a nexus of medical homicide plus organ donation, the debate then concerns the limiting principle, if any.

### *5.2.1 Organ harvesting after euthanasia*

A 2017 research letter titled "Potential Number of Organ Donors After Euthanasia in Belgium" appeared in JAMA drawing on 2015 national data [99]. Although Belgium has population-wide presumed consent donation since1986 (*opting out systeem*) [100], 1288 people were still wait-listed for organs in 2015. Medical lethality presents new sourcing opportunities – as in China, the date of availability is clear, but under color of autonomy. Among 2022 lethally dispatched individuals, 204 (10.1%) were identified as potential sources of minimally 1 organ, up to 684 in all, in a year producing only 260 conventional dead-donor kidneys. The authors surmised "if 400 kidneys were donated by patients undergoing euthanasia ...".

Non-terminal Belgians comprised 15.3% in 2014 and 14.8% in 2015 of facilitated deaths. Of these 19% had primary *psychische stoornissen en gedragsstoornissen* - psychic disturbances and behavior disturbances – and a new nonterminal *polypathologie* category comprised 29.2 and 35.8% of the nonterminal for the 2 years [101]. Social valorization of organ donation under the color of patient autonomy could influence a decision to end one's life for a psychiatric patient struggling with depression or other condition.

Bollen et al. however characterize donation after euthanasia as "the same as for any patient donating an organ - to enable patients to carry out their last will of donating organs to help other people, after their own death" [99]. Calling it "pure altruism" also a 2017 letter [102]. errantly cited a systematic review and ethnographic analysis concerning dignity, autonomy, and control at end of life [103] not mentioning *organ*, *donation,* or *transplantation* as warrant that "[t]he fact that they have the possibility to donate organs has a positive influence on their suffering and has been shown to reduce ongoing chronic pain, potential low mood, and diminished quality of life" [102]. In Belgium there was also a strongly gendered dimension that manifested in a series of 100 consecutive psychiatric patient requests for death: females exceeding males by a 3.4 to 1 [104]. Offered as explanation: "women fulfil the diagnostic criteria for mental disorders more often than men" and have higher mental healthcare demand and utilization.

In 2016 Bollen et al. also published "Organ Donation After Euthanasia: A Dutch Practical Manual" as a Special Article in the American Journal of Transplantation [105]. Its introduction informed "[a] discussion of ethical considerations is not included in this paper, but this is not intended to dismiss the necessary ethical discussions to be held in this domain" (nonetheless it was followed by a section "Ethical Issues Regarding Euthanasia and Organ Donation").

They note standard lethal practice is often without severe organ ischemia pointing to a possibility of DCD (after circulatory death donation) within the Euthanasia Act while dying *in order to donate organs* lies outside the Act. A treating physician, they state, should investigate whether a patient has been solicited to consider dying to make organs available or were attempting that. If denied (who would admit?) the gate is open: "it is ethical for the patient to donate organs". Still, as valorized in popular media, the social conclusion is clear: 'While you no longer value your life, we value your organs.'

### *5.2.2 Euthanasia by explantation*

The 'dead donor rule' originated in USA: the organ source must be dead before retrieval *and* retrieval cannot cause the death. A fundamental question is 'how dead is dead?' but the new twist suggested is: perhaps it does not matter. Already at risk is the 'dead donor rule' in part via redefinition, although here without pretense.

The final efficiency step is death by organ explantation, broached in 2012 by Savulescu and Wilkinson subtitled "Alternatives for maximizing the number and quality of organs for transplantation" [106] and acronymed ODE (Organ Donation Euthanasia). By reification through acronym (RTA) an object is generated for consideration while distancing from its explicit semantic content. What was perhaps previously unthinkable becomes a thing.

Lethal procurement minimizes ischemia whether in the back of a mobile execution van in China or in Belgium. Ironically where *directed donation* is desired, it is intoned by Bolen et al., legal constraints *'require'* living donation as Eurotransplant

DCD allocation is nondirected only. This Bolen et al. call 'heart-beating euthanasia' ("to perform euthanasia *by* removing the heart, under general anesthesia") [105]. However "[in] addition to this legal threshold, practice has shown that, occasionally, relatives insist on seeing the patient die before being brought to the operating room."

As with execution of prisoners in China, a unique feature of institutionalized lethality is availability of vital organs on precise schedule and location. In 2018 Bollen et al. published another exploratory article in the *Journal for Heart and Lung Transplantation* "Euthanasia through living organ donation: Ethical, legal, and medical challenges" [107] – challenges being hurdles to be overcome, including retiring the 'dead-donor rule' altogether in a singular act of conflation. Specifically, the article "addresses whether it is legally and ethically sound to donate organs, especially the heart, as a living donor and to perform euthanasia in the same procedure in a patient who fulfills the due diligence requirements for euthanasia". Ethos with an epsilon can simply mean customs and habits.

"Organ donation euthanasia (ODE) would then cause death by the associated surgical procedure, and in addition would improve the quality of the other donated organs, a procedure that would fully respect the patient's autonomy" [107]. ODE increases medical specialties directly performing an intentionally lethal act by one: surgeons. A body absent a heart is presumed to instantaneously satisfy (de-) cardiac death with or without cardioplegia [108] - yet the sourcing person, if perfused, could receive another heart and continue living - the functional logic of heart transplantation.

In Belgium and the Netherlands 2019 guidelines indicate "the patient should pose the question of organ donation, and only *after* a positive response to the euthanasia question, thus keeping both procedures strictly separated" – however Bollen et al. hold otherwise: "it is our belief that a physician should always inform a patient who is medically suitable about the possibility of organ donation, even if this could disrupt the trust relationship." Supply side altruism (socialization) is driving the issue: "In the experience of the authors, requests to be anesthetized with subsequent removal of organs – including the heart – in a "living organ donation" procedure, are voiced by an increasing number of patients" [107]. The affective dimension: feeling better about the lethal choice. Grounds for conscientious objection by practitioners are myriad [109].

The authors claim no greater harm is done to the organ source by killing through explantation or by killing first and explanting second, offering a pretzeled exegesis that the procedure "respects the Hippocratic Oath, which mandates taking care of the organ donor and the recipient in the best possible way." However, the Hippocratic Oath, which prohibits administering a lethal substance or advising such a course, in extension prohibits lethal organ extraction [110]. Caution is utilitarian: negative publicity in the imagination of the public at large might lead to a net loss of willingness to donate generally in the total population ("prohibitive from a utilitarian point of view" [107]).

In 2022 a highly illuminating and revealing scoping review by Mulder et al. appeared in the *American Journal of Transplantation* on "Practice and challenges for organ donation after medical assistance in dying" [111]. Expanding organ harvesting to intentional, planned deaths could pressure PAS jurisdictions to expand to direct medical homicide. However *Table B6 Research gaps and further actions* includes: "Research into the option of self-administration through the 'stopcock procedure' might overcome jurisdiction-dependent ethical and legal impediments, increasing access to ODE." The patient opens the valve in clinical control for explanting her organs.

Additionally of physiological interest: "Research into the application of cardioplegics might reduce the occurrence of undesirable autoresuscitation and could reduce warm ischemia time, in the interests of the recipient, without harming the MAiD patient or their interests." Autoresuscitation (called "Lazarus phenomeon") per Gordon et al. [112] is "the return of spontaneous circulation after termination of resuscitation (TOR) following cardiac arrest (CA)". The scoping review found of 63 patients who autoresuscitated: 22 recovered to hospital discharge (82% with good neurological results); two recovered from cardiac arrest but died of other causes before discharge.

Autoresuscitation, generally a ground for rejoicing, is clinical failure when the primary clinical goal is a permanently dead patient and secondary goal accessing their organs ("[t]he aim of the 'MAiD-patient care pathway' is a controlled, comfortable, and swift death" [111]). The patient wills to die but the body wills to live. Mulder et al. confess, "[u]pholding the dead donor rule and the need for viable organs lead to the 'permanent' death definition within DCDD. However, permanent does not equal irreversible, leaving a window for rare, undesired autoresuscitation" [111]. "Oh death where is thy sting? O grave where is thy victory?" (I Cor 15:55, KJV). For delay perhaps a second lethal dose "after a predefined fixed period and for the OPO providers to wait for permanent death to occur (or reoccur)" [111].

### *5.2.3 Right of first and last refusal*

Grounds for conscientious objection by practitioners are myriad [109].

Not discussed is the right of conscientious objection for a would be recipient: to refuse an organ obtained after or through medicalized homicide. (including recipient opt-out during registration). This right implies a system duty to mark such organs. A system refusal to mark such organs giving weight of objections may motivate to decline to place themselves on a transplant list. A cooperation in evil analysis is implied (with classical distinctions: formal/material, immediate/mediate, proximate/remote cooperation). This is not comparable to one wishing to pass on an organ due to, say, donor ethnicity - save where ethnicity is a proxy for genocidal exploitation (e.g. organs from Uighurs in Xinjiang Province in China).

A systemwide rejection of medical homicide plus or through organ harvesting would mean fewer organs to transplant and fewer lives extended, implying it is preferable morally and societally even if patients die sooner (including the most sympathetic child) than to live longer with organs obtained under such circumstances. This is certainly the view I hold.

## 6. Medical homicide as backstop for nonresponsive bureaucracy

Canada's 2023 MAiD report (minus Yukon and Northwest Territories) indicates 19,660 lethal treatment requests and 15,434 MAiD deaths (2906 dying otherwise, 915 ineligible, 496 withdrawn) – the highest count in the world [113].

So-called Track I deaths (natural death forseeable) comprised 95.9% and Track 2 (not foreseeable) 4.1% with a gender disparity: +3.2% male for Track 1 but +17.0% female Track 2. 4.7% of 2023 deaths were MAiD (2.0% in 2019). In 2021 Bill C-7 established so-called "Track 2" without 'foreseeable death' [114] and Track 1's 10-day waiting period was rescinded.

The planned 2023 introduction of lethality as treatment for nonterminal psychiatric indications alone, presently postponed, raised broad concerns [115, 116] and strained a value-free professional association statement: "The Canadian Psychiatric Association (CPA) did not and does not take a position on the legality or morality of MAiD. Provision of MAiD is a decision reflecting current Canadian ethical, cultural and moral views" [117] - a remarkable flexibility of ἔθος [118] (custom, habit) after abandoning ἦθος [119] (custom plus moral discernment), with an unavoidable conundrum as Coehlo et al. point out: which suicides to actively prevent or which to abet when, per Mental Health Commission of Canada, less than 1/3 of adult care need is met? [11]. Additionally, while MAD (Medically Assisted Death, their acronym) was fully funded, Canadian healthcare allocations lagged OECD averages with palliative, chronic specialty, and disability support care services. Median specialist wait times between 1993 and 2021 doubled in Ontario (9.2–18.5 median weeks) and over quadrupled in Nova Scotia (11.5–53.2 median weeks) [120]. Median housing program wait time in 2021 was 25 weeks.

Both Quebec and federal governments declined appealing a Quebec Superior Court's decision striking the "reasonably foreseeable" death requirement [121]. On 17 March 2021 revised MAID legislation Bill C-7 ("An Act to amend the Criminal Code (medical assistance in dying)") entered into force, amending Criminal Code 241.2 to include 241.2(3.1) "Safeguards – natural death not foreseeable" [114].

In April 2022 Canada's CTV News reported a 51 year old Ontario woman ("Sophie") with multiple chemical sensitivities (MCS) died from MAiD on February 22 after 2 years of written appeals to government channels failed to secure low-allergen housing despite increased cigarette and marijuana smoke wafting through ventilation and hallway chemical cleansers [122]. This period included at-home COVID restrictions, likely with increased common area disinfection [123]. CTV Newsgave poor marks to the charity location's housing manager although minimal mitigation was attempted (blocking vent flow but not addressing loss of heating/cooling). In a privately shared video 8 days before ending her life, Sophia's ire was not at the charity: "The government sees me as expendable trash, a complainer, useless and a pain in the a*" [122]. Before her lethal appointment friends raised $12,000 Canadian. Sophie emailed: "If nothing turns up before FEB 22 please know that it is ok, I already have a way out. I don't have the energy to fight anymore." Sophie embodied limited autonomy (unjustly restricted options, internalized bias, hopelessness/despair) [124] yet she also framed her death as a policy intervention: "If my death helps to show the government that those of us with MCS will keep on having MAID if they don't act soon, then I'm glad I could help someone else not have to suffer the way I have."

Rohini Peres, president of the Environmental Health Association of Québec (ASEQ-EHAQ), which served Ontario, confirmed post-mortem Sophia's two-year effort to gain relief. ASEQ-EHAQ launched an online letter campaign to specific bureaucracy recipients (Provincial Premier; Housing Minister; ...) and established a GoFundMe campaign to raise housing relocation resources with click field text "OUR CANADA? / IS IT EASIER TO ELIMINATE A PERSON THAN PROVIDE HEALTHY HOUSING?" [125]. It appears yes. With Sophie's lethal solution approaching, four doctors (including a MAID provider) wrote a support letter to federal officials without success. After the story went viral several people contacted Peres inquiring about MAID as a possible solution for their intractable housing problems.

Two weeks later a 31-year-old wheelchair user, 'Denise', likewise with MCS, likewise seeking nonallergenic housing, was likewise approved for death on the same basis [126]. In a report video 'Denise' states: "When people are backed into a corner, living in poverty, it doesn't feel like a choice anymore." An environmental health physician commented: "These people are given the easy way out to alleviate their suffering by the government as opposed to having their needs met [....] These patients can easily return to wellness if they are given the right environment to live. It's a simple equation." Horrified strangers genned up $65 K Canadian via GoFundMe for emergency respite at a low scent hotel with an openable window rekindling hope [127].

In 2022, 65-year-old Canadian Les Landry, with qualifying comorbidities, applied for death stating his primary reason was poverty. The first doctor approved it, informing were he turned down by the second he could shop around [128]. Mr. Landry called the ease of application "bizarre" pointing out "home visits by doctors ceased to be the norm decades ago"but "they're willing to do a house call to kill you [...] I told it to the [second] doctor, I want to live. I don't want to die'" who approved the application like the first. Coehlo et al.: "However, the reality is that MAD costs less than state-supported health and community care for the disabled, which deliberately or not can create a perverse incentive to guarantee access to MAD, despite no guarantee for access to care or community support." The Track 2 death wait period is 90 days while delay for disability support after lost capacity to work is often much longer [129].

In March 2025 the UN Committee on the Rights of Persons with Disabilities issued observations criticizing Canada's MAiD practices under article 10 (Right to Life) of the Convention on the Rights of Persons with Disabilities [130] noting criticism of Track 2 MAiD also by the Committee on the Elimination of Discrimination against Woman and by the Special Rapporteur on Extreme Poverty and Human Rights, among others. The Committee rejected disability as grounds to expand MAiD (Quebec's unchallenged Truchon decision), noting disproportionate deaths for women with disabilities, marginalized disabled people, and a general "upward trajectory of persons with disabilities killed through Track 2 MAiD" plus "systematic failures" to address social determinants of health. Consequently it recommended repeal of Track 2 MAiD entirely, rejecting also proposed expansions for 'mature minors' or advance requests.

An April 2023 by Wiebe and Mullen article explores "Choosing death in unjust conditions: hope, autonomy and harm reduction" [124]. Harm reduction trailblazed by methadone (easing heroin withdrawal) and needle exchange (reducing hepatitis/HIV) is framed to include a lethal *pharmakon*. Certainly harm reduction as trope has long been embedded in popular discourse for assisted suicide (a less bad death). The article claims first-person autonomy, not public good (raised by Dugdale and Callahan [12]), as a "more appropriate moral and political framework for the consideration of AD [assisted death]." Wiebe and Mullin include *hope* as a necessary dimension for autonomy - 'active hope' or 'engaged hope' - requiring pursuable goals that matter personally and motivation to act. (By contrast despair is "from Latin desperare 'to despair, to lose all hope', from de 'without' (see de-) + sperare 'to hope,' from spes 'hope' [131]). Individuals choosing a lethal solution per Wiebe and Mullin are sufficiently autonomous even would they not were unjust circumstances otherwise. Oddly: "persons requesting MAiD are arguably acting with engaged hope in seeking what the consider to be the best option of the options available to them." That the time horizon to amelioration is long is taken as further warrant for validity of the lethal choice as harm reduction: Death as treatment for social malady without reform.

An unjust circumstance however is not only difficult but implies external responsibility: interpersonal, bureaucratic, ethnic (racism), or diffuse ('society'). *Unjust* implies responsibility to act even when not ascribing intent. To choose death is tragic; the ongoing contexts atrocious. Among the grotesque effects of such deaths are decreased social benefit costs and net increase (one unit each) in available public housing. Might this constitute a perverse incentive (a final backstop) to not address the most difficult cases or most unpleasant clients in a system?

## 7. Conclusion: The trouble with normal

Since Hippocrates medicine has been considered a holy art, one safeguarded by limiting principles including refusal to participate in lethal application of related skills. Homicide, suicide and medical lethality are matters of public concerns also involving public wrongs. Governments in particular have sought to medicalize lethal practices including execution; 'medical' practitioners have participated under banners of humanity and technical expertise. Putative goods such as transplantation have increasingly been tied to lethal intent, imposed or requested, which alters the nature of practices. Proposed expansions of lethal practices now include killing through organ extraction not as rogue criminality (China) but as standard practice (Netherlands/Belgium). Per Bruce Coburn, the trouble with normal is it can always get worse [132]. Elements brought to light above show this to be the case as requesting death functionally becomes a backstop for failed bureaucratic systems tasked to meet basic needs. In totalitarian societies, medicalized lethality can simply be a tool of repression providing resources and income flow under medical demand curves. In liberal democracies the introduction of medically mediated lethal solutions intersect a variety of social problems with conflicted incentive structures while corrupting basic public health and medical culture. Ultimately these issues concern just or unjust ends and means, worth an admonition [133]:

*Das Z i e l nicht zeige, zeige auch den Weg.*
*Denn so verwachsen ist hienieden Weg und Ziel,*
*Daß eines sich stets ändert mit dem andern.*
*Und andrer Weg auch Andres Ziel erzeugt.*

*Point not the goal until you plot the course.*
*for ends and means to man are tangled so.*
*that different means quite different aims enforce.*
*Conceive the means as end in embryo.*

## Acknowledgements

No funding to acknowledge.

## Conflict of interest

The author declares no conflict of interest.

## Author details

Kirk C. Allison
College of Saint Scholastica, Duluth, Minnesota, USA

*Address all correspondence to: kallison0001@gmail.com

## References

[1] Harper D. Etymology of homicide. In: Online Etymology Dictionary. n.d. Available from https://www.etymonline.com/word/homicide [Accessed: January 02, 2023]

[2] Harper D. Etymology of medicine. In: Online Etymology Dictionary. n.d. Available from: https://www.etymonline.com/word/medicine [Accessed: January 13, 2023]

[3] Blackstone's Commentaries on the Laws of England: 1765-1769. Yale Law School Avalon Project. pp. I.39-I.41. (book.[chapter].page). Re Justinian: Turis praecepta funt haec, honefte vivere, alterum non laedere, fuum cuique tribuere. Inft. 1. 1. 5. Available from: https://avalon.law.yale.edu/subject_menus/blackstone.asp [Accessed: January 15, 2023]

[4] Transl. of Latin in [3] (IV.14.189) frp, Lonang Institute https://lonang.com/library/reference/blackstone-commentaries-law-england/bla-414/#fn62d [Accessed: April 29, 2023]. Quote derives from Menenius 3 de re milit. attributed to Emperor Hadrian, found in Justinian's Digest (Dig. 49.16.6.7). Available from: https://www.thelatinlibrary.com/justinian/digest49.shtml [Accessed: April 29, 2023]

[5] Nótári T. Some remarks on the issue of suicide in Roman criminal law. Acta Universitatis Sapientiae Legal Studies. 2019;**8**(1):75-87. Available from: https://acta.sapientia.ro/content/docs/some-remarks-on-the-issue-of-suicide-in-.pdf [Accessed: April 29, 2023]

[6] Bennett RE. A fate worse than death? Dissection and the criminal corpse. In: Capital Punishment and the Criminal Corpse in Scotland, 1740-1834. Palgrave Historical Studies in the Criminal Corpse and its Afterlife. Cham, Switzerland: Palgrave Macmillan; 2018. pp. 159-185. DOI: 10.1007/978-3-319-62018-3_6 [Accessed: May 03, 2023]

[7] Houston RA. Introduction. In: Punishing the Dead? Suicide, Lordship, and Community in Britain, 1500-1830. online ed. Available from:. Oxford; 2010. DOI: 10.1093/acprof:oso/9780199586424.003.0001 [Accessed: May 01, 2023]

[8] Houston RA. Punishing the Dead? Suicide, Lordship, and Community in Britain, 1500-1830. Oxford: Oxford University Press; 2010. p. 23 FN 106

[9] Wax JW, An AW, Kosier N, Quill TE. Voluntary stopping eating and drinking. Journal of the American Geriatrics Society. 2018;**66**(3):441-445. DOI: 10.1111/jgs.15200

[10] Gert B, Culver CM, Clouser KD. An alternative to physician-assisted suicide. In: Battin MP, Rhodes R, Silvers A, editors. Physician Assisted Suicide: Expanding the Debate. New York: Routledge; 1998. pp. 182-202

[11] Coelho R, Lemmens T, Gaind KS, Maher J. Normalizing death as "treatment" in Canada: Whose suicides do we prevent, and whose do we abet? World Medical Journal. 2022;**70**(3):27-35

[12] Dugdale LS, Callahan D. Assisted death and the public good. Southern Medical Journal. 2017;**110**(9):559-561

[13] National Academies of Sciences, Engineering, and Medicine. Physician-Assisted Death: Scanning the Landscape: Proceedings of a Workshop. Washington, DC: The National Academies Press; 2018. p. 31. DOI: 10.17226/25131

[14] Jack B. Goethe's Werther and its effects. Lancet Psychiatry. 2014;**1**(1):18-19. DOI: 10.1016/S2215-0366(14)70229-9 [Accessed: February 04, 2023]

[15] Lutter M, Roex KLA, Tisch D. Anomie or imitation? The Werther effect of celebrity suicides on suicide rates in 34 OECD countries, 1960-2014. Social Science & Medicine. 2020;**246**:112755. DOI: 10.1016/j.socscimed.2019.112755 [Accessed: February 04, 2023]

[16] Gallagher R, Passmore MJ. Deromanticizing medical assistance in dying. CMAJ. 2021;**193**(26):E1012-E1013. DOI: 10.1503/cmaj.78845

[17] Frei A, Schenker T, Finzen A, Dittmann V, Kraeuchi K, Hoffmann-Richter U. The Werther effect and assisted suicide. Suicide and Life-Threatening Behavior. 2003;**33**(2):192-200. DOI: 10.1521/suli.33.2.192.22768 [Accessed: February 04, 2023]

[18] Johnston WG. Before the Legislature of the State of California Declaration of Williard Johnston MD in re SB 128. 2015. Available from: https://choiceisanillusion.files.wordpress.com/2015/05/willard-johnston-maynard-decl.pdf [Accessed: February 05, 2023]

[19] Sikora A, Fleischman AR. Physician participation in capital punishment: A question of professional integrity. Journal of Urban Health. 1999;**76**(4):400-408. DOI: 10.1007/BF02351498

[20] Harper D. Etymology of integrity. Online Etymology Dictionary. n.d. Available from: https://www.etymonline.com/ word/integer [Accessed: March 20, 2023]

[21] Harper D. Etymology of integer. Online Etymology Dictionary. n.d. Available from: https://www.etymonline.com/word/integer [Accessed: March 20, 2023]

[22] Harper D. Etymology of fraction. Online Etymology Dictionary. n.d. Available from: https://www.etymonline.com/word/fraction [Accessed: April 27, 2025]

[23] Kershaw A. A History of the Guillotine. New York: Barnes and Noble Books; 1993. pp. 14, 34-37, 45-47, 80-83, 86-89

[24] φάρμακον. In: Liddell HG, Scott R, editors. A Greek-English Lexicon. Revised and Augmented throughout by. Sir Henry Stuart Jones. With the Assistance of. Roderick McKenzie. Oxford: Clarendon Press; 1940. p. 1917

[25] Dixon RD. Execution by Lethal Injection Procedures. [Letter and Document.] 2025. Available from: https://fdc-media.ccplatform.net/content/download/1561/file/FDC-Execution-by-Lethal-Injection-Procedures.pdf [Accessed: May 02, 2025]

[26] Waisel D. Physician participation in capital punishment. Mayo Clinic Proceedings. 2007;**82**(9):1073-1082. DOI: 10.4065/82.9.1073. Available from: https://www.mayoclinicproceedings.org/article/S0025-6196(11)61369-4/fulltext [Accessed: March 05, 2023]

[27] Pancuronium Bromide. Wikipedia. Updated 30 April 2025. Available from: https://en.wikipedia.org/wiki/Pancuronium_bromide; [Accessed: April 30, 2025]

[28] Export Control Joint Unit. Export Controls: Torture and Capital Punishment Goods. 2012. Last update 7 May 2024. Available from: https://www.gov.uk/guidance/controls-on-torture-goods [Accessed: April 30, 2025]

[29] AP News. Idaho Governor Signs Firing Squad Execution Bill into Law. 2023. Available from: https://apnews.com/article/death-penalty-executions-firing-squads-idaho-law-de6a68243433a4f58f70256c03891adb [Accessed: April 21, 2025]

[30] American Medical Association Code of Medical Ethics Opinion 9.7.3 Capital Punishment. Available from: https://code-medical-ethics.ama-assn.org/ethics-opinions/capital-punishment [Accessed: June 17, 2023]

[31] World Medical Association. WMA Resolution on Physician Participation in Capital Punishment. 2018. Available from: https://www.wma.net/policies-post/wma-resolution-on-prohibition-of-physician-participation-in-capital-punishment/ [Accessed: June 20, 2023]

[32] World Medical Association. WMA Declaration on Euthanasia and Physician-Assisted Suicide. 2019. Available from: https://www.wma.net/policies-post/declaration-on-euthanasia-and-physician-assisted-suicide/ [Accessed: June 20, 2023]

[33] Gahagan J. Genevieve Lhermitte: Belgian mother who killed her five children euthanised. BBC. 3 Mar 2023. Available from: https://www.bbc.com/news/world-europe-64835051 [Accessed: March 05, 2023]

[34] CBS News. Spain allows suspected gunman to be euthanized before trial, angering victims. CBS/AP. 24 Aug 2022. Available from: https://www.cbsnews.com/news/eugen-sabau-spain-suspected-gunman-euthanized/ [Accessed: June 20, 2023]

[35] Franke I, Urwyler T, Prüter-Schwarte C. Assisted dying requests from people in detention: Psychiatric, ethical, and legal considerations-a literature review. Frontiers in Psychiatry. 2022;**13**:909096. DOI: 10.3389/fpsyt.2022.909096. Available from: https://europepmc.org/article/med/35966491 [Accessed: June 21, 2023]

[36] Favaro A. The number of medically-assisted deaths in Canada's prisons a concern for some experts. CTVNews. 2023. Available from: https://www.ctvnews.ca/health/the-number-of-medically-assisted-deaths-in-canada-s-prisons-a-concern-for-some-experts-1.6380440 [Accessed: June 21, 2023]

[37] Shaw J, Driftmier P. "Dying with a smile, just knowing that somebody's listened to me": End-of-life care and medical assistance in dying in Canadian prisons. Omega (Westport). Epub December 31, 2021. 2024;**88**(4):1290-1313. DOI: 10.1177/003022282110523 [Accessed: June 21, 2023]

[38] PubMed.gov. Homicide. 2024. Available from: https://pubmed.ncbi.nlm.nih.gov/?term=homicide&filter=dates.1000%2F1%2F1-2024%2F12%2F31 [Accessed: January 18, 2024]

[39] Watson A. Three medico-legal cases of homicide, in which insanity was pleaded in exculpation. The Edinburgh Medical and Surgical Journal. 1832;**38**(112):45-58

[40] PubMed.gov. Homicide. Results by Year. Download CSV. 2024. Available from: https://pubmed.ncbi.nlm.nih.gov/?term=homicide&timeline=expanded [Accessed: January 18, 2024]

[41] PubMed.gov. Medical Homicide. 2023. Available from: https://pubmed.ncbi.nlm.nih.gov/?term="medical+homicide" [Accessed: January 04, 2024]

[42] Duncanson E, Richards V, Luce KM, Gill JR. Medical homicide and extreme negligence. The American Journal of Forensic Medicine and Pathology. 2009;**30**(1):18-22. DOI: 10.1097/PAF.0b013e3181873824

[43] Syme R. Necessity to palliate pain and suffering as a defence to medical homicide. Journal of Law and Medicine. 2009;**17**(3):439-451

[44] Statement of the American Association of Suicidology: "Suicide" is not the same as "Physician Aid in Dying". 2017. [Retired on 24 February 2023]: AAS Executive Committee. AAS Update on Physician Assisted Death Previous Statement. February 24, 2023. Available from: https://suicidology.org/aas-update-on-physician-assisted-death-previous-statement/ [Accessed: February 18, 2025]

[45] Battin MP. Development of the AAS statement on "suicide" and "physician aid in dying". Suicide and Life-Threatening Behavior. 2019;**49**(3):774-776. DOI: 10.1111/sltb.12453

[46] Oregon Health Authority. Death with Dignity Annual Reports (1998-2024). Available from: https://www.oregon.gov/oha/ph/providerpartnerresources/evaluationresearch/deathwithdignityact/Pages/ar-index.aspx

[47] State of Oregon. Psychiatric/psychological consultant's compliance form (if required) - Revised 05/2018. Available from: https://www.oregon.gov/oha/ph/providerpartnerresources/evaluationresearch/deathwithdignityact/Documents/psyform.pdf [Accessed: February 18, 2025]

[48] Question 15 (p. 5). Oregon Death with Dignity Act Attending Physician Follow-up Form. https://www.oregon.gov/oha/ph/providerpartnerresources/evaluationresearch/deathwithdignityact/Documents/mdintdat.pdf [Accessed: February 18, 2025]

[49] CEJA Report 5-A-18. Subsequently voted on by the American Medical Association House of Delegates on June 10, 2019 under REPORT 2 OF THE COUNCIL ON ETHICAL AND JUDICIAL AFFAIRS 2-A-19. Available from: https://www.ama-assn.org/system/files/2019-05/a19-ceja2.pdf [Accessed: February 07, 2023]

[50] AMA Code of Medical Ethics. Opinion 5.7 Physician Assisted Suicide. Available from: https://code-medical-ethics.ama-assn.org/ethics-opinions/physician-assisted-suicide [Accessed: February 07, 2023]

[51] AMA Code of Medical Ethics. Opinion 1.1.7 Physician Exercise of Conscience. Available from: https://code-medical-ethics.ama-assn.org/ethics-opinions/physician-exercise-conscience [Accessed: February 07, 2023]

[52] AMA Code of Medical Ethics. Opinion 5.8 Euthanasia. Available from: https://code-medical-ethics.ama-assn.org/ethics-opinions/euthanasia [Accessed: February 07, 2023]

[53] Harper D. Etymology of euthanasia. Online Etymology Dictionary. n.d. Available from: https://www.etymonline.com/word/euthanasia [Accessed: February 10, 2023]

[54] Dolan JM. Is physician-assisted suicide possible? The Duquesne Law Review. 1996;**35**:355-393. Available from: https://dsc.duq.edu/dlr/vol35/iss1/15 [Accessed: February 10, 2023]

[55] Jusjurandum [Oath]. Hippocrates Collected Works I. Hippocrates. W. H. S. Jones. Cambridge. Harvard University Press. 1868. Available from: http://data.perseus.org/texts/

urn:cts:greekLit:tlg0627.tlg013 [Accessed: February 20, 2023]

[56] Miles SJ. The Hippocratic Oath and the Ethics of Medicine. Oxford: Oxford University Press; 2005

[57] American Clinicians Academy on Medical Aid in Dying. 2023. Available from: https://www.acamaid.org/ [Accessed: March 02, 2023]

[58] Austin JL. How to Do Things with Words. Oxford: Clarendon Press; 1962. p. 4n2

[59] CDC. Physician's Handbook on the Medical Certification of Death. 2003. . Available from: https://www.cdc.gov/nchs/data/misc/hb_cod.pdf [Accessed: January 11, 2023]

[60] Centers for Disease Control. U.S. Standard Certificate of Death-Rev 11/2003. Available from: https://www.cdc.gov/nchs/data/dvs/death11-03final-acc.pdf [Accessed: January 11, 2023]

[61] Confirmed as "recommendation", not requirement in 2 emails to author. Oregon Health Authority. Available from: dwda.info@dhsoha.state.or.us . Emails (2). 2023 Jun 26

[62] Oregon Health Authority. Death with Dignity Act. Reporting forms and instructions. Death certificate recommendations. Available from: https://www.oregon.gov/oha/PH/PROVIDERPARTNERRESOURCES/EVALUATIONRESEARCH/DEATHWITHDIGNITYACT/Pages/pasforms.aspx [Accessed: June 23, 2023]

[63] Washington State Department of Health. Instructions for physicians and other medical certifiers of death certificates: Compliance with the Death with Dignity Act. Available from: https://doh.wa.gov/sites/default/files/legacy/Documents/Pubs//422-151-DWDInstructionsForPhysicians.pdf [Accessed: June 23, 2023]

[64] Washington State Medical Association. As I-1000 signatures are counted, Washington state medical association opposition to physician-assisted suicide reiterated. 2008 Jul 2. In: Allison KC. Public health, populations, and lethal ingestion. Disability and Health Journal. 2010;**3**(1):56-70. DOI: 10.1016/j.dhjo.2009.09.005

[65] RCW 70.58A.590 Penalties. In: Chapter 70.58A RCW. Vital Statistics. Available from: https://app.leg.wa.gov/RCW/default.aspx?cite=70.58A&full=true [Accessed: July 03, 2023]

[66] Tucker KL. Aid in dying in Montana: Ten years after state v. Baxter. Montana Law Review. 2020;**81**:207-212

[67] Brown J, Thorpe L, Goodridge D. Completion of medical certificates of death after an assisted death: An environmental scan of practices. Healthcare Policy. 2018;**14**(2):59-67. DOI: 10.12927/hcpol.2018.25685

[68] Downie J, Oliver K. Medical certificates of death: First principles and established practices provide answers to new questions. CMAJ. 2016;**188**(1):49-52. DOI: 10.1503/cmaj.151130. Epub 2015 Dec 14. Available from: https://pmc.ncbi.nlm.nih.gov/articles/PMC4695354/

[69] Harper D. Etymology of incentive (n./Adj.). Online Etymology Dictionary. n.d. Available from: https://www.etymonline.com/word/incentive [Accessed: May 03, 2023]

[70] Ord T. Practical Ethics Blog. Oxford University. Euthanasia and perverse incentives; 2008. Available from: http://blog.practicalethics.ox.ac.uk/2008/10/

euthanasia-and-perverse-incentives/ [Accessed: January 15, 2023]

[71] Richardson B. Insurance companies denied treatment to patients, offered to pay for assisted suicide, doctor claims. Washington Times. 31 May 2017. Available from: https://www.washingtontimes.com/news/2017/may/31/insurance-companies-denied-treatment-to-patients-o/ [Accessed: April 26, 2025]

[72] Sanchez A. Insurer offers to pay for assisted suicide but not chemotherapy. InsuranceBusiness. 2016. Available from: https://www.insurancebusinessmag.com/us/news/breaking-news/insurer-offers-to-pay-for-assisted-suicide-but-not-chemotherapy-39441.aspx [Accessed: April 26, 2025]

[73] Potter W. Exclusive: 'Disgusting' slideshow offering assisted suicide 'is emailed to HEALTHY patients by Canadian healthcare provider,' as unease grows over country's euthanasia program. The Daily Mail. 2023. Available from: https://www.dailymail.co.uk/news/article-12239765/Disgusting-Canadian-healthcare-provider-offers-assisted-suicide-thousands-healthy-patients.html

[74] The Transplantation Society. "To TTS members:" 2006. https://www.tts.org/images/stories/pdfs/StatementMembs-ChineseTXProg.pdf [Accessed: May 22, 2023]

[75] Allison KC, Caplan A, Shapiro ME, Els C, Paul NW, Li H. Historical development and current status of organ procurement from death-row prisoners in China. BMC Medical Ethics. 2015;**16**(1):85. DOI: 10.1186/s12910-015-0074-0. Available from: https://bmcmedethics.biomedcentral.com/articles/10.1186/s12910-015-0074-0 [Accessed: February 08, 2023]

[76] Paul NW, Caplan A, Shapiro ME, Els C, Allison KC, Li H. Human rights violations in organ procurement practice in China. BMC Medical Ethics. 2017;**18**(1):11. DOI: 10.1186/s12910-017-0169-x. Available from: https://bmcmedethics.biomedcentral.com/articles/10.1186/s12910-017-0169-x [Accessed: February 08, 2023]

[77] Allison KC. Transplant ethics. Minneapolis Star Tribune. 7 Oct 2012. Available from: https://www.startribune.com/ transplant-ethics/172892541/ [Accessed: May 22, 2023]

[78] The Independent Tribunal into Forced Organ Harvesting from Prisoners of Conscience in China. Judgment. 2021. Available from: https://chinatribunal.com/wp-content/uploads/2020/03/ChinaTribunal_JUDGMENT_1stMarch_2020.pdf [Accessed: February 08, 2023]

[79] Allison KC. China's execution transplantation system and international institutions. A too-sticky wicket? In: Trey T, Chu T, editors. An Unprecedented Evil Persecution. Taipei: Clear Insight Pub; 2016. pp. 132-150. Available from: https://dafoh.org/an-unprecedented-evil-persecution-chinas-execution-transplantation-system-and-international-institutions-a-too-sticky-wicket/ [Accessed: May 22, 2023]

[80] Steering Committee of the Istanbul Summit. Organ trafficking and transplant tourism and commercialism: The declaration of Istanbul. The Lancet. 2008;**372**(9632):5-6

[81] Schwarz A. Responsibilities of international pharmaceutical companies in the abusive Chinese organ transplant system. In: Matas D, Trey T, editors. State Organs. Woodstock ON: Seraphim Editions; 2012. pp. 27-34. Author translation

[82] Ramzy A. China sets Jan. 1 deadline for ending transplants from executed prisoners. New York Times. 2014. Available from: https://archive.nytimes.com/sinosphere.blogs.nytimes.com/2014/12/04/china-sets-jan-1-deadline-for-ending-transplants-from-executed-prisoners/ [Accessed: May 2022, 2023]

[83] Li Y. Organizations praise China's progress in organ donation. Global Times. 2017. Available from: http://www.ecns.cn/news/society/2017-07-27/detail-ifytetzm3040736.shtml [Accessed: May 22, 2023]

[84] Robertson MP, Hinde RL, Lavee J. Analysis of official deceased organ donation data casts doubt on the credibility of China's organ transplant reform. BMC Medical Ethics. 2019). Available from:;**20**:79. DOI: 10.1186/s12910-019-0406-6

[85] Guttman E. The Slaughter. Amherst: Prometheus Books; 2014

[86] Matas D. Organ harvesting in China is real, here are the smoking guns. Bitter Winter. 17 May 2022. Available from: https://bitterwinter.org/organ-harvesting-in-china-is-real-smoking-guns/ [Accessed: May 22, 2023]

[87] Foursquare City Guide. Kashgar Airprort (KHG). Photos. Special Passenger Human Organ Transplant Channel. Amber Z. 2021. Available from: https://bit.ly/42VREO8 & https://4sq.com/3ooPQhD [Accessed: May 22, 2023]

[88] European Parliament resolution on the reports of continued organ harvesting in China (2022/2657(RSP)). 2022. Available from: https://www.europarl.europa.eu/doceo/document/RC-9-2022-0250_EN.pdf [Accessed: May 22, 2023]

[89] Independent Tribunal into Forced Organ Harvesting of Prisoners of Conscience in China. China Tribunal Full Judgement. 2020. Available from: https://chinatribunal.com/final-judgment/ [Accessed: May 05, 2023]

[90] Holm AM, Fedson S, Courtwright A, Olland A, Bryce K, Kanwar M, et al. International Society for Heart and Lung Transplantation statement on transplant ethics. The Journal of Heart and Lung Transplantation. 2022;**41**(10):1307-1308. DOI: 10.1016/j.healun.2022.05.012

[91] Paul NW, Allison KC, Li H. Cases abusing brain death definition in organ procurement in China. Cambridge Quarterly of Healthcare Ethics. 2022;**31**(3):375-389

[92] Robertson MP, Lavee J. Execution by organ procurement: Breaching the dead donor rule in China. American Journal of Transplantation. 2022;**22**(7):1804-1812. DOI: 10.1111/ajt.16969. Available from: https://www.ncbi.nlm.nih.gov/pmc/articles/PMC9542006/ [Accessed: May 22, 2023]

[93] Panna AS. Determination of death: Ethical and biomedical update with international consensus. In: Clark PA, editor. Bioethical Issues in Healthcare. London, UK: IntechOpen; 2022. DOI: 10.5772/intechopen.100604

[94] Ding ZY, Zhang Q, Wu JW, Yang ZH, Zhao XQ. A comparison of brain death criteria between China and the United States. Chinese Medical Journal. 2015;**128**:2896-2901. Available from: https://www.ncbi.nlm.nih.gov/pmc/articles/PMC4756902/ [Accessed: February 08, 2023]

[95] Brain Injury Evaluation Quality Control Centre of National Health and Family Planning Commission. Criteria and practical guidance for determination

of brain death in adults (BQCC version). Chinese Medical Journal. 2013;**126**(24):4786-4790

[96] Wijdicks EF, Varelas PN, Gronseth GS, Greer DM, American Academy of Neurology. Evidence-based guideline update: Determining brain death in adults: Report of the quality standards Subcommittee of the American Academy of neurology. Neurology. 2010;**74**:1911-1918

[97] Slomski A. Another 'brain dead' patient wakes up just in time. Medscape. 16 Oct 2018. pp. 1-3. Available from: https://www. medscape.com/viewarticle/902143 [Accessed: February 08, 2023]

[98] Glazier A, Capron A. Normothermic regional perfusion and US legal standards for determining death are not aligned. American Journal of Transplantation. 2022;**22**(5):1289-1290. Available from: https://onlinelibrary.wiley.com/doi/10.1111/ajt.17002 [Accessed: June 10, 2023]

[99] Bollen J, van Smaalen T, ten Hoopen R, van Heurn E, Ysebaert D, van Mook W. Potential number of organ donors after euthanasia in Belgium. Journal of the American Medical Association. 2017;**317**(14):1476-1477. DOI: 10.1001/jama.2017.0729 [Accessed: May 19, 2023]

[100] Federal Public Service. Organ Donation – Citizens. 2016. Available from: https://www.health.belgium.be/en/organ-donation-citizens [Accessed: May 19, 2013]

[101] FCEE Euthanasie Verslag. 2016. Available from: https://overlegorganen.gezondheid.belgie.be/nl/documenten/fcee-euthanasie-verslag-2016 [Accessed: May 19, 2013]

[102] Bollen J, de Jongh W, Hagenaars H, van Dijk G, Ten Hoopen R, Ysebaert D, et al. Organ donation after euthanasia: A pure act of altruism fulfilling the patient's last wish. American Journal of Transplantation. 2017;**17**(3):843-844. DOI: 10.1111/ajt.14167

[103] Rodríguez-Prat A, Monforte-Royo C, Porta-Sales J, Escribano X, Balaguer A. Patient perspectives of dignity, autonomy and control at the end of life: Systematic review and meta-ethnography. PLoS One. 2016;**11**(3):e0151435. DOI: 10.1371/journal.pone.0151435

[104] Thienpont L, Verhofstadt M, Van Loon T, Distelmans W, Audenaert K, De Deyn PP. Euthanasia requests, procedures and outcomes for 100 Belgian patients suffering from psychiatric disorders: A retrospective, descriptive study. BMJ Open. 2015;**5**(7):e007454. Published 2015 Jul 27. DOI: 10.1136/bmjopen-2014-007454. Available from: https://bmjopen.bmj.com/content/bmjopen/5/7/e007454.full.pdf [Accessed: February 08, 2023]

[105] Bollen J, de Jongh W, Hagenaars J, van Dijk G, Ten Hoopen R, Ysebaert D, et al. Organ donation after euthanasia: A Dutch practical manual. American Journal of Transplantation. 2016;**16**(7):1967-1972. DOI: 10.1111/ajt.13746. Epub 2016 Mar 10 [Accessed: May 19, 2023]

[106] Wilkinson D, Savulescu J. Should we allow organ donation euthanasia? Alternatives for maximizing the number and quality of organs for transplantation. Bioethics. 2012;**26**(1):32-48. DOI: 10.1111/j.1467-8519.2010.01811.x [Accessed: May 20, 2023]

[107] Bollen JAM, Shaw D, de Wert G, Ten Hoopen R, Ysebaert D, van Heurn E, et al. Euthanasia through living organ

donation: Ethical, legal, and medical challenges. The Journal of Heart and Lung Transplantation. 2019;**38**(2):111-113. DOI: 10.1016/j.healun.2018.07.014. Epub 2018 Jul 27

[108] Carvajal C, Goyal A, Tadi P. Cardioplegia. In: StatPearls. Treasure Island (FL): StatPearls Publishing; 2023. Excerpt in PubMed. Available from: https://pubmed.ncbi.nlm.nih.gov/32119350/ [Accessed: May 20, 2023]

[109] Ely EW. Death by organ donation: Euthanizing patients for their organs gains frightening traction. Intensive Care Medicine. 2019;**45**:1309-1311. DOI: 10.1007/s00134-019-05702-1 [Accessed: June 10, 2023]

[110] Boudreau JD, Somerville MA. Euthanasia is not medical treatment. British Medical Bulletin. 2013;**106**(1):45-66. DOI: 10.1093/bmb/ldt010 [Accessed: June 05, 2023]

[111] Mulder J, Sonneveld H, Van Raemdonck D, Downar J, Wiebe K, Domínguez-Gil B, et al. Practice and challenges for organ donation after medical assistance in dying: A scoping review including the results of the first international roundtable in 2021. American Journal of Transplantation. 2022;**22**(12):2759-2780. DOI: 10.1111/ajt.17198

[112] Gordon L, Pasquier M, Brugger H, Paul P. Autoresuscitation (Lazarus phenomenon) after termination of cardiopulmonary resuscitation - A scoping review. Scandinavian Journal of Trauma, Resuscitation and Emergency Medicine. 2020;**28**:14. DOI: 10.1186/s13049-019-0685-4

[113] Health Canada. Fifth Annual Report on Medical Assistance in Dying in Canada 2023. Santé Canada: Health Canada; 2024. Available from: https://www.canada.ca/en/health-canada/services/publications/health-system-services/annual-report-medical-assistance-dying-2023.html [Accessed: May 03, 2023]

[114] Parliament of Canada. Bill C-7 [An Act to Amend the Criminal Code (Medical Assistance in Dying)]. 2021. Available from: https://parl.ca/DocumentViewer/en/43-2/bill/C-7/royal-assent [Accessed: May 26, 2023]

[115] Alt A. Concern grows over 'medical aid in dying for mental illness' law. Medscape. 23 Jan 2023. pp. 1-5. Available from: https://www.medscape.com/viewarticle/987350 [Accessed: February 23, 2023]

[116] Statement by Ministers Lametti, Duclos and Bennett on medical assistance in dying in Canada. Department of Justice Canada. 2022. Available from: https://www.canada.ca/en/department-justice/news/2022/12/statement-by-ministers-lametti-duclos-and-bennett-on-medical-assistance-in-dying-in-canada.html [Accessed: February 23, 2023]

[117] Chaimowitz G, Freeland A, Neilson GE, Mathew N, Rasasingham R, Snelgrove N, et al. Medical Assistance In Dying: Aide médicale à mourir. Canadian Journal of Psychiatry / Revue canadienne de psychiatrie. 2020;**65**(9):664-667. Available from: https://journals.sagepub.com/doi/epdf/10.1177/0706743720919299 [Accessed: May 29, 2025]

[118] ἔθος , εος, τό, (ἔθω). In: Liddell HG, Scott R. A Greek-English Lexicon. revised and augmented throughout by. Sir Henry Stuart Jones. with the assistance of. Roderick McKenzie. Oxford. Clarendon Press. 1940. Perseus Digital Library. Available from: http://

www.perseus.tufts.edu/hopper/morph?l=e%29%2Fqos&la=greek&can=e%29%2Fqos0 [Accessed: February 23, 2023]

[119] ἦθος , εος, τό (cf. ἔθος). In: Liddell HG, Scott R. A Greek-English Lexicon. revised and augmented throughout by. Sir Henry Stuart Jones. with the assistance of. Roderick McKenzie. Oxford. Clarendon Press. 1940. Perseus Digital Library. Available from: http://www.perseus.tufts.edu/hopper/text?doc=Perseus%3Atext%3A1999.04.0057%3Aentry%3Dh)%3Dqos [Accessed: February 23, 2023]

[120] Moir M, Barua B. Waiting your Turn: Wait times for healthcare in Canada, 2021 Report. Fraser Institute. Available from: https://www.fraserinstitute.org/sites/default/files/waiting-your-turn-2021.pdf [Accessed: June 12, 2023]

[121] Truchon c. Procureur général du Canada, 2019, QCCS 3792

[122] Favaro A. Woman with chemical sensitivities chose medically-assisted death after failed bid to get better housing. CTV News. 13 Apr 2022. Available from: https://www.ctvnews.ca/health/woman-with-chemical-sensitivities-chose-medically-assisted-death-after-failed-bid-to-get-better-housing-1.5860579 [Accessed: May 24, 2023]

[123] Canadian Institute for Health Information. Canadian COVID-19 Intervention Timeline. 2022. Available from: https://www.cihi.ca/en/canadian-covid-19-intervention-timeline [Accessed: May 26, 2023]

[124] Wiebe K, Mullin A. Choosing death in unjust conditions: Hope, autonomy and harm reduction. Journal of Medical Ethics. 2023;**50**(6):407-412. DOI: 10.1136/jme-2022-108871

[125] ASEQ-EHAQ. Take Action Now. 2023. Available from: https://aseq-ehaq.ca/en/take-action-now/ [Accessed: May 26, 2023]

[126] Favaro A. Woman with disabilities nears medically assisted death after futile bid for affordable housing. CTV News. 2022. Available from: https://www.ctvnews.ca/health/woman-with-disabilities-nears-medically-assisted-death-after-futile-bid-for-affordable-housing-1.5882202 [Accessed: May 26, 2023]

[127] Kilander G. Canadian woman, 31, who applied for assisted suicide pauses request after well-wishers donate $65k to her. The Independent. 2022. Available from: https://www.independent.co.uk/news/world/americas/assisted-suicide-canada-toronto-gofundme-b2091802.html [Accessed: May 26, 2023]

[128] Pennock L. EXCLUSIVE: 'I don't want to die, but I don't want to be homeless': Canadian man, 65, has a doctor's approval for euthanasia despite admitting becoming POOR is a main reason he's applying to die. DailyMail.com. 2022. Available from: https://www.dailymail.co.uk/news/article-11516989/Canadian-man-doctors-approval-euthanasia-despite-admitting-POVERTY-main-factor.html [Accessed: June 14, 2023]

[129] Cheese T. Quadriplegic Ontario woman considers medically assisted dying because of long ODSP wait times. CBC News. 2023. Available from: https://www.cbc.ca/news/canada/toronto/rose-finlay-medically-assisted-dying-odsp-1.6868917 [Accessed: June 24, 2023]

[130] Committee on the Rights of Persons with Disabilities. Concluding observations on the combined second and third periodic reports of Canada. CRPD/C/CAN/CO/2-3. 2025. Available

from: https://tbinternet.ohchr.org/_layouts/15/treatybodyexternal/Download.aspx?symbolno=CRPD%2FC%2FCAN%2FCO%2F2-3&Lang=en [Accessed: April 03, 2025]

[131] Harper D. Etymology of Despair. Online Etymology Dictionary. n.d. Available from: https://www.etymonline.com/word/despair [Accessed: June 02, 2023

[132] Coburn B. The trouble with normal [Recording]. On: The Trouble With Normal. True North/Columbia; 1983. 3:35. Lyrics available from: https://www.allthelyrics.com/lyrics/bruce_cockburn/the_trouble_with_normal-lyrics-1072647.html [Accessed: June 03, 2023]

[133] Lassalle F. Franz von Sickingen. Eine historische Tragoedie. Berlin: Verlag von Franz Duucker; 1859. p. 63. Translation in: Bondurant J. Conquest of Violence. Revised ed. Berkeley: University of California Press; 1965, p. xiii.

Chapter 9

# Reflections on the Role of the Family in Euthanasia and Medical Decision-Making

*Francis Pamela Molina Sabogal*
*and Giovanny Armando Argoty Chamorro*

## Abstract

Euthanasia comes from the Greek word for "good death." It is considered a medical procedure, intentional and voluntary at the explicit request of the patient; death is caused by a third party. This concept is widely debated from the perspective of medical bioethics, and in terms of approval, legal regulation, and application, it varies considerably in different regions of the world. The debate remains open and depends on various psychosocial and cultural determinants in which the family plays a fundamental role, accompanying the patient during the process, from decision-making to the performance of the procedure. This document describes, through a narrative review, the general panorama of euthanasia in Colombia, considering the legal framework, which has been regulated in the country for almost 30 years. It also highlights the importance of the bioethical elements that impact the doctor-patient-family relationship, the needs in the interdisciplinary approach, informed decision-making, and the approach to grief.

**Keywords:** euthanasia, personal autonomy, grief, family, attitude to death, health care professionals

## 1. Introduction

Euthanasia comes from the Greek word for "good death," in which a doctor intentionally ends the life of a patient by administering medication in response to a voluntary request from a person with decision-making capacity. In a Latin manuscript from 1826, euthanasia is described as the "skillful relief of suffering" in relation to all those conditions that facilitate a peaceful and painless death. Although it is an individual decision, this practice is closely linked to a broad social context, exerting an impact on the family, community, and social level [1].

The increase in longevity, the greater prevalence of chronic diseases, and scientific advances make evident the need to have palliative care teams when the management is not curative. This in turn leads to ethical and legal debates on critical interventions at the end of life, understood as active pain control, adequacy of therapeutic effort, euthanasia, and physician-assisted suicide [2, 3].

In this context, decision-making regarding end-of-life interventions, respecting the autonomy and dignity of the patient, influences the quality of life and directly impacts the subjective experience of their final days and the relationship with their caregivers and family members. It is essential that these decisions are based on a comprehensive approach that combines palliative care, ethical support, and emotional accompaniment, both for the patient and their family [4].

The frequency of euthanasia varies throughout the world, given the complexity of the socio-cultural and legal contexts existing in the different regions of the world. Currently, euthanasia and physician-assisted suicide are legal only in a few countries, such as the Netherlands, Belgium, Switzerland, Luxembourg, Canada, and 11 jurisdictions in the USA (California, Colorado, District of Columbia, Hawaii, Montana, New Jersey, New Mexico, Oregon, Vermont, and Washington), which makes it evident that normative, ethical, and cultural differences influence its adoption [3–5].

At the Latin American level, Colombia, Cuba, and Ecuador are the countries in which a favorable evolution has been evident with regard to the legal frameworks for physician-assisted death, with Ecuador being the most recent country to decriminalize the request for euthanasia but which still has to build a protocol by the Ministry of Health of this country to adequately regulate this practice [6].

In Colombia, up to the year 2022, 322 cases of euthanasia were officially registered, which were carried out in accordance with current regulations and legislation, following the protocol implemented since 2015, the year in which the registration of procedures began [6].

Acceptance of euthanasia has grown both in society in general and among medical professionals. However, differences continue to be observed in the attitudes of both groups in relation to the interventions to be carried out at the end of life and what constitutes a "good death." This last concept, understood in a dynamic context, evolves over time and is influenced by cultural, social, and even religious values, which are of utmost importance to recognize within the doctor-patient-family relationship since they influence decision-making and support during the end-of-life process [3].

It is a multidimensional relationship in which essential aspects such as empathy and respect interact, which are indispensable components for the health professional, since they allow him to offer support and a comprehensive approach based on bioethical principles for decision-making, thus guaranteeing informed and humanly responsible decisions [7].

In the following chapter, based on a bibliographic review of narrative characteristics, we intend to generate reflections on the role of the family during the accompaniment of the patient in decision-making at the end of life, considering different psychosocial dimensions in relation to the fundamental bioethical principles such as autonomy, beneficence, non-maleficence, and justice.

## 2. General overview in Colombia

Latin America is experiencing a demographic transition toward an increasingly aging population, with a mortality pattern whose main cause is chronic diseases, diseases caused by unnatural causes, and communicable diseases. This phenomenon is a crucial factor that must be considered by the medical community and society in general, raising awareness about the importance of end-of-life care and informed decision-making in this area [4].

*DOI: http://dx.doi.org/10.5772/intechopen.1009763*

For its part, Colombia was one of the first countries to adopt a regulation on euthanasia. Since 1997, the right to die with dignity has been recognized as a fundamental right because it is closely linked to the principles of autonomy and human dignity enshrined in the 1991 Constitution. The right to die with dignity is a complex right because it depends on circumstances to be verified. Currently, in the framework of bioethical, legal, and regulatory discussions, this right includes palliative care and interventions aimed at improving the quality of life of patients and their families, considering different options regarding the adequacy of therapeutic effort and/or euthanasia [2, 6, 8].

Since 2015, the euthanasia application protocol has been describing different recommendations for the adequate application of the procedure, establishing criteria for its request: making a request in a voluntary, informed, and persistent manner by the patient, who must have the capacity to understand and be able to express his or her will in a free and informed manner. This can be expressed directly, either verbally or in writing [2, 6, 9].

The request for euthanasia according to Resolution 971 of 2021 can be received by any medical professional, not necessarily the attending physician, to initiate the processing of the request in a timely manner; that is, all physicians are responsible for receiving all requests. After that, it is the physician's responsibility to verify according to the clinical history that the patient has a serious or incurable injury or illness, that it is a free decision, and that it is made by the patient himself [6, 10, 11].

The physician must provide specific information about the right to die with dignity, the possibility of accessing palliative care, and activating within the following 24 hours the Scientific-Interdisciplinary Committee that healthcare entities must have [6, 10, 11].

This committee must be made up of professionals from various areas, such as doctors specializing in palliative care and psychiatry, as well as experts in bioethics and clinical psychology. These professionals are responsible for evaluating the patient's clinical and mental state, the treatments administered, and their effectiveness, ensuring that consent is free, informed, and unequivocal. In addition, they must corroborate that the patient suffers from a serious and incurable injury or illness. Once the request has been studied, the committee must issue a response within a maximum period of 10 calendar days, counting from the date on which the petition was filed [6, 10, 11].

Since 2021, access to euthanasia has been extended to patients with non-terminal pathologies, and in 2022 the Constitutional Court included assisted suicide as a route to medically assisted death [2, 6, 9].

In our country, studies have been carried out that explore the relationship between access to palliative care and decision-making regarding euthanasia, listing the limitations that may exist for access to this service in some regions; according to data for the year 2021 in the Colombian Observatory of Palliative Care, it was described that 41% of people who die in Colombia need this type of care, with a rate of specialized services of 0.5/100,000 inhabitants and with a coverage of 51% [2, 4, 12].

Although there is no direct causal relationship between the interventions of the palliative care team and the death of people who make the request for euthanasia, it is important to strengthen access to these services in order to reduce the inequality represented, comply with national regulations, and continue the support by this interdisciplinary group until the last days of life in patients who submit the request [2, 4, 6].

By 2022, 322 euthanasia procedures had been carried out in Colombia, adhering to the protocol; it should be noted that this figure does not include euthanasias carried out between the period from 1997 to 2015, nor those carried out outside the system (at home, with the help of relatives or doctors who charge for it); according to DescLAB (Laboratory of Economic, Social and Cultural Rights), for the year 2023 alone, 271 euthanasia procedures were carried out, which represents a significant increase compared to previous years [6, 11].

Taking these data into account, the integration of teams made up of palliative care and other specialties such as family medicine and psychiatry should be considered, which allows for ensuring support in decision-making, trying to alleviate suffering, and offering emotional support, both individual and family, thus guaranteeing the provision of high-quality services, a challenge that must be considered within the Colombian health system and that requires the strengthening of health care networks, especially in those more remote areas, where the primary care physician would play a fundamental role.

## 3. Bioethical principles, doctor-patient and family relationships

Autonomy is the ability to decide and act with the support of others so that these decisions can be taken into consideration and put into practice for the benefit of the patient. This bioethical principle is essential in the euthanasia process because it indicates the right of the patient to request a dignified death. And to guarantee that this request is considered with respect and priority by the family and health personnel [13].

According to the protocol for the application of euthanasia in Colombia, informed consent must be based on voluntariness, without any type of coercion and persistence over time, and the ability to understand the pertinent information that demonstrates competence to make decisions about one's own life. Therefore, the autonomy of the patient, in the face of the decision of euthanasia, requires priority medical support, which must provide detailed information about his diagnosis, prognosis, and therapeutic alternatives, guaranteeing decision-making in a free and informed manner [9, 14].

Many still consider the role of the doctor to be paramount in euthanasia, as they are the ones who could guarantee a dignified and painless end of life, and there are those who believe that the patient's autonomy could be expressed as a unique aspect. However, it has been shown that without the support of loved ones, the process toward euthanasia could be even more complex, as they are crucial for a death chosen by the patient to be configured as a good death [13].

A study published in 2019 evaluated the principle of autonomy regarding euthanasia decision-making in the Netherlands and estimated that human decisions are not totally autonomous; they are always made in circumstances of great impact and complexity and in the presence of people relevant to the patient's life, such as their family; therefore, during the path to euthanasia, decisions could be modified and reconsidered on more than one occasion [13].

Likewise, it is essential to consider other bioethical principles such as beneficence, through which the patient is offered the opportunity to receive integrative palliative care that allows him to make his decisions calmly. Although it is not mandatory for the patient to inform his family of his decision, respecting confidentiality and self-determination, it is recommended that he communicate it himself, since an open dialog will favor emotional accompaniment and support throughout the process [9].

If this is the case, the principle of beneficence could extend to the family when, by the decision of the patient, they become participants and must receive support before, during, and after the loss, creating an environment of serenity, privacy, and respect. In this process, the relatives of the person requesting euthanasia can benefit from various types of support, which are mentioned below [14]:

1. *Informational support:* This consists of having a communication strategy that allows the patient and the family to have clear concepts, in addition to a broad overview of alternatives and the limitations in their management.

2. *Instrumental support:* This is based on providing the patient and their family with tangible tools for decision-making, such as timely services, multidisciplinary management, and assistance both in the outpatient and inpatient settings.

3. *Emotional support:* Taking a caring approach toward the patient and their family, providing trust, empathy, and support in the process of a dignified death.

4. *Evaluation support:* Allowing the patient to achieve a self-evaluation of their situation while their family understands and supports this decision. This process includes feedback to the family based on mutual respect and equality.

In this way, it is intended that the health team be closer to both the patient and the family, serving as facilitators of active communication and involving the family in the euthanasia process.

It is also important to consider the principle of non-maleficence, which contemplates "do no harm" and encourages shared decision-making between the patient and his/her family, ideally, free of therapeutic obstinacy, understood as the continuation of treatments and interventions that, instead of benefiting the patient, can prolong his/her agony without the possibility of improvement [8].

Addressing these challenges requires a comprehensive evaluation and an interdisciplinary team that considers clinical, emotional, and spiritual aspects, with a humanized approach that alleviates suffering. Studies have shown that feeling better prepared and having the support of the family is related to greater tranquility, allowing one to say goodbye consciously, in an act of joint decision-making, and without stigma [1, 14].

In addition, it was shown that the earlier the family could get involved in the processes toward a dignified death, the greater the acceptability, understanding, and clarity to request the support of health professionals were, making it easier for the patient to be at peace with his/her decision [14].

The bioethical principle of justice, for its part, is related to universal access to palliative care and euthanasia, as well as the possibility of deciding on interventions at the end of life. However, this principle is conditioned by the particularities of each region and the availability of such services, a controversial situation in Colombia, given the limitations in access, since there are areas of the country where the interdisciplinary and integrated care required for euthanasia is not available [2]. In other words, these particularities demonstrate the regional inequalities experienced in health services, which are concentrated in urban and centralized areas, which limit access to remote regions due to their geographic location, and economic, social, or war vulnerability.

These limitations highlight the need to strengthen health infrastructure, expand specialized training, and establish mechanisms for investment in economic resources to contribute to the development of systems that guarantee care for the application of the euthanasia protocol.

## 4. Perspectives from the request for euthanasia

Euthanasia is associated with a profound ethical, religious, legal, and emotional debate. Various studies have analyzed the motives and reasons that justify its request, identifying elements related to the impact on quality of life, for example, the difficulty in alleviating certain symptoms such as pain or suffering (dyspnea, diarrhea, fatigue) and the loss of functionality, conditions that generate feelings of hopelessness and helplessness, or the desire not to be a burden. In addition, other factors have been highlighted, such as being able to choose the way of dying, having the presence of the family, and avoiding losing one's own essence in the progression of the disease [2, 3].

Therefore, the reasons that justify critical interventions at the end of life are dynamic and can vary as patients and their families progress through the disease process. In this context, the role of the caregiver influences attitudes toward such procedures. These situations should be systematically explored by treating physicians, given that different studies show that patients, families, and health professionals agree more frequently on the implementation of management aimed at active pain control and the adequacy of therapeutic effort. However, greater discrepancies are observed in relation to the implementation of euthanasia, which shows the need to expand research in this area and, based on the results, provide respective interventions [2, 3].

Regarding the proportion of positive attitudes of the population toward euthanasia, there are differences between countries; for example, in Korea they generally support conservative treatment options at the end of life, unlike in the Netherlands, the United States, or Canada, where the percentage of approval is usually higher. Even in countries with greater acceptance of euthanasia, there are internal disagreements within the different population groups, where educational, cultural, economic, social, emotional, and affective factors play an important role in shaping these attitudes [3].

DescLAB reported a greater favorability of euthanasia in Colombian public opinion; for 2021, 70% of the population indicated that they agreed with the possibility of accessing euthanasia when experiencing physical and psychological suffering secondary to serious and incurable diseases [11].

In this order of ideas, obstacles have been found, that call into question the patient's decision when requesting euthanasia; these obstacles are, for example, the paternalistic attitude of the doctor when "measuring the amount of pain" or "measuring the amount of suffering" that could justify or not the request for euthanasia, the complexity of decision-making in situations involving the family in addition to the loss of autonomy that can occur in the context of aging and fragility, which together translates into leaving decisions in the hands of others [13].

All of the above highlights the importance of the physician taking into account the psychosocial context and addressing each case individually when carrying out specific interventions aimed at joint decision-making; this approach will facilitate an open dialog in which the meaning of illness and death is explored for both the patient and his/her family, allowing for the emotional expression of all those involved, and consequently, comprehensive and personalized support.

## 5. Approaching grief before, during, and after euthanasia

Although the construction of an "anticipatory grief" (understood as the anticipatory phases that facilitate emotional detachment before death occurs) experienced by the family before the euthanasia of their loved one is frequently addressed, it is equally crucial to consider how the family unit faces grief months or years after their loss. Research has shown that the risk groups for developing "pathological grief" are those who, even from the beginning, sought less support. For this reason, it is essential to provide a step-by-step accompaniment that allows the family to be guided before, during, and after their loss, with the help of a multidisciplinary and transmural team, that is, one that goes beyond the hospital and evaluates the family dynamics in grief after euthanasia [1, 15].

This is how grieving family members may require subsequent conversations and interventions. A study conducted in the Netherlands in 2024 showed that there were three main topics discussed with the family sometime after euthanasia; these include the following [16]:

i. The retrospective look at the technical aspects of the path to euthanasia.

ii. The emotional experience during this path.

iii. The mental well-being of the family sometime after euthanasia.

The study revealed that in addition to addressing grief, it is important to consider other aspects that could affect the family dynamics and the mental well-being of everyone, such as the barriers to care, time from the request for euthanasia to its implementation, empathy of the health personnel and support from the palliative phase [16].

In addition, it has been shown that, during the approach to grief, the intervention of the primary care physician is essential, since he or she has been able to establish, even from the initial diagnosis, a solid relationship between the doctor, patient, and family and is closely familiar with the needs of the family group regarding the decision of euthanasia, and the accompaniment of the mourning in each of its phases [14, 16].

Although there are currently no established programs for family care after euthanasia, it continues to represent a great challenge for health personnel and institutions, since the support and follow-up of each member of the family translates into the interest of providing all the necessary help in time, managing to work positively on their loss [14, 16].

Therefore, it is vital to contribute to the construction of an anticipated mourning process for the patient and their family. This mourning will be facilitated by a serene environment, which will help create good memories in the face of the death of their loved one [14, 16].

A study in Belgium that analyzed the experiences of families and assisted grief revealed that feeling prepared for a process such as euthanasia is characterized by three dimensions [16]:

i. *Cognitive:* It covers all the tools of medical, spiritual, legal, and psychosocial knowledge.

ii. *Affective:* It involves emotionally preparing for anticipated grief, and making guilt-free decisions.

iii. *Behavioral:* It refers to the organization of each of the steps of euthanasia.

Finally, addressing a grieving process after euthanasia requires a multidimensional approach that allows not only a dignified death but also welcomes the acceptance and emotional well-being of those involved.

## 6. Conclusions

Individual and social behavior, the structure of institutions, and the legal framework established in each country for regulating interventions associated with the end of life have an impact on the doctor-patient-family relationship, as well as on informed decision-making.

In this context, psychosocial factors and the concept of death are often more closely associated with positive or negative attitudes toward end-of-life interventions than demographic factors per se. In fact, the attitude toward death is linked both to the way of dying and to the implementation of specific interventions [3].

Therefore, exploring, addressing, and strengthening the doctor-patient-family relationship allows health professionals to identify and manage specific needs that arise during this process, offering adequate support for decision-making [3].

For some time now, the importance of the relationship between health professionals and the patient's family has been recognized to create an atmosphere of serenity during a process full of questions and emotions. An atmosphere of serenity is defined as one that allows both the patient and his family the necessary tranquility to decide, achieving connection, and thus focusing on the process of death, allowing in turn the health personnel to have a role of support and guidance, but without disturbing the intimate and fraternal moment of the family nucleus [14].

The connection relationship between the family and the health personnel is crucial for the euthanasia request to be accepted. During this process, the health personnel must use clear and detailed communication that allows finding the correct way to be present: using the most appropriate words and adopting the most empathetic positioning and emotions. Also, the health personnel have an important mission, since they must guide the patient to be the one to inform his family of the decision of euthanasia and not to be informed as a medical indication [14].

Clear language must be used, allowing each step of the process to be explained, describing medications, steps, times, and places. In addition to using a checklist so that the family has clarity about the accompaniment and the role that the doctor fulfills at the time of euthanasia.

Using an open dialog, the different attitudes and positions of patients and family members must be addressed, recognizing requests for both euthanasia and the desire to continue receiving palliative care, understanding these as a dynamic and modifiable process over time, and providing the necessary support to those involved, given that both practices are based on the autonomy and dignity of patients [2].

At the Colombian level, the strengthening and expansion of access to the pertinent specialties that allow the needs of each patient to be addressed in a comprehensive manner is projected. The collaboration of interdisciplinary teams will facilitate objective consensus and deliberations in each case, supporting decision-making and alleviating physical and emotional suffering.

In addition, the significant increase in euthanasia procedures recorded in the country opens a new paradigm on the favorability of the procedure in public opinion, which intensifies the debate and underlines the need to strengthen the academic training of health professionals in issues related to the end of life [4]. Medical education must continue to evolve to adapt the therapeutic effort, properly manage the interruption and non-start of certain treatments, and ultimately change the perception of death, considering it not as a negative outcome but as a fundamental right of the patient to die with dignity.

## Author details

Francis Pamela Molina Sabogal[1,2*] and Giovanny Armando Argoty Chamorro[3,4]

1 Family Medicine, Armenia, Quindío, Colombia

2 Colombian Society of Family Medicine, Colombia

3 Psychiatry, Armenia, Quindío, Colombia

4 Colombian Society of Psychiatry, Colombia

*Address all correspondence to: fpmolina@fucsalud.edu.co

## References

[1] Boven C, Van Humbeeck L, Van den Block L, Piers R, Van Den Noortgate N, Dillen L. Bereavement care and the interaction with relatives in the context of euthanasia: A qualitative study with healthcare providers. International Journal of Nursing Studies. 2023;**140**:104450

[2] Erazo-Munoz M, Borda-Restrepo D, Benavides-Cruz J. Euthanasia in Colombia: Experience in a palliative care program and bioethical reflections. Developing World Bioethics. 2024;**24**(4):310-317

[3] Yun YH, Kim K-N, Sim J-A, Yoo SH, Kim M, Kim YA, et al. Comparison of attitudes towards five end-of-life care interventions (active pain control, withdrawal of futile life-sustaining treatment, passive euthanasia, active euthanasia and physician-assisted suicide): A multicentred cross-sectional survey of Korean patients with cancer, their family caregivers, physicians and the general Korean population. BMJ Open. 2018;**8**(9):e020519

[4] De Vries E, Leal Arenas FA, van der Heide A, Gempeler Rueda FE, Murillo R, Morales O, et al. Medical decisions concerning the end of life for cancer patients in three Colombian hospitals—A survey study. BMC Palliative Care. 2021;**20**:1-12

[5] Observatorio de Bioetica UCV. El estado de Maine en los Estados Unidos de América Aprueba el Suicidio Asistido y la Eutanasia. Universidad Católica de Valencia; 2022. Available from: https://www.observatoriobioetica.org/2022/01/el-estado-de-maine-en-los-estados-unidos-de-america-aprueba-el-suicidio-asistido-y-la-eutanasia/37730

[6] Tabakman R. Evolución Favorable de los Marcos Legales para la Muerte Asistida por Médicos en Ecuador, Cuba y Colombia. Medscape; 2024. Noticias y Perspectivas. Available from: https://espanol.medscape.com/verarticulo/5912308

[7] Atuesta Fajardo J, Argoty Chamorro G, Diaz J. Relación médico paciente en tiempos de pandemia por covid-19. Revista Latinoamericana de Psiquiatría: Órgano Oficial de la Asociación Psiquiátrica de América Latina. 2020;**1**(19):22-25

[8] Corte Constitucional de Colombia. Sentencia T-970/14. Bogotá: Corte Constitucional de Colombia; 2014

[9] Ministerio de Salud y Protección Social. Protocolo para la aplicación del procedimiento de eutanasia en Colombia. Bogotá: Ministerio de Salud y Protección Social; 2015

[10] Ministerio de Salud y Protección Social. Resolución número 971 de 2021. Bogotá: Ministerio de Salud y Protección Social; 2021

[11] Correa L. Eutanasia en Colombia: Cifras y Barreras para Ejercer el Derecho a Morir Dignamente en Colombia. DescLAB; 2024. Available from: https://www.desclab.com/post/eutanasiacifras#:~:text=Desde%202015%20%E2%80%93a%C3%B1o%20en%20el,de%20la%20eutanasia%20en%20Colombia

[12] Sánchez Cárdenas MA, León Delgado MX, Rodríguez Campos LF, Parra SL, et al. Estado Actual de los Cuidados Paliativos en Colombia: Reporte Técnico 2021 Observatorio Colombiano de Cuidados Paliativos

[Internet] (Investigación). 2022. Available from: https://hdl.handle.net/20.500.12495/7656

[13] van der Geest S, Satalkar P. Autonomy and dying: Notes about decision-making and "completed life" euthanasia in the Netherlands. Death Studies. 2021;**45**(8):613-622

[14] Boven C, Dillen L, Dierickx S, Van den Block L, Piers R, Van Den Noortgate N, et al. Relatives' experiences of being involved in assisted dying: A qualitative study. Qualitative Health Research. 2023;**33**(13):1154-1164

[15] Sancho MG. El Duelo y el Luto. 1st ed. Editorial El Manual Moderno; 2017. p. 97; 8

[16] Renckens SC, Pasman HR, van der Heide A, Onwuteaka-Philipsen BD. Aftercare provision for bereaved relatives following euthanasia or physician-assisted suicide: A cross-sectional questionnaire study among physicians. International Journal of Public Health. 2024;**69**:1607346

Chapter 10

# Terminal Illness, Intolerable Suffering, a Bad Death, Loss of Autonomy: Where to Next for Assisted Dying's Burgeoning Inclusion Criteria – A Duty to Die?

*Una P. Canning*


## Abstract

This work explores the arguments by those favouring a change in the law in support of physician assisted suicide (PAS) in England and Wales. It focuses on the criteria most often cited for justifying a change in the law, notably terminal illness, intolerable suffering, a bad death and autonomy. Definitions of terminal illness are investigated along with data reporting on death rates for a range of conditions including cancer, Parkinson's disease, Motor Neuron Disease, suicide and those designated as "public health funerals". The paper questions the notion of a mechanical definition of suffering that is equated with physical pain and argues that more weight needs to be given to the social gradient in health and that autonomy is a social achievement achieved through our network of relationships. The paper concludes by arguing that the normative choices we are expected to make in the effort to "die well" should not take precedence over efforts to enable all citizens to "live well" in the intervening years.


**Keywords:** euthanasia, physician assisted suicide, eligibility criteria, terminal illness, intolerable suffering, a bad death, autonomy

## 1. Introduction

The word euthanasia is taken from Greek and is composed of two parts - *eu* meaning good and *thanatos* meaning death. That diverse typologies of euthanasia have existed throughout history can be seen in the practice of selective infanticide in the classical Graeco-Roman era when newborn babies deemed not worthy of existence were killed [1]. The underlying assumptions that influenced this practice says Wyatt [1] "was the belief that the value of life lay primarily in its usefulness, partly to the parents, but especially to the state as a future citizen". Kure [2] identifies what he calls "social euthanasia" and were killings directed at those with incurable diseases or handicaps who, for the good of the community, were abandoned or directly killed because of the social good it bestowed. Along with social euthanasia there was also a form of euthanasia called *mors voluntaria* (voluntary death) where one could demonstrate bravery and moral excellence by choosing death over foreseeable humiliation brought about by old age or a serious illness [2].

These diverse types of euthanasia have led to an absence of a universally agreed definition of euthanasia, with the word left open to "semantic substitutions" that are often not distinguished from one another and include terms such as "assisted dying", "physician assisted dying", "physician assisted suicide" [2]. Contemporary debates on euthanasia centre around the assisted dying debate where the terms euthanasia and physician assisted suicide (PAS) are both used [3]. In today's language the word euthanasia is understood to involve a doctor or other professional, administering a lethal drug by intravenous injection at the patient's request, to intentionally bring about death: it is also referred to as "voluntary active euthanasia" [3]. The difference between euthanasia and PAS is that it is the patient who self-administers the lethal medication and not the doctor. However in countries such as the UK where PAS is currently illegal, it can also refer to a relative or friend helping someone travel to another jurisdiction to die such as *Dignitas* in Switzerland [4].

In the period after World War Two (WW2) and following the successes of medicine in prolonging life, the concept of euthanasia was invoked to avoid suffering caused by medical technology. Euthanasia in this context typically involved the with-holding of treatment that in the case of non-competent patients was called non-voluntary euthanasia, or the withdrawal from treatment by competent patients, and described as voluntary euthanasia. Distinguishing between PAS and euthanasia, the philosopher Gerald Dworkin sees euthanasia as the final act "in which the physician performs the last casual step leading to the death of the patient, and thus can be said to kill the patient" [5]. Referring to the "withdrawal" from treatment by a competent patient, Dworkin discerns no difference between PAS and "voluntary euthanasia", which allows competent patients to refuse or withdraw from treatment, even if it will result in death [5]. Writing in the late 1990s in the period immediately after the first US state, Oregon introduced lawful PAS, Dworkin argued that the values of "autonomy and relief of suffering" are the cornerstones for his and he believes, wider society's support for PAS so death can be "as painless and dignified as possible" [5].

Medical involvement in assisted dying is legal in Australia, Belgium, Canada, Colombia, Ecuador, Luxembourg, the Netherlands, New Zealand, Portugal, Spain and parts of the United States. It is not legalised in Switzerland and occurs outside of the healthcare system in organisations such as *Dignitas*. Although assisted dying is illegal in Switzerland, assisting a suicide is not, and while doctors are involved in prescribing the lethal chemical used, its administration is usually left to lay volunteers [6]. In 1997 the US state of Oregon was the first jurisdiction in the world to make PAS lawful. The law stipulates that certain conditions need to be fulfilled including: the patient be of sound mind; have less than six months to live; make a request both orally and in writing; get two doctors to agree to the request and confirm that the patient is not suffering from depression and obscuring their judgement [5]. In 2002 the Netherlands was the first country in the world to allow both "termination of life on request" carried out by a physician and "assisted suicide" where the physician supplies the drug, but the person administers it. The term euthanasia is used to refer to both types of death in the Netherlands and is not confined to those diagnosed with a terminal illness but requires six "due care" criteria to be fulfilled if a doctor is to avoid criminal proceedings [7]. Three of the due care criteria necessitate the responsible doctor to: "be satisfied the patient's request is voluntary and well considered; be equally satisfied the patient's suffering is 'hopeless' and 'unbearable'

[and] arrived at the conclusion, together with the patient, that there is no reasonable alternative to relieve the suffering" [7].

In Canada the term "medical assistance in dying "(MAiD) is used for both physician assisted suicide (where lethal drugs are provided by a physician and the patient self-administers the drug), and euthanasia, (where lethal drugs are directly administered by the physician at the patient's request) [8]. Since MAiD was legalised in 2016, euthanasia has been the method of choice for those requesting death and accounts for over 99 per cent of such deaths in Canada [8]. Following a legal challenge, Canada expanded its law in 2021 to include anyone with a physical medical condition or disability, and whose death need not be reasonably foreseeable [6]. Though Canadian law legislates for PAS or euthanasia to be offered on these grounds, Maher [9] a Canadian psychiatrist, writes that Canadians are being approved for PAS primarily for reasons of poverty, inadequate housing, or social exclusion with a third of the population supporting PAS for people who are homeless or in poverty. Within months of passing the initial PAS legislation in 2016, Canadian health economists had estimated that tens of millions of dollars of the healthcare budget would be saved by the legislation, compared to meeting treatment and care costs [6] that are paid for through a publicly funded healthcare system.

Unlike Canada, Belgium, and the Netherlands which all offer euthanasia, Oregon restricts its laws to PAS. Data reveal that when given a choice between PAS and euthanasia, the majority choose euthanasia. In the US state of California which introduced PAS the same year as Canada legalised PAS and euthanasia, there were 407 PAS deaths in California compared to 2838 in Canada [10]. In 2022 California reported 853 PAS deaths, whereas Canada reported 13,241 with all deaths occurring because of euthanasia, apart from seven [10].

## 2. Physician assisted suicide (PAS) in the UK

### 2.1 A safe and peaceful death

To obtain "a safe and peaceful death" as described by the UK organisation *Dignity in Death (DiD)*, UK citizens currently have to travel to *Dignitas* in Switzerland. The fact that "many cannot travel" is the reason given for "risk[ing] a painful and gruesome death by ending their lives at home" because the choice of "dying safely and comfortably at home" is denied under current UK legislation [11]. The cost of travelling to *Dignitas* from the UK is estimated to be in the region of £15,000: the cost for a Swiss national is estimated to be 7500 Swiss Francs (SF) or 11,000 SF if *Dignitas* make all the necessary funeral and administrative arrangements (VAT not included) [4]. With 4000 SF paid in advance, the brochure also states: "no guarantee of an accompanied suicide can be linked to this payment". In 2023, data from *Dignitas* puts UK membership of the organisation at 1900 people, a 24 per cent rise on the previous year—to join *Dignitas* a one off joining fee along with an annual fee is required [4]. According to the organisation, 40 people from the UK ended their lives at *Dignitas* in 2023, the highest level since 2019 [12].

Calling for a change in the UK law, the campaign group *Dignity in Dying* (DiD) [11] argue the case to legalise assisted dying could not be clearer with "300 dying people end[ing] their own lives in this country every year". Until 1961 suicide had been a criminal act in the UK and a person who survived an attempt could be prosecuted. With the introduction of the Suicide Act, 1961 suicide was decriminalised meaning that charges would not be brought against those who attempted it. The Act however did not legalise suicide and campaigners are currently seeking to change the law because in their view, current legislation is not working. The group argue that the low numbers of prosecutions of persons accused of assisting a suicide compared to the number of "terminally ill people [...] taking measures into their own hands by attempting to end their lives" is no comfort for those who assist someone on compassionate grounds because they cannot be assured of immunity from prosecution [13].

Following a freedom of information request by DiD to Directors of Public Health in England in 2014 asking for data on the number of suicides involving people diagnosed with a terminal illness, the organisation calculated 332 terminally ill people took their own lives in 2012 [13]. In April 2021, the then British Secretary of State for Health and Social Care, Matt Hancock MP, called for more data on suicides by the terminally ill and the possible impact the ban on assisted suicide was having on such people. Hancock's intervention came as a result of new figures from the Office of National Statistics (ONS) which suggested that one in seven suicides are by people with experience of cancer, neurological, heart or lung disease. According to the *All Party Parliamentary Group* (APPG) on *Choice at the End of Life* the Health Secretary had written to the ONS asking for more data and noted that "anyone who believes in high-quality public discourse would want to see an independent and impartial set of facts on which we can have a discussion" [11].

Recent suicide data for England (2023) reported 5656 suicides, with male suicide rates at 17.1 per 100,000, compared to a female suicide rate of 5.6 per 100,000 [14]. Regional variations in suicide exist with the highest rate and biggest increases seen in the north west of England (14.7 deaths per 100,000 people, compared with 12.5 deaths per 100,000 in 2022) with London having the lowest rate (7.3 per 100,000). Data from the Office of Health Improvement and Disparities [15] reports that the leading cause of death for men and women aged 20–34 years in the north west of England in 2020, was suicide and injury. In the devolved nation of Northern Ireland, 31 per cent of suicides occurred in the most deprived areas, which was over three times higher that of the least deprived areas (9.4%). A similar picture was reported in Scotland with people in Scotland's most deprived areas two and a half times more likely to die by suicide, than those living in the least deprived areas.

### 2.2 The Oregon model - "Best fit" for the UK

In October 2024, the Labour Member of Parliament (MP) Kim Leadbeater for Spen Valley in West Yorkshire, introduced her Terminally Ill Adults (End of Life) Private Member's Bill to the House of Commons [16]. The contents of the Bill propose allowing terminally ill adults with a prognosis of six months or less to live, to end their lives and to exclude individuals experiencing "intolerable suffering" but not facing imminent death. To safeguard against misuse, approval from two doctors who must confirm the patient's diagnosis along with a judge, is needed before any decision to proceed is granted. Safeguards, such as a mandatory cooling-off period to ensure decisions are made with full consideration and without external pressure, are also included.

### 2.3 Eligibility criteria

The first jurisdiction in the world to make PAS lawful was the US state of Oregon in 1997: euthanasia is prohibited by US federal law [17]. The Oregon model is considered to be a possible "best fit" for adoption in the UK with the attraction that the rates of death by PAS has remained low, although there was a 28 per cent increase in 2021 [17]. Terminal illness with a prognosis of less than six months are included in Oregon's eligibility criteria. According to the available data, most people accessing PAS in Oregon tend to be well educated and have sufficient funds to cover the costs that are estimated to be US$ 5000 raising questions about equity of access [17]. The issue of cost is yet to be decided in the UK, which offers a universal health service, paid for out of taxation and free at the point of need. However Section 32 of the Bill proposes the "Secretary of State's powers to ensure assistance is available [to] enable the provision of such assistance as part of the health service in England and the health service in Wales" [16].

### 2.4 Age

In Oregon, the age of eligibility for PAS is 18 years, with the proposed UK legislation following suit: 82 per cent of those accessing PAS in Oregon were 65 years or older. A similar pattern for age has been identified in the Netherlands where 78.5 per cent of euthanasia deaths are amongst people in the sixties to eighties age group [18]. However, the Dutch *Termination of Life on Request and Assisted Suicide Act* 2002 has enabled euthanasia to be conducted on children 12–16 years if the parent's consent. This was extended to children below 12 years in 2023 with the Dutch government expressing the belief that it would apply to around 5–10 children a year who suffer unbearably from their disease and with no hope of improvement [1]. The Belgium law on euthanasia was also amended in 2014 to remove any age restriction with minors requesting euthanasia needing parental consent and to meet the criteria of having "a terminal or incurable disease, or be near to death, or suffering from chronic pain" [1]. In Canada in 2023 the Special Joint Committee on Medical Assistance in Dying (MAiD) recommended expanding MAiD to "mature minors" under the age of 18 years whose death was "reasonably foreseeable". It recommended parents be involved in the process but ultimately the decision should rest with the child, provided they have legal capacity according to an independent assessor [1].

### 2.5 Decisional capacity

Amongst the eligibility criteria for PAS in Oregon is the requirement of competency along with the ability to perform the task of self-administering the lethal medication. In the Netherlands commentators have noted a shift away from the termination of life in the competent patient, towards termination of life in non-competent patients who lack "decisional capacity" [7]. Article 2.2 of Dutch law stipulates that an "advanced euthanasia directive" (AED) can replace a patient's oral request as a means to fulfilling the first criterion of "due care" and the need for the doctor to be satisfied that the "request is voluntary and well considered." Canada legalised PAS for patients with mental capacity and a terminal illness in 2016 but less than five years later dropped the requirement that a patient's natural death be reasonably foreseeable following a legal challenge. Kim [19] sees this burgeoning of inclusion criteria for PAS as linked to the laws on equality and is "limited only by the ingenuity of 'equality technicians'". The expansion in eligibility he sees as a result of prioritising the private reasons of patients - a process that is not open to scrutiny:

> *"As the appeal to addressing suffering is the most common rationale for assisted dying, it is not difficult to imagine how this would go. Once a society deems it permissible for a private citizen to terminate the life of someone at their request because they belong to a group defined by suffering X, an equality technician can surely ask: 'what about the others in the group defined by Y who seem to share salient features with those in group X. After all, it seems dehumanizing to rank one person's suffering over another's in terms of their moral significance" [19].*

The "widespread strategic use of equality arguments" has given rise to a "dystopian equality" which qualifies anyone who asks for PAS regardless of other characteristics such as age, disability, decisional capacity etc [19]. In the proposed Bill for England, Section 15 allows for someone else other than the patient to sign the relevant document as a proxy [16]. Critics believe this opens up the possibility of abuse from family members with ulterior motives and unscrupulous doctors.

## 3. The elusive and tenuous eligibility criteria for PAS

### 3.1 Terminal illness

The current Bill before the UK Parliament stipulates that a person is terminally ill if:

a. the person has an inevitably progressive illness, disease or medical condition which cannot be reversed by treatment, and

b. the person's death in consequence of that illness, disease or medical condition can reasonably be expected within 6 months [16].

Proponents of PAS have argued that assisting individuals with mental capacity and a terminal illness whose natural death is reasonably foreseeable is not self-killing or murder:

> *"If we assist people who are not suffering from a terminal illness to end their lives we are assisting suicide; whereas if we assist a terminally ill person out of this world, we are only assisting his or her dying – because we are hastening a death which is approaching from natural causes" [13].*

But this is disputed by those against changing the law on suicide who argue that:

> *"If you end your own life deliberately, in law that is suicide; and a doctor or anyone else who knowingly supplies you with the means, or otherwise helps you to do so, is assisting suicide" [13].*

In the book *Death by Appointment* [13] the authors argue that advocating for a law that allows those who are terminally ill some form of assistance to end their lives, is a law offering differing levels of protection to people in different health states. Using the examples of Multiple Sclerosis (MS) or Parkinson's disease that are incurable and potentially life-limiting, the difference between a diagnosis of Parkinson's and a diagnosis of "terminal illness" is one of timeframe. In the case of Parkinson's, which is a progressive, neurological disease that involves physical, cognitive, and psychological symptoms, the disease itself does not cause death but the symptoms related to the disease can, such as having a fall. And a law that distinguishes between someone with a terminal illness with months to live and someone who has to cope with an incurable condition for much longer, such as Parkinson's is potentially discriminatory [13]. This view is echoed by Sir Nicholas Mostyn a former high court judge diagnosed with Parkinson's disease; Mostyn has attacked the current bill before Parliament by arguing that because people with neurodegenerative diseases are not terminally ill, and therefore not covered by the proposed change in the law "the Bill is no f***ing use to us at all" [20].

That there is no set list of terminal illnesses is confirmed by the Marie Curie website which describes terminal illness as "an illness or condition which cannot be cured and is likely to lead to someone's death. It's sometimes called a life-limiting illness" [21]. The website gives some examples of diseases that can be classified as terminal such as: advanced cancer, dementia (including Alzheimer's), Motor Neurone Disease (MND), lung disease, neurological diseases such as Parkinson's, and advanced heart disease. The information provided by the website goes on to say that these illnesses are not always terminal and that advanced cancer for example, which is defined as cancer which has spread, or is at a later stage, can potentially be treated to control its growth or spread. In the case of terminal cancer this usually means the cancer cannot be controlled and is likely to be the cause of someone's death (a recent example of this in the UK is the Olympic cyclist Sir Chris Hoy who recently revealed he has terminal cancer and has a prognosis of between two and four years to live [22]. In the UK around 167,000 cancer deaths occur every year with approximately 78,000 in females and 89,200 male [22]. With one in two people expected to get cancer at some point in their lifetime, more than half (54%) of those who die every year are aged 75 and over, with mortality rates for all cancers highest in people aged 90 plus [23].

The list of terminal illnesses identified by the Marie Curie website includes diseases other than cancer, such as Motor Neurone Disease (MND) and Parkinson's. Unlike cancer, MND is an uncommon condition that mainly affects people in their 60s and 70s but can impact people of all ages and affects around 5000 people in the UK at any one time [24]. The condition can significantly shorten life expectancy and eventually leads to death with an estimated six people dying each day from the disease [24, 25]. Parkinson's UK estimates 145,000 people have been diagnosed with the disease and while it does not itself cause death, its symptoms can. With an ageing population, it is expected that 1 in 37 people will be diagnosed with the disease in their lifetime [26].

The use of a timeframe to prognosticate in the case of terminal illness is open to doubt. Providing an exact diagnosis may not always be possible with diagnostic error remaining a major source of preventable harm. Studies have revealed that the practice of prognosticating is riddled with inaccuracies and clinicians' predictions vary for cancer and non-cancer patients from 23 per cent to 78 per cent [27]. The difficulties prognosticating are associated in the mind of Cassell [28] with medicines total embrace of science. This is because scientific methods are only suited to generalities, and "it is an uncomfortable fact that doctors do not treat disease they treat patients". This "uncomfortable fact" means that the same disease in different individuals may present differently and have different treatment and outcomes because "the scientific basis of medicine does not recognise nor provide a methodology to deal with such individual variations on the level of patient-doctor interactions" [28]. That science and medicine are inextricably bound is undeniable says Cassell [28] but the paradoxes and strains produced by believing they are the same has led to a conception "of the ideal physician as a scientist" that is unsustainable.

## 4. Intolerable suffering

The website of the UK group *Dignity in Death* (DiD) [11] argues that "assisted dying allows a dying person the choice to control their death if they decide their suffering is unbearable. It is illegal in the UK." Favouring a change in the law to make assisted dying legal, the group contend:

> *"Dying people deserve the choice to control the timing and manner of their death [and that] dying people are already ending their lives to avoid painful and undignified deaths. Many pay thousands of pounds to travel abroad to guarantee a safe and peaceful death. They do so to access a proven and safe way to control their death with medical supervision. Many cannot travel so risk a painful and gruesome death by ending their lives at home. Many are suffering and dying without dignity because they have no choice. We believe dying people should have the means to control their death safely and comfortably at home" (DiD) [11].*

In *The nature of suffering and the goals of medicine,* Cassell [28] argues the concept of suffering is rarely discussed in the medical literature because of its preoccupation with the body and the identification of physical disease. Although physical pain remains a major source of human suffering the two concepts are not synonymous. This is because suffering extends beyond the physical and into realms "that threaten the intactness of the person" [28]. Medicines lack of concern for suffering is associated with its persistent dichotomy between mind and body. For medicine, the person, along with the mind, is problematic because it is not identifiable in objective terms and therefore lacks:

> *"An alternative place in medicine's objective categories. Therefore as long as the mind-body dichotomy is accepted, suffering is either subjective and thus not truly "real" - not within medicine's domain - or identified exclusively with bodily pain. [...] That bodily pain causes personal suffering cannot itself be understood until the dichotomy between mind and body is rejected" [28].*

Suffering is ultimately a personal matter that exists, and often only understood, in the context of others. As such, there can be no mechanical simplicity in any definition of suffering, as all aspects of person are open to damage and loss as a result of the lived experience of the person. Diversity of suffering means that reductionist scientific methods, so successful in other parts of human biology, are not useful for understanding whole persons, or the potential for injury and suffering that exists in all of us:

> *"We all recognise certain injuries that almost invariably cause suffering: the death or suffering of loved ones, powerlessness, torture, the loss of a life's work, physical agony, memory failure and unremitting fear. Each is both universal and individual. Each touches features common to us all, yet each contains features that must be defined in terms of specific persons at a specific time" [28].*

In Cassell's view [28] problems of staggering complexity arise when we attempt to understand all the known dimensions of person and their relationship to illness and suffering.

## 5. A bad death

Use of the word "good" in euthanasia creates controversy with arguments persisting as to what precisely constitutes the kind of death considered good. For Kure

[2] the word "good" is related to fundamental values associated with philosophical views, and metaphysical and religious beliefs, amongst others. With the advent of Christianity the act of suicide which previously had been accepted in Antiquity, came to be deemed as reprehensible. Augustine of Hippo regarded it as the "most grievous sin of all since it alone could never be repented during the lifetime of the sinner [5]. In Christianity failure to repent for mortal sin constituted a "bad death" because the sin condemned the person to the worst possible afterlife [2]. This condemnation is evident in the book *Reading in the Dark* by Seamus Deane. The narrator, a young boy in 1950s Derry, is reluctant to sit with his sick grandfather. Finding it difficult to hold a conversation, his older brother Liam suggests a list of possible topics:

> *"'Just talk about football,' Liam advised. [...] Or the priests. He's good value on them, but now he's getting nervous, so he mightn't be as good as he used to be. Like Constantine.'*
>
> *Great-uncle Constantine, on my mother's side, was the sole family heretic. He had been a know-all, we were told, a man who read too many books and disagreed with everybody, especially the priests. In his thirties, he had started to read a notorious French writer called Voltaire, who was on the Catholic index of forbidden authors. [...] Then he went blind, became ill and caved in by being restored to the bosom of the Church before he died. The blindness was a judgement and a warning, we were told. Thank God he had heeded it, but no wonder, for his sainted mother, Isabella – or Bella, for short – had worn out her knees praying for his soul. Lord, she was the happy woman when he died, escorted into heaven by the Last Sacraments and wee Father Gallagher from the Long Tower parish who had personally burnt the Voltaire book page by page in the kitchen fire, saying better far that these pages should burn, like Voltaire himself, rather than the soul of the man who had read them and been blinded body and soul by their evil glare" [29].*

Constantine's family we are told, is assured by the clergy that he had a "good death" having avoided hell in the afterlife following his repentance for reading banned books. But in chastising his grandson for doing his French language homework rather than studying the Irish language, the grandfather reveals the story was cooked-up by well meaning relatives:

> *"'And look at what the French did to Constantine. Lost him his sight, then they say, his soul.'*
>
> *'Constantine? Sure he died a Catholic.'*
>
> *'He did not. He didn't. He died a heretic. Refused to see the priest and died holding that French book across his chest that they tried to get off him.'*
>
> *'I heard diff [erently].'*
>
> *'Of course you did. They cooked up the story so's not to give a bad example. But old Con, he's down there roasting with all the other atheists, God rest him [29].'"*

Deane's book has been described as a hybrid between two modes of writing - autobiography and fiction. Before he became blind, great uncle Constantine had been a printer/compositor for the local newspaper, the *Derry Journal*, and was an avid reader of all types of literature, including those on the banned list: Constantine died in 1946, aged 69 years [30].

With advances in medical technology and science in the decades after WW2 came a new concept of the "good death". This new understanding included the notion of "assistance" or "mercy killing" that arose in reaction to the prolongation of life resulting from a technologized and dehumanising medicine, which denied a natural death [2]. The concept operated on two basic precepts: the first involved the concept of "letting die" so as to make possible a dignified dying, while the second included the notion of "mercy killing" (killing upon request or without request) [2]. There also emerged around this time the existence of a number of organisations favouring euthanasia such as *The Dutch Society for Voluntary Euthanasia*, 1976.

Sissela Bok [5] notes how use of the word "assistance" has made the debate on assisted dying less "jarring" and is a term preferred when compared to that of "mercy killing" or euthanasia. With the primary moral focus for those who support PAS "on the liberty of persons to commit suicide if that is their considered choice" Bok sees the word "assistance" as adding two further additional factors to the concept:

> *"The element of helpfulness or assistance and the singling out of physicians, not relatives or others, as providing such assistance. Both the emphasis on helpfulness and the restriction on physicians as alone permitted to offer such help have proved reassuring to many who remain wary of active euthanasia" [5].*

In arguing for a dignified death, advocates of PAS set out a model statute for how physicians should be involved in assisted dying that was written it 1996: "Ending one's life in solitude can be a lonely and frightening undertaking, fraught with uncertainty, ambivalence and opportunities for failure. We hope that the responsible physician will be present at the patient's death in order to reassure the patient" [5]. Having a physician involved is considered reassuring because there is always the possibility for failure, whereas with medical assistance, it is possible that the process be "carried out effectively" [5]. But given the uncertainties as to what should be done in the event of an unsuccessful suicide attempt and whether "further assistance" by a physician or others who may be present, is permissible, the word "assistance" has been circumscribed in discussions of PAS. This is the case in Oregon where the word "assistance" refers to physicians assessing and prescribing the medication but are absent at the suicide, therefore avoiding the need to intervene in an unsuccessful suicide attempt [5]. As Bok observes there is nothing to say how physicians should act in such cases and whether assisting to finish the act of suicide, physicians are crossing the line in doing so. There are those who argue that assisted dying should be completely separated from healthcare [6].

In Oregon, patients have to first find a physician willing to assess a patient's competency and write the prescription, then find a pharmacist willing to dispense the required medicines [17]. According to Regnard [31] the number of studies evaluating the adverse effects of lethal medications is poor or non-existent. Data from Oregon indicates that the number of doctors willing to prescribe such drugs is very low meaning that "most doctors practising AS&E do so with little experience" [31].

With the UK seeking to follow in the footsteps of Oregon, the "medical supervision" seen as vital to DiD for dying people to "control their death" will require the approved substance to be provided directly and in person by the coordinating doctor to that person. The "coordinating doctor" in the Bill is described as a registered medical practitioner "who has such training, qualifications and experience as the Secretary of State may specify by regulations". According to Section 18 of the Bill, *Provision of Assistance*:

(5) The coordinating doctor may be accompanied by such other health professionals as the coordinating doctor thinks necessary.

(6) In respect of an approved substance which is provided to the person under subsection (2), the coordinating doctor may:

a. prepare that substance for self-administration by that person,

b. prepare a medical device which will enable that person to self-administer the substance, and

c. assist that person to ingest or otherwise self-administer the substance [16].

It also requires the coordinating doctor "to remain until the person has died, or has determined that the procedure has failed, or the person has decided not to self-administer the approved substance". In other jurisdictions where PAS is lawful, the doctors who prescribe the medication tend to be volunteers and not the doctor who normally treats the patient [16]. In Switzerland where assisting suicide is not illegal, doctors prescribe the lethal chemical, with its administration performed by lay volunteers [6]. The term "accompanied suicide" is used to describe the presence of a *Dignitas* escort team and for people who live in Switzerland, the act generally occurs at home. Because the substance is officially listed as a narcotic, the prescription is only handed over to *Dignitas*, never directly to the patient [4]. For legal reasons, the patient must be able to undertake the last act—that is "to swallow, to administer via the gastric tube, or to open the valve of the intravenous access tube" and if the patient is incapable of doing any of the required actions, then the *Dignitas* escort team cannot help [4].

### 5.1 End of life and palliative care

In 1995 a large scale study of five US medical centres investigating the treatment of patients at the end of life, reported neglect and maltreatment of the dying [5]. The study found patients experienced considerable suffering and pain, along with poor communication and that patients' preferences for cardiopulmonary resuscitation (CPR) was misunderstood in 80 per cent of cases. A UK study by Pollock et al. [32] reported that patients and the public risk being "deceived and badly served by uncritical peddling of the idealised notion, or 'imaginary' of 'the good death'" and the need for it to be at home. This "peddling" they say, works as a way of disciplining and constraining patient and public perspectives:

> *"The discourse of the good death is a largely professional and policy construct combining ideology and pragmatism, and purveying assumptions about the purported homology between public policy and private preferences [32].*

The study found that narratives about the "good death" privileges some issues such as "personal choice, control and individual autonomy" and sidelines others, notably:

> *"The consequences for informal caregivers but also the wider structural determinants of opportunity such as socioeconomic status, material circumstances and social resources, diagnosis, or the variable quality and availability of health and social services" [32].*

The existing narrative assumes palliative and end-of-life care is available, and that all dying persons do so in comfort, and free from pain, a claim that is not consistent with the study's findings or from data on the number of public health funerals (PHF) that occur in England. In the year 2023/24, an estimated 4,400 public health funerals (PHF) were arranged in England. These are funerals provided by local government because of a lack of family or funds. From March to April 2024, the Local Government Association (LGA) conducted an online survey of district councils, unitary councils, metropolitan districts and London boroughs regarding their PHF provision [33]. Under the Public Health (Control of Disease) Act 1984, when a resident passes away outside of a hospital, and/or it appears to the council that no suitable arrangements for the disposal of the body have been made, the council will make the necessary arrangements for a PHF. Responses were used to estimate the overall number of PHF across England, by assigning the number of the most similar available council to each council where there was no response. In the 2022/23 financial year, an estimated 4,400 PHF were arranged by councils in England, an increase of around 500 from the estimated figure for 2021/22 (3,900). According to the data, around 1,700 PHF were conducted for those aged between 16 to 64 years old, and 2,600 for those aged 65 and over. An estimated six million pounds was spent on public health funerals (PHF): an increase of around £324,000 in costs since 2021/22.

In a table of 80 nations, Britain has been rated first in its provision of end of life care [10]. But there is evidence that palliative care is not equally distributed throughout society with those less likely to receive palliative care being older people, people with non-cancer conditions, people from ethnic minorities, and those from lower socio-economic groups living in deprived areas [34]. In the Netherlands there are those who wonder whether the strength of support for assisted dying would have been as strong, if palliative care had been more prominent and available earlier. In Canada where palliative care is relatively rare and inadequate, similar arguments have been proposed [9, 35]. There is also evidence that the purpose of palliative care is misunderstood by the general public with Maher [9] reporting a lack of awareness amongst Canadians who conflate PAS with palliative care and not as a specialty of medicine in which experts are trained for the purposes of alleviating physical suffering [9]. In the UK there is a perception amongst some members of the general public that specialist palliative care services such as hospices, are places where people go to get "bumped off" [6].

## 6. Loss of autonomy

Today the words "person" and "individual" are used interchangeably. Yet the idea of an individual did not come into existence until around about the twelfth century. The idea of individual as free-standing and autonomous has arisen "in the larger sense of political, in that they are equal to other individuals, with rights, obligations, and the ability to redress injury by others" [28]. The field of bioethics which emerged in the 1970s sees individual freedom of choice and independence as more important than "the disease, the doctor, the relationship with the doctor and the social setting [or] recovery from illness" [28].

Schneewind in his book *The Invention of Autonomy* [36] describes how use of the word autonomy was not "discovered" but "invented" during a period when new ways of conceptualising humanity emerged in the period known as the *Enlightenment.* The outlook that emerged centred on the belief that all normal individuals are equally able to live together in a morality of self-governance. This conception of morality according to Schneewind [36] "provides a conceptual framework for a social space in which each might rightly claim to direct our own actions without interference from the state, the church, the neighbours or those claiming to be better or wiser than we". This framing is different to the original use of the term which was used in a political and constitutional context. According to Onora O'Neill, it was originally used by the Ancient Greeks for matters of jurisprudence "and the Greeks would not have spoken of individuals (who do not make laws at all) either as autonomous or as lacking autonomy" [13]. Writing on the topic, the philosopher Alasdair Macintyre [37] concludes that "autonomy is not a property of every rational agent. It is an achievement, a social achievement, as is rationality itself. It is in and through our network of relationships that we achieve or fail to achieve, rational control of our lives".

With the success of medical science seemingly providing equality for all in its pursuit of disease theory and in the treatment of disease, other factors associated with sickness, such as cultural and social factors, are neglected [28]. That sickness cannot be completely understood apart from the personal lifestyle and the social setting in which it occurred, tends to be ignored by physicians enthralled by the scientific and technological progress of medicine. The existence of a social gradient in health [38] demonstrating that the poor have more sickness and illnesses that are more severe, when compared to socio-economic groups further up the gradient, is evidence that medicine has artificially circumscribed its task. Focusing as it does on science and technology, medicine has failed to develop a methodology to deal with individual variations so as to treat different individuals or groups, who may have a different presentation, course, treatment, and outcome for their disease [28].

The values of autonomy and the desire for a relief of suffering, are values according to Dworkin, which speak to "the liberty of persons to commit suicide if that is their considered choice" [5]. Advocates of assisted dying are often described as "highly determined [and] accustomed to a life of control" [13]. But with a social gradient in health, the liberty of persons in exercising choice will be decidedly circumscribed according to their socio-economic group. For the highly determined individual accustomed to a life of control, there is always the possibility of a legal challenge if the criteria don't fit (this has already occurred in Canada where legal challenges have expanded eligibility criteria). For those whose autonomy is circumscribed because of poverty, social isolation, marginalisation, legal challenge will rarely be an option. But with a third of the Canadian population supporting PAS for people who are homeless or in poverty, the knowledge that others outside of their socio-economic group are advocating for them, means that finding the resources to mount a legal challenge will not be necessary.

### 6.1 A duty to die

A further group under-represented in the PAS debate is that of disabled people: 16 million people in the UK are reported to have a disability [39]. Inspired by Darwinism a new interpretation of a "good death" emerged at the beginning of the twentieth century which called for "undesirable" and "unfit" persons to be euthanised—usually intellectually or physically disabled people [2, 40]. Questioning the proposed new law in Britian for assisted dying that is premised on terminal illness, the Paralympian Tanni Grey-Thompson along with Flora Klintworth [39] argue that legislators need to consider how such a law would affect every member of society including "not just the terminally ill celebrities of Britain but also the everyday citizens". With evidence that attitudes towards death were coarsened following the introduction of the *Liverpool Care Pathway* and during the Covid-19 pandemic with a blanket "Do not Resuscitate" (DNR) order placed on disabled people, those opposed to the law feel there are good grounds for caution [17, 39]. In *Disability – a duty to die?* [39] the authors argue that changing the law on suicide so that "people who possess certain characteristics or symptoms of pain – creates a value judgement on those who resolve to live with these same traits". Cassell [28] notes how the political dimension of illness and the actions of others can increase the fears of the sick along with judgements which say "some people – disabled people – are 'better off dead' that dying lives are 'fundamentally unliveable' or that the elderly and infirm have a 'duty to die'" [39].

## 7. Conclusion

That persons cannot be reduced to their parts so that they can be better understood—the approach used in reductionist scientific methods—dispels any suggestion of mechanical simplicity in the definition of suffering. For Cassell [28] suffering is ultimately a personal matter and is something that exists and often only understood, in the context of others. And when all aspects of person are open to damage and loss as a result of the lived experience, a law that allows persons to actively pursue death on an arbitrarily defined definition of terminal illness and suffering, is not only unfair but reckless. We already have evidence from other jurisdictions that such arbitrary definitions are open to legal challenge—Canada being a prime example. In a relatively short period of time, Canada has witnessed a burgeoning of its inclusion criteria due to both legal challenges, and to applicants being approved for PAS primarily for reasons of poverty, inadequate housing, or social exclusion. To think that a similar scenario does not await the UK is surely naïve. The aptly named "equality technicians" are doubtless waiting in the wings and, in a manner of speaking, keen to make a "killing" in the process. And as the equality technicians strive to confirm the value of autonomy while vying to trump the suffering of the "highly determined [individual] accustomed to a life of control" versus the "terminally ill celebrities of Britain" ordinary citizens can only hope there will be enough money left in the public purse to pay for the normative choices we are expected to make in the effort to "die well" but also and more importantly, to "live well" in the intervening years.

*DOI: http://dx.doi.org/10.5772/intechopen.1009397*

## Author details

Una P. Canning
Independent Researcher, London, England

*Address all correspondence to: u.canning1@gmail.com

## References


[1] Wyatt J. Vulnerable lives—Euthanasia in the newborn and paediatric populations. In: Hughes J, Finlay I, editors. The Reality of Assisted Dying: Understanding the Issues. Maidenhead: Open University Press; 2025. pp. 155-161

[2] Kure J. Good death within its historical context and as a contemporary challenge: A philosophical clarification of the concept 'euthanasia'. In: Kure J, editor. Euthanasia: The "Good Death" Controversy in Humans and Animals. London, UK: InTechOpen; 2011. pp. 22-44

[3] Finlay I, Hughes J. Introduction. In: Hughes J, Finlay I, editors. The Reality of Assisted Dying: Understanding the Issues. Maidenhead: Open University Press; 2025. pp. 1-13

[4] Dignitas Brochure. [Accessed: 25 January 2025]

[5] Dworkin G, Frey RG, Bok S. Euthanasia and Physician-Assisted Suicide. Cambridge: Cambridge University Press; 1998

[6] Thomas HL. De-medicalization: Why we should completely separate assisted dying from health care and what this would achieve. In: Hughes J, Finlay I, editors. The Reality of Assisted Dying: Understanding the Issues. Maidenhead: Cambridge University Press; 2025. pp. 131-138

[7] Hertogh C. Making euthanasia legal in the Netherlands: Implications for the doctor-patient relationship. In: Hughes J, Finlay I, editors. The Reality of Assisted Dying: Understanding the Issues. Maidenhead: Cambridge University Press; 2025. pp. 38-44

[8] Coelho R, Herx L. The rapid expanion of euthanasia and assisted suicide: The view from Canada. In: Hughes J, Finlay I, editors. The Reality of Assisted Dying: Understanding the Issues. Maidenhead: Cambridge University Press; 2025. pp. 51-58

[9] Maher J. The euthanasia paradox. In: Hughes J, Hughes I, editors. The Reality of Assisted Dying: Understanding the Issues. Maidenhead: Cambridge University Press; 2025. pp. 167-171

[10] Preston C. Assisted dying: The evidence from abroad. In: Hughes J, Finlay I, editors. The Reality of Assisted Dying: Understanding the Issues. Maidenhead: Cambridge University Press; 2025. pp. 28-37

[11] Dignity in Dying (DiD). [Accessed: 1 November 2024]

[12] BBC News. Assisted Dying: Family Shares Experience of Dignitas - BBC News. Available from: https://www.bbc.uk/news/articles/ced3ngwp3g5o [Accessed: 1 November 2024]

[13] Finlay I, Preston R. Death by Appointment: A Rational Guide to the Assisted Dying Debate. Newcastle Upon Tyne: Cambridge Scholars Publishing; 2020

[14] Samaritans. Latest suicide data. 2024. Available from: https://www.samaritans.org/about-samaritans/research-policy/suicide-facts-and-figures/latest-suicide-data/ [Accessed: 1 November 2024]

[15] Office for Health Improvement and Disparities (OHID). Office of Health Improvement and Disparities (OHID).

Health Profile for the North West of England. 2021. Available from: https://fingertips.phe.org.uk/static-reports/health-profile-for-england/regional-profile-north_west.html [Accessed 1 November 2024]

[16] Terminally Ill Adults (End of Life) Bill—Parliamentary Bills—UK Parliament. Available from: https://bills.parliament.uk/bills/3774 [Accessed: 25 January 2025]

[17] Ost S, Preston N. Should assisted dying be part of mainstream healthcare? In: Hughes J, Finlay I, editors. The Reality of Assisted Dying: Understanding the Issues. Maidenhead: Cambridge University Press; 2025. pp. 125-130

[18] Hughes J. Older people and those living with dementia. In: Hughes J, Finlay I, editors. The Reality of Assisted Dying: Understanding the Issues. Maidenhead: Cambridge University Press; 2025. pp. 162-166

[19] Kim SYH. Instability of eligibility criteria for assisted death and its implications. In: Hughes J, Finlay I, editors. The Reality of Assisted Dying: Understanding the Issues. Maidenhead: Cambridge University Press; 2025. pp. 188-193

[20] The Express and Star. Ex-High court judge says parkinsons suffers left out of assisted dying debate. 2024. Available from: https://www.expressandstar.com/news/uk-news/2024/10/13/ex-high-court-judge-says-parkinsons-sufferers-left-out-of-assisted-dying-debate/ [Accessed: 25 January 2025]

[21] Marie Curie What are examples of terminal illnesses? Is advanced cancer always terminal? Available from: https://www.mariecurie.org.uk/who/terminal-illness-definition [Accessed: 1 November 2024]

[22] BBC News. Cyclist Sir Chris Hoy announces his cancer is terminal. Available from: https://www.bbc.co.uk/news/articles/cj4dr9xdxgro [Accessed: 1 November 2024]

[23] Cancer Research UK. Cancer statistics for the UK 2024. Available from: https://www.cancerresearchuk.org/health-professional/cancer-statistics-for-the-uk#heading-One [Accessed: 1 November 2024]

[24] Brain and Spine Foundation. Motor Neurone Disease-Fact Sheet. Available from: https://www.brainandspine.org.uk/health-information/fact-sheets/motor-neurone-disease/ [Accessed: 1 November 2024]

[25] NHS. Motor Neuron Disease. Available from: https://www.nhs.uk/conditions/motor-neurone-disease/ [Accessed: 1 November 2024]

[26] Parkinson's UK. Number of people with Parkinson's rising. Available from: https://www.parkinsons.org.uk/news/number-people-parkinsons-rising [Accessed: 1 November 2024]

[27] MacCormick F. Challenges in diagnosis and prognosis. In: Hughes J, Finlay I, editors. The Reality of Assisted Dying: Understanding the Issues. Maidenhead: Cambridge University Press; 2025. pp. 108-113

[28] Cassell E. The Nature of Suffering and the Goals of Medicine. 2nd ed. Oxford: Oxford University Press, Kindal Edition; 2004

[29] Deane S. Reading in the Dark. London: Vintage, Kindal Edition; 1996

[30] Doherty C. Doherty Family History. Self-published. Dublin: Duffy Bookbinders; 2006

[31] Regnard C. The enigma of lethal drugs. In: Hughes J, Finlay I, editors. The Reality of Assisted Dying: Understanding the Issues. Maidenhead: Open University Press; 2025

[32] Pollock K, Caswell G, Turner N, Wilson E. Beyond the reach of palliative care: A qualitative study of patient and public experiences and anticipation of death and dying. Qualitative Health Research. 2024;**34**(14):1428-1441. DOI: 10.1177/10497323241246705

[33] Local Government Association (LGA). Public Health Funerals, Public health funerals 2024 research report. 2024. Available from: https://www.local.gov.uk/publications/public-health-funerals-2024-research-report

[34] Sleeman LE, Williamson KE. Palliative care: Need, provision and evidence. In: Hughes J, Finlay I, editors. The Reality of Assisted Dying: Understanding the Issues. Maidenhead: Open University Press; 2025. pp. 114-119

[35] Huxtable R. A journey through the contested terriority of assisted dying: How law can go wrong - and right. In: Hughes J, Finlay I, editors. The Reality of Assisted Dying: Understanding the Issues. Maidenhead: Open University Press; 2025. pp. 96-101

[36] Schneewind JB. The Invention of Autonomy: A History of Modern Moral Philosophy. Cambridge: Cambridge University Press; 1998

[37] Macintyre A. Medicine aimed at the care of persons rather than what ...? In: Cassell M, Siegler E, editors. Changing Values in Medicine. Frederick, Maryland: University Publications of America; 1979. pp. 83-96

[38] Graham H, Kelly MP. Health inequalities: Concepts, frameworks and policy. [Online]. Available from: www.hda.nhs.uk/evidence

[39] Grey-Thompson T, Klintworth F. Disability - a duty to die? In: Hughes J, Finlay I, editors. The Reality of Assisted Dying: Understanding the Issues. Maidenhead: Open University Press; 2025. pp. 145-149

[40] Yuill K. The humanist case against assisted suicide and euthanasia. In: Hughes J, Finlay I, editors. The Reality of Assisted Dying: Understanding the Issues. Maidenhead: Open University Press; 2025. pp. 205-210

Chapter 11

# The Future of Euthanasia in the Netherlands

*Wim Graafland*

## Abstract

The Netherlands has played a pioneering role in the legalization of euthanasia, which has resulted in both international recognition and criticism of the Netherlands. In other countries, assisted suicide rather than euthanasia was central. The doctor plays a central role in the Netherlands while this is much less the case in countries where assisted suicide is involved. More experience has now been gained through legislation in other countries with another important theme as to whether patients must be in a terminal phase to be eligible for euthanasia. The questions are which is better: the Dutch euthanasia model or assisted suicide and whether the terminal phase is a condition for euthanasia or assisted suicide. In the Netherlands, the call for an amendment to the law is becoming increasingly stronger, the question being whether it is further distancing itself from international practice or whether it is seeking more rapprochements.

**Keywords:** euthanasia, assisted suicide, the Netherlands, the Dutch history of euthanasia, future developments

## 1. Introduction

The Netherlands has had a euthanasia law[1] since 2002, together with Belgium and Luxembourg. This makes these countries the first with euthanasia legislation. Switzerland and some US states already had legislation regarding assisted suicide. The number of countries with legislation on euthanasia and assisted suicide is steadily increasing. **Table 1** lists the countries with legislation in the field of euthanasia and assisted suicide [2, 3].

In the late sixties, social discussion about euthanasia began in the Netherlands. In 1969, psychiatrist van den Berg published 'Medical power and medical ethics' [4]. In this book, illustrated with shocking images, the writer concludes that if the doctor goes too far in prolonging life, he must also be the one who must be able to end this life mercifully. This immediately gave the doctor a central position in the implementation of the euthanasia practice that followed, and, despite the legalization of the euthanasia debate, he has never lost this position. This development is in stark contrast to practice in other countries, where the doctor is much less prominent. In this chapter, we will discuss this in detail and describe the current

[1] "Wet toetsing levensbeëindiging op verzoek en hulp bij zelfdoding" (WTL, 2002) [1] called the euthanasia law.

| | Euthanasia | Assisted suicide |
|---|---|---|
| Australia (all six states) | * | * |
| Austria | - | * |
| Belgium | * | * |
| Canada | * | * |
| Colombia | * | - |
| Germany (awaiting regulation) | - | * |
| Luxembourg | * | * |
| the Netherlands | * | * |
| New Zealand | * | * |
| Portugal (awaiting regulation) | * | * |
| Spain | * | * |
| United Kingdom (in process, not definitive) | - | * |
| United States (California, District of Columbia, Colorado, Hawaii, Maine, Montana, New Jersey, Oregon, Vermont, Washington) | - | * |
| Switzerland | - | * |

**=possible*
*-= not possible*

**Table 1.**
*Countries in which euthanasia or assisted suicide are legal or in the process (2024).*

euthanasia situation in the Netherlands. To understand this properly, we also must go back in history. Finally, we would like to consider the future of euthanasia in the Netherlands. Which scenarios are conceivable?

## 2. Short history of euthanasia in the Netherlands

Since the early 1970s, there has been discussion about euthanasia in the Netherlands. At that time, but certainly in the time before that, there was little knowledge among general practitioners in the Netherlands to alleviate terminal suffering. In many situations, they found themselves with their backs against the wall and had no other means available except morphine and especially the conversation with and attention for their patient. Today's palliative care is not even in its infancy. The Netherlands lagged behind in this regard compared to, for example, the U.K. where palliative care developed strongly. General practitioners also often did not have a clear picture of what exactly euthanasia entailed, and all kinds of terms were still discussed, such as active, passive, direct, indirect, voluntary and involuntary euthanasia. Many were not yet familiar with Leenen's [5] definition.[2]

Spreeuwenberg [6] notes that the biggest opponents of euthanasia among his interlocutors liberally treated patients with severe pain or shortness of breath in the terminal stage with substances that could be associated with a shortening of life, but that they did not call this euthanasia. In the strict sense, there was often no question of euthanasia

[2] Definition of euthanasia: "intentional life-ending action by someone other than the person concerned, but at his or her request".

in its current meaning because there was almost always a lack of a discussion about this and an explicit question or expression of wishes from the patient in this regard. Doctors were allowed to do anything if killing was not the explicit goal of the treatment. "There were also general practitioners who actively ended the patient's life without consulting the patient. Sometimes it was sufficient to act to end life if a patient had once expressed that he did not want to continue living. Distressing were the situations in which general practitioners came to such a decision based on the emotional bond with their patient or in which they had no idea at all how they could bring about the death of their patient in an acceptable manner. This even led to a general practitioner confessing to having killed his patient with a pillow" [7]. General practitioners at the time showed such a variety of motives, attitudes and practices and such a lack of knowledge that it was clear to Spreeuwenberg [6] that this situation absolutely did not serve the interests of people who have to face death, reason for him to contribute to the development of the authoritative position of the Royal Dutch Society for the Promotion of Medicine from 1984 on euthanasia [8]. This position did not imply that euthanasia was one of the professional duties of a doctor, but that an authoritative guideline supported by the KNMG had to be offered to doctors who were prepared to act to end life in situations where there was clearly hopelessness, intolerability and voluntariness. With this position of the KNMG, the Netherlands has created an irreversible situation that ultimately led to the acceptance of the euthanasia law in 2002, while in our neighboring country Germany, the opposite was the case and their doctors' organizations turned against euthanasia.

The euthanasia discussion began, as mentioned, in 1969 after the publication of 'Medical power and medical ethics' by psychiatrist van den Berg [4]. Van den Berg [9] makes a connection between treatments that have gone too far by the doctor, who must therefore take responsibility for ending the unviable life. With this he championed euthanasia. In addition, the social discussion was fed, among other things, by case law (including Postma, 1973, Schoonheim 1984, see the appendix for an overview), the establishment of the Dutch Association for Voluntary Euthanasia (NVVE) in 1973, which later changed its name to the Dutch Association for a Voluntary End of Life, and the media, such as Henk Mochel, who presented euthanasia as a mild death in 4 episodes for the television in 1972 [10]. Key players in this process are lawyers and ethicists, the Royal Dutch Society for the Promotion of Medicine (KNMG), the Public Prosecution Service (OM), politicians and public opinion, but not so much the doctors. Rather, they felt overruled by lawyers, ethicists and policymakers, people who, like the doctor, did not have their feet in the daily clay. The prevailing central motif among doctors, mercy, was replaced by the legal right of self-determination, which was understandable during the emancipation period in the 1970s: mercy and compassion had become old-fashioned, they reminded of the faith that people wanted to get rid of. There was talk of a euthanasia elite that was in charge.

According to Kennedy [11], this elite consisted of: Piet Muntendam, physician and policymaker, Henk Leenen, health lawyer, Heleen Dupuis, theologian-ethicist and Harry Kuitert, theologian-ethicist. Doctors felt restricted on all fronts: their old position of power was being undermined. It was a power struggle [12]. For the most part, doctors stayed out of the discussion. However, this also devoid of emotion from the euthanasia discussion and arrangements could be made. Definitions of termination of life and euthanasia are developing, as are the due care criteria (see **Table 2**) that euthanasia requires if a doctor wants to remain free from punishment for euthanasia.

In 1986, a national consultation group consisting of representatives of the Public Prosecution Service (OM) and the State Supervision of Public Health developed a reporting procedure. Doctors who complied with the criteria stated in this

| |
|---|
| The doctor has become convinced that there was a voluntary and well-considered request from the patient |
| The doctor became convinced that the patient's suffering was hopeless and unbearable |
| The doctor informed the patient about the situation he was in and about his prospects |
| The doctor concluded with the patient that there was no reasonable other solution for the situation in which he found himself |
| The doctor has consulted at least one other independent doctor, who has seen the patient and given his written opinion on the above-mentioned due care requirements |
| The doctor carried out the termination of life or assisted suicide with medical care. |

**Table 2.**
*The legal due care requirements of the Euthanasia Act (2002).*

procedure and reported their actions could count on a smooth handling by the Public Prosecution Service. In 1994, this growing practice was enshrined in law with an amendment to one article of the Mortuary Examination Act. Euthanasia remained in the Criminal Code, but doctors who complied with the criteria had nothing to fear from the Public Prosecution Service.

From 1998 onwards, five Regional Euthanasia Review Committees (RTE) examined the reports before they were sent to the Public Prosecution Service. All this resulted in the euthanasia law of 2002. In 2024, this law is still in force after four legal evaluations, the last in 2023. This law reinforces a situation that had existed for several decades before, namely, the situation that doctors, when their backs were against the wall, had no choice but to help their patients by relieving their suffering using substances that caused them to die. We would now characterize part of this practice as palliative care, which means that immediate and active termination of life is no longer always necessary. But about 30–40 years ago, when palliative medicine was still in its infancy, this knowledge and resources were not yet available. Despite the major involvement of lawyers in their profession in the Netherlands, the Euthanasia Act of 2002 has given doctors a lot of peace and freedom in their actions regarding their patients with a wish for euthanasia.

All things considered, most doctors think it is a good thing that society has made euthanasia possible in the Netherlands. Due to the openness about the subject, there is more knowledge about the best way to perform euthanasia and intercollegial consultation has also become commonplace. This has led to a significant improvement in practice. However, not all doctors agree with this. The context of dying is not the same for every patient and is difficult to capture in arrangements and paperwork. A paper reality is created that differs from practice. If the euthanasia case is presented correctly to the assessing committee, no problems will arise. Meyler, professor of cardiology, says in an interview with The [12]: "As long as there have been doctors, they have helped patients die. It is part of the doctor's profession to give patients a gentle death. No two people die in the same way and no two people are alike in euthanasia. You can't arrange that. This means that assistance with dying, including euthanasia, must be left to the doctor."

Houtepen [13] recently supplemented this with his statement to move away from the narrower concept of 'medical basics' in terms of medically classifiable causes and to exchange this for a broader description of the medical domain. Only then is there sufficient professional scope for a doctor to follow up on the practical medical judgment that a patient is really 'spent' and can no longer continue, by honoring a euthanasia request. This is also evident in the discussion about existential suffering as a refractory symptom to justify continuous palliative sedation: the doctor's practical judgment is central to whether there is not only 'no longer wanting to', but also 'no longer being able to do it'. '. We must leave it to doctors to determine which part of the group that requests euthanasia due to 'tiredness of life'. If 'on' means 'really on' according to a doctor, this concerns an assessment of the patient's health options and therefore falls within the medical domain.

## 3. The current situation of euthanasia in the Netherlands

Since then, there have been several developments: the first is a further improvement of all kinds of techniques, increase in knowledge and support within palliative medicine, which makes it possible to effectively alleviate most physical complaints in terminal patients, such as pain, shortness of breath, confusion. This means that, medically speaking, doctors feel less likely to have their backs against the wall than before. The largest group with a wish for euthanasia, patients with cancer in the terminal phase, can be better guided with palliative care. The share of this so far largest group of patients for euthanasia is therefore (relatively) smaller (4th WTL law evaluation, 2023). In addition, in the Netherlands there is a shift toward patient groups with a longer life expectancy, such as psychiatric patients and patients with so-called multi-layered age-related conditions who do not want to wait for an end that is meaningless for them but want to take control into their own hands (4th WTL law evaluation, 2023). And then also the growing group of dementia, who can also request euthanasia based on a living will, and finally the usually older patient with a so-called completed life.

The amount of euthanasia in the Netherlands, 9068 in 2023 (4th WTL law evaluation, 2023), is increasing. Euthanasia has become the new standard of humane dying for many and is increasingly experienced as a basic right. The fact that so far there have been 'only' approximately 9000 euthanasia per year is due to the unpredictability of the final phase of life. This means that you can easily end up back in the hospital from your home, the place where most people want to die. There is also the moral compass of general practitioners to exercise restraint and postpone euthanasia as long as possible. The doctor functions as a funnel containing a moral filter for the wish that exists widely in society: that you can choose when you want to leave this life based on self-determination. The expectation of most commentators is that a further increase will occur in the coming years due to the aging of the Dutch population and the autonomy paradigm of the baby boom generation (4th WTL law evaluation, 2023).

Furthermore, attempts are being made by politicians to include 'completed life' in a law (a new law or an extension of the current euthanasia law), making it possible to help people with 'finished life' problems to die. Recently, in 2023, the liberal party D66 (Amended Completed Life Act) submitted a new bill to this end. This entails a new type of dying counselor. In addition, there are people who want to express a wish to end their life outside the euthanasia law. These people can do this entirely on their own and, for example, take advice from existing literature [14, 15]. They can also seek professional guidance from the various Right-to-die organizations in the Netherlands. Finally, natural death has almost completely disappeared from contemporary culture and the terminal phase is becoming increasingly medicalized. An important example of this is palliative sedation, which has been used in approximately a quarter of the deaths in the Netherlands in 2023. To date, in the Netherlands, continuous sedation (until death) has usually been chosen, which can be seen as disproportionate and where the difference with euthanasia, despite the theoretical differences between euthanasia and palliative sedation, is not always clearly visible, certainly not for the patient and his loved ones. The KNMG [16] recently published a new protocol for palliative sedation, in which more attention is paid to proportionality.

### 3.1 The role of the doctor

The question is whether our society is served by an increasing medicalization of people's dying and what place the doctor will take in dying and in future euthanasia practice. Doctors play an important role in terminal and palliative care and in euthanasia. She/he has four roles in this: She/he is a consultant/counselor for his patient, she/he is the decision maker and decides whether euthanasia will proceed, she/he is the prescriber of the medication and ultimately also the executor of the euthanasia. This can make it complex, also because she/he is also the one who provides palliative care.

In addition, the doctor-patient relationship has changed due to contemporary practice (larger practices with collaborating doctors, many part-timers, general practitioners' offices) in end-of-life guidance. There is no longer 7/24 care by your own doctor. The increasing use of the Dutch Euthanasia Expertise Center in termination of life also gives a different, more functional meaning to the doctor-patient relationship. This could result in a change in the role of the doctor in euthanasia. The developments from euthanasia performed by doctors to suicide performed by the patient themselves also play a role in this. As mentioned above, there is a shift in patient groups with a wish to end their lives who are not terminal and who are well able to carry out their own death by suicide within the framework of the euthanasia law. In other countries such as Switzerland and the US, where life is only ended by assisted suicide, the doctor is even absent. I have defended the position elsewhere [17] that the choice for euthanasia in the Netherlands, together with the focus on the doctor in this process, has been a historical mistake. This is due to doctors themselves, such as van den Berg in 1969, the case law conducted by doctors, by doctors' organizations such as the KNMG in 1984, the method of administering a lethal injection, promoted by the Dutch anesthetist Pieter Admiraal, together with the delayed development of palliative care in the Netherlands. All this has unnecessarily put the ball in the doctor's court. More than 97% of life terminations under the euthanasia law in the Netherlands consist of euthanasia by means of euthanasia administered intravenously by the doctor and in only just under 3% the patient takes the drug himself. It should make you think that in a country like the Netherlands it is self-evident that doctors are the executors of euthanasia, while in several other countries with a long history of assisted suicide it is not the doctors who carry it out. Certainly, if you take into account that a larger proportion of requests for euthanasia no longer come from people with a terminal condition, in which doctors are involved anyway, and who are well capable of ending their own lives, it will be questionable whether doctors, better trained in palliative care, will continue to handle a growing number of euthanasia requests from non-terminal patients.

Another aspect that must be considered is the large difference in the amount of euthanasia in the Netherlands (5.1% of deaths in 2022) and of assisted suicides in the state of Oregon (0.66% of deaths in 2020), both countries which already have a long-standing practice of ending life [18]. In the Netherlands, the percentage of active life ending by assisted suicide or euthanasia is more than seven times higher than in the state of Oregon. There are a few contextual reasons for this. First, the role and attitude of the doctor. Where public agreement with the possibility between the Netherlands and the state of Oregon is equal [18], the participation of doctors differs considerably. In the Netherlands, 78% of general practitioners have actively participated in ending a patient's life (and 13% can imagine doing so), while in Oregon 51% of general practitioners support the law and 34% of them are willing to issue a prescription to write. In 2020, all prescriptions were written by 142 doctors (out of more than 6000 registered doctors). In the Netherlands, 55% of euthanasia requests have been approved, in Oregon only 18%. Another difference is the place of death in our lives. Since people in the Netherlands quickly think of the possibility of euthanasia when they hear the diagnosis of incurable cancer, Americans exclude death from their considerations. But perhaps the most important is the central role of the doctor in the Netherlands, who is easily accessible to a euthanasia wish and therefore quickly takes on co-responsibility for this wish, which relieves the patient. As a priest-physician, he thus sanctions euthanasia and the patient does not have to commit suicide, albeit with the help of the doctor, which is still considered morally reprehensible. The Netherlands can call itself a spoiled country because of the role of the doctor.

Also technically speaking, any euthanasia using intravenously administered substances can be completely replaced by suicide, either by ingesting substances or by turning on an intravenously installed (so-called elastomer) pump [14]. This leads to the question of whether the role that the doctor has in carrying out euthanasia remains solely with the doctor or whether other professional groups are given a role in this, such as the trained volunteers in Switzerland or the death attendants envisaged by D66 in the initiative law for completed life.

## 4. The future of euthanasia in the Netherlands

After four legal evaluations, the last in 2023, the euthanasia law has remained sustainable and unchanged. Despite the fact that there is a lot of criticism to be made about this, the overall conclusion is that this law has created peace and clarity in the regulation of Dutch euthanasia practice, both for doctors and for people with a euthanasia wish, and that at the same time this law left room for developments, e.g. that of new patient groups, such as the group of elderly people with multiple ailments of old age.

Then the question is whether the Euthanasia Act (Wtl) will need to be amended in the coming years. The latest legislative evaluation of 2023 outlines five scenarios for future end-of-life regulation. These scenarios are lines of thought for future regulation of end-of-life questions in light of discussions and developments in recent years. Over a longer period, the need within society for more say and control for citizens over the end of life appears to be increasing and it is therefore important to continue the social debate about this, also for the position and perception of the Wtl. I will give a brief overview of the above five scenarios.

The first three scenarios relate to the Wtl, while scenarios four and five relate to possible legislation in addition to that law. The scenarios are as follows:

1. Leave the Wtl as it is

2. Adjust parts of the Wtl

3. Replace the Wtl with a new law

4. In addition to the Wtl, create a 'completed life' law for the elderly

5. Expand options for assisted suicide, including by non-physicians

### 4.1 Leave the Wtl as it is

This scenario assumes that there are no (convincing) arguments for amending the Wtl, or for opting for additional forms of regulation in addition to the Wtl. The idea is that the Wtl generally functions well, and that society is familiar with this law. In addition to the Wtl, there is a humane alternative to physician assistance in terminating life, namely stopping eating and drinking, but this alternative does not require further regulation.

### 4.2 Adjust parts of the Wtl

In this scenario, it is decided to retain the Wtl as such but to amend this law on one or more points. These may be larger or smaller adjustments in line with contemporary developments and views.

First, one may consider the criminal law anchoring of the Wtl. The position of the doctor and the carefulness of the euthanasia practice will be done more justice if the criminalization is structured differently. A second theme is the retrospective assessment by the RTCs and the way this has been done since the entry into force of the Wtl in 2002. Doctors largely assess the entire reporting procedure as 'neutral', but one in five doctors does find this procedure 'burdensome'. However, the ever-increasing number of annual reports raises the question of whether the existing system remains sustainable (in terms of the required capacity and resources) and what its substantive added value is. It can be argued that the costs of the current assessment system no longer outweigh the benefits and that, unlike in the initial period of the law, this system is no longer necessary to guarantee careful practice. Examples from other countries show that forms of care and assessment are also possible that do not require the extensive RTC organization that currently exists in the Netherlands. This could also involve a shift in emphasis to prior assessment.

### 4.3 Replace the Wtl with a new law

This scenario differs from the previous scenarios: in this scenario, the central question is whether the Wtl, which is currently functioning well, will also prove to be future proof in the longer term. The Wtl, which came into effect in 2002, is based on developments that occurred in the eighties and nineties of the last century. Afterwards, there are discussion points and new insights that, if we were to make a euthanasia law now, might lead to a different regulation than the Wtl. A second reason for this scenario can be found in the experiences gained abroad. These arrangements demonstrate choices and insights that can also be meaningful for the Netherlands in certain respects. For example, involving other healthcare providers in addition to doctors, such as nurse practitioners (Canada, New Zealand), removing the age limit of 12 years, a broader implementation of Advance Care Planning (Australia), clarifying or specifying criteria for legal capacity (New Zealand and Australia), including in the law that the patient determines the unbearable and reasonableness of alternatives (Canada, New Zealand and Australia), including in the law requirements for the training that an independent consultant must have received (Australia), or in law one include further description of the required independence of the consultant (Canada, Spain).

### 4.4 In addition to the Wtl, create a 'completed life' law for the elderly

This scenario leaves the Wtl as such intact but responds to the political desire to create a separate arrangement for elderly people above a certain age limit that makes it easier to have a request for termination of life granted than is the case under the Wtl, with less dependency from the doctor, which provides the possibility of receiving assisted suicide from an end-of-life counselor, if there is a voluntary, well-considered and sustainable request made by a competent person. This bill assumes that the person concerned determines when his or her life is complete and does not impose the further requirement that there must be suffering. The liberal political party D66 recently sent a revised bill to the House of Representatives on this matter. The social and political developments surrounding 'completed life' can be seen as a call for more citizen autonomy regarding end-of-life issues. The idea behind the bill is that it is reasonable to shape the right to self-determination of older people in such a way that they have broader options to realize an end-of-life wish than what currently results from the Wtl. For many doctors, performing euthanasia or assisted suicide in a 'completed life' situation is unthinkable. There is more support for this among citizens.

### 4.5 Expand options for assisted suicide, including by non-physicians

This scenario can be seen as a variant of the previous scenario but chooses a different starting point in which the options for assisted suicide are expanded. First, the voluntary, well-considered and sustainable wish to die of a competent person is not linked to a minimum age and, furthermore, room is created for assisted suicide by persons who are not a doctor or (legally recognized) end-of-life counselor, such as relatives. Arguments for this scenario can be found in the case law of the European Court of Human Rights (ECtHR) and the much more explicit (constitutional) case law and further legal formation in Germany and Austria. The ECtHR speaks in general terms of a right to a self-chosen end of life and does not attach an age limit to this. However, there will of course be a need for legal safeguards to prevent abuse and protect vulnerable groups. Even according to Dutch case law, such a scenario is not entirely impossible. After all, the Supreme Court has expressly considered, especially in the Heringa case, that a loved one may be able to appeal to impunity due to a state of emergency, although the scope for this is very limited. This scenario would put an end to the situation in the Netherlands of equating euthanasia and assisted suicide, regarding the person who may carry out the termination of life (currently only the doctor) and the applicable standards and (assessment) procedures. Scenario 5 is not about removing all procedures and safeguards, making lethal means freely available without any form of control.

## 5. Conclusion

If you were to make a euthanasia law in 2024 based on the current social reality in the Netherlands, it would look different than in 2002. In my opinion, now is the time to prepare a new euthanasia law. The following principles could be used for this:

- First, gradually replacing euthanasia with assisted suicide. For the time being, this is still a utopia given the current predominance of euthanasia over assisted suicide in the Netherlands, but it is the goal in the long run.
- Furthermore, completed life must be integrated into this law. Two different laws next to each other are confusing.
- No age limit should be included in the law.
- Requiring a medical cause to be the basis for a request for termination of life is too restrictive. Sustainable existential factors also play an important role.
- The doctor's duties are those of terminal and palliative care and not of killing people. In this law, he has an important role as a counselor for his patient and in informing the end-of-life counselor about medical aspects and possible alternative solutions. He no longer plays a role in the execution of the termination of life, other than as a prescriber of the medication.

The end-of-life counselor becomes the central figure in this process. His training and qualifications should be included in the law.

- Assisted suicide should become possible and non-punishable for non-physicians, which also offers more scope for the autonomous route of ending life.
- Criteria in the new law will be sustainability and well-considering of the request. The criteria of unbearable and hopeless disappear.
- The patient's wishes are central: it is a patient law.
- A waiting period is recommended for non-terminal patients, as is also the case in some foreign countries.
- And finally, testing, whether before or after, continues to exist.

The Netherlands will have to make a choice whether to bring its euthanasia legislation closer to the international community or to choose its own path again, just as in 2002. If the above principles are used in a new law, there is a high chance of the latter, unless the Netherlands can replace euthanasia with assisted suicide.

## Appendix

*Overview of 'key judgments' contributing to the forming of (the practice of) the Termination of life on request and assisted suicide review procedures Act [19].*

### A.1 Postma-Boven (1973)

A 78-year-old nursing home occupant who was physically seriously ill and suffered among other ailments from a half-sided paralysis, incontinence and pneumonia expressed her wish to end her lift to her treating physician and family members. The treating physician was not willing to help, after which her daughter, Mrs. Postma-Boven, a physician, ender her mother's lift by injecting a lethal dose of morphine. The physician was sentenced to one-week imprisonment with a probation period of one year seen the "purity of her motives". Contrary to the judgment of the court in 1952- when a Dutch physician appeared before court for the first time of violating Article 293 of the Penal Code and it was decided not to be the task to create grounds for a legal exclusion—in the Postma court case the judge formulated conditions about in which circumstances it could be justified to terminate life on request of the patient. These conditions were (a) the patient was sick because of an incurable illness or disease, (b) the physical or mental suffering was subjectively serious and unbearable for the patient, (c) the patient had clearly expressed the wish to end life or be relieved from his or her suffering, and (d) the treating physician (or another physician in consultation with the patient) had ended the life of the patient. The Lower Court had specifically not mentioned the necessity of the dying phase of the patient, so non-terminal patients could also obtain this assistance from a physician.

## A.2 Schoonheim (1983–1986)

A 95-year-old disabled, and bedridden woman had repetitively, during a decade, requested her physician, Mr. Schoonheim, to end her suffering. The week preceding her death her situation deteriorated. After pronouncing again, she did not wish to experience such a situation, her physician granted her wish and ended her life. The physician reported the termination of life on request of the patient. Initially, he was dismissed from prosecution in Lower Court but found guilty without punishment in Higher Court. The supreme Court held that the invocation of a situation of "force majeure" (or necessity)—resulting from a conflict of duties—was justifiable when the physician (a) carefully balanced the duty to alleviate hopeless suffering and the duty to preserve the patient's life, (b) acted according to the norms of medical ethics and medical-professional standards, and (c) made a decision that objectively seen was justified, taking into account the exceptional circumstances of the case. Factors that could play a role were further decline of already unbearable suffering, not being able to die in a dignified manner and possibilities to alleviate the suffering. The Higher Court of the Hague concluded that Schoonheim had reasonably concluded the suffering of the patient was unbearable, that no other possibilities were available to relief her suffering, that he acted in a situation of "force majeure", and he therefor was acquitted.

## A.3 Chabot (1993–1994)

A 50-year-old woman lived a life full of sad and traumatic events, among others an unhappy and violent marriage, and the deaths of both her sons of whom one intentionally ended his own life. After many years of psychiatric help and several attempts to end her own life, another attempt was to be foreseen. The psychiatrist Chabot—involved through Right-to-Die Netherlands—determined she suffered intensely, that the suffering was durable, unbearable and hopeless. After he consulted seven experts in writing and concluded that through her objection to further treatment a "realistic perspective" not was available, he assisted in her suicide by providing the lethal medication. Both the Lower and Higher Court honored his appeal for "force majeure". The Supreme Court, however, ruled guilty without punishment. The major criticism was that he did not consult experts who met the patient in person. Beforehand the requirement for consultation was less stringent. Essentials from the verdict were that it was not the source of the suffering (either being psychiatric, somatic of otherwise) but the unbearableness and hopelessness of it. This implied that suffering from a psychiatric disease could also be ground for assistance in dying from a physician, and that psychiatric patients also had a free and autonomous will.

## A.4 Brongersma (2000–2002)

The 86-year-old former Dutch senate member Brongersma primarily suffered—beside several problems related to old age—from his physical and social deterioration, the loneliness, dependency and feelings of uselessness. His physician established his unbearable and hopeless suffering, his voluntary and well-considered request and consulted another physician after which the physician provided Brongersma with lethal medication to intentionally end his own life. Initially, the Lower Court of Haarlem acquitted him as a result of conflict of duties ("force majeure"), and the Higher Court of Amsterdam guilty without punishment. Interestingly, contrary to the former court cases concerning physicians assisting in dying, the High Court of Amsterdam did not take a casuistic approach but looked for more general norms. Finally, The Supreme Court held that questions about life and existential suffering (such as hopelessness, despair, loneliness and existential suffering caused by the inability to adapt to a new situation) were beyond the doctor's professional competence. They further specified that unbearable suffering should originate from a medically classifiable condition, either somatic or psychiatric.

## A.5 Advanced dementia case (2019–2020)

A nursing home physician ended the life of a 74-year-old deeply demented woman based on her advance directive. Her written advance directive was drafted after she received the diagnosis for dementia in 2012. She re-confirmed the written advance directive in 2015, and at regular basis during several years confirmed her wish she did not want to live deeply demented in a nursing home. When she was transferred to a nursing home in 2016, the nursing home physician read her medical file, talked to and observed the patient, talked to her former treating physician, her husband and daughter, consulted the treatment team of the nursing home, the psychologist of the patient, a consultant from the Euthanasia Expertise Centre and two independent physicians who both judged the nursing home physician met all criteria of due care. After ending the life of the patient, the Regional Disciplinary Board of The Hague and the Central Disciplinary Board judged that the nursing home physician did not meet the criteria of due laid out in the Termination of life on request and assisted suicide review procedures Act and received a formal warning (93, 94). The following court case was aimed at answering the question if the physician had the duty to confirm the current wish to live or die from a deeply demented incompetent patient. The Court of The Hague judged the physician did not need to verify the current wish to die of a deeply demented and completely incompetent patient, that the nursing home physician had met all criteria of due care in the situation of a deeply demented incompetent patient and therefor was acquitted. (95) The Supreme Court confirmed that the advance directive was clear and reversed the judgment of the Central Disciplinary Board. Nevertheless, the Supreme Court did not judge about the need for the physician to consult with the patient.

## A.6 Wertheim-Elink Schuurman (1981)

Mrs. Wertheim-Elink Schuurman (1981) helped an acquaintance by supplying a lethal medication, mixing the medication with chocolate custard, feeding it to the acquaintance and offering alcohol to enhance the lethal effect. She did not inform the authorities. Something she had done before in 1974 when she assisted an aunt, something which did not result in any juridical consequences. This time she was sentenced to a half-year suspended sentence with a one-year probation period and two weeks of house-arrest. While the way she assisted was judged uncareful on all criteria the judge formulated (for example not involving a physician), she did not have to go to prison due to the physical and psychological burden because of her old age. (82) Note: Mrs. Werheim-Elink Schuurmans 'husband and a friend were also present at the assisted suicide and were not prosecuted. This indicates that that being present at an assisted suicide is neither punishable nor that there is a duty to intervene, in the sense to prevent a suicide. Also, the option of non-physicians being able to assist was judged permissible if a physician was involved.

## A.7 Heringa (2013–2018)

Albert Heringa had conversations with his 99-years old (step)mother (Mrs. Moek) about her wish to end life and eventually provided her the lethal medication to take her own lift. He filmed the suicide. This film was aired as a documentary after which Heringa was prosecuted. The Lower Court of Gelderland ruled guilty without punishment, motivated by the long trial period and the intimate bond between son and mother, and despite the absence of "medical or mental force majeure" and acting in uncareful ways. In appeal, the Higher Court of Arnhem applied the criteria of due care from the Termination of life on request and assisted suicide review procedures. Act to the assistance he offered. The Court concluded that the request of the mother was well-considered and voluntary, that she was informed about her situation, that she did not have reasonable alternatives at that time, and that the son had carefully acted. During her ingesting the lethal medication as far as his position as non-physician allowed for. He even was acquitted due to acknowledging a conflict of duties ("force majeure") between adhering to Article 294 and the unwritten moral duty to help his mother with realizing her wish to end life in a peaceful and dignified manner. However, in 2017 the Supreme Court overruled this verdict by stating that the criteria of due care from the Termination of life on request and assisted suicide review procedures Act were incorrectly applied to a non-physician, as they were specifically designed for physicians. In 2018, the Higher Court of 's Hertogenbosch sentence him to six months conditional imprisonment with a two year probation period. Despite acknowledging that the son had acted out of compassion, and the long duration of the trial, several aspects of the case negatively influenced the sentence: not enough efforts to change his mother's mind, being motivated by his conviction that the law on assistance in dying should be changed, leaving his mother alone after she fell asleep but before she passed away (and not recognizing the possibilities of complications), and not being transparent about his role in his mother's death in the years before the airing of the documentary in 2019, The Supreme Court upheld this judgment.

## Author details

Wim Graafland
PHD Protestants Theological University, Utrecht, the Netherlands

*Address all correspondence to: w1.graafland@gmail.com

## References

[1] Fourth legislative review of the Act review of termination of life upon request and assisted suicide (WTL). National Government. 2023

[2] Kono M, Arai N, Takimoto Y. Identifying practical clinical problems in active euthanasia: A systematic literature review of the findings in countries where euthanasia is legal. Palliative and Supportive Care. 2023;**21**(4):705-713. DOI: 10.1017/S1478951522001699

[3] Mroz S, Dierickx S, Deliens L, Cohen J, Chambaere K. Assisted dying around the world: A status quaestionis. Annals of Palliative Medicine. 2021;**10**(3):3540-3553

[4] Boer TA. Eind Goed, een protestantse kijk op euthanasie in Nederland. Utrecht: Kok Boekencentrum Uitgevers; 2021

[5] Leenen HJJ. Euthanasie in het gezondheidsrecht. In: Muntendam P, editor. Euthanasie. Boom: Leiden; 1977. pp. 72-146

[6] Spreeuwenberg C. Huisarts en stervenshulp. Rijksuniversiteit Utrecht, Utrecht: Academisch Proefschrift Utrecht; 1981

[7] Spreeuwenberg C. Huisartsen over hun zorg voor mensen in de laatste levensfase. Veranderingen tussen 1980 en 2020. Amsterdam: Amazon; 2023

[8] KNMG. Standpunt Euthanasie. Utrecht: KNMG; 1984

[9] Van den Berg JH. Medische macht en medische ethiek. Nijkerk: Callenbach; 1969

[10] Mochel H. Een milde dood. Kampen: Kok b.v; 1972

[11] Kennedy JC. Een weloverwogen dood: Euthanasie in Nederland. Amsterdam: Prometheus; 2002

[12] The AM. Verlossers naast God, dokters en euthanasie in Nederland. Houten: Bohn Stafleu Van Loghum; 2009

[13] Houtepen R. Verruim het medisch domein voor euthanasie en geef arts het vertrouwen. Utrecht: Medisch Contact; 2023

[14] Chabot B, Graafland W. Uitweg, een waardig levenseinde in eigen hand. Amsterdam: Nijgh & Van Ditmar; 2023

[15] Nitschke P, Stewart F. The Peaceful Pill Handbook. Independently published; 2019

[16] KNMG. Guideline Palliative Sedation. Utrecht; 2022

[17] Graafland W. Stop euthanasie en maak ruim baan voor Hulp bij Zelfdoding, Medisch Contact. Dordrecht: Springer uitgeverij; 2021

[18] Den Hartogh den G. What Kind of Death, the Ethics of Determining one's Own Death. New York: Routledge; 2023

[19] Hagens M. Non-punishable Assistance in Intentionally Ending one's Own Life outside the Termination of Life on Request and Assisted Suicide Review Procedures Act. Amsterdam, the Netherlands: Ipskamp Printing. 2022

Chapter 12

# Euthanasia: In Search of the Most Appropriate Approach

*Francesco Allegri*

## Abstract

After defining "euthanasia" and its various cases, I will analyze four normative approaches that try to answer the question: "is euthanasia right?". They are the sanctity of life approach, the liberal approach, the utilitarian approach, and the Kantian approach. I will defend the Kantian approach by arguing that it is the most balanced. The Kantian approach appears to be the most balanced from the moral point of view because it rejects the excesses of the other three positions (traditional, utilitarian, and liberal). In a particular way, against the liberal approach that ascribes an absolute relevance to autonomy, Kantians point out that in ethics, there are other important moral principles. For liberals, it is sufficient that an action concerning ourselves is freely chosen and in full awareness to be morally justified. But such action could harm us or not respect our value as persons. Like when a subject hugely harms his body with drugs. Instead, the Kantian approach prescribes that an individual ought to respect the value of his person and therefore not irreparably harm his body or mind. But respecting the value of person does not mean that we are never justified in anticipating our own death. There are anticipations of death that do not violate the respect for the value of our person. For example, in cases of altruistic suicide or when the level of suffering is unbearable and we are at the end of our existence (and therefore we have no more important chapters of our life to write).

**Keywords:** ethics, bioethics, euthanasia, the sanctity of life approach, the liberal approach, the utilitarian approach, the Kantian approach

## 1. Introduction

In this chapter I set myself the following tasks: (a) to outline a definition of euthanasia that can satisfy both those who are in favor of euthanasia and those who are against it; (b) to indicate how many and what forms of euthanasia there can be; (c) to identify and analyze four normative approaches that try to answer the question: "is euthanasia right?"; and (d) to argue in support of what I think is the most balanced approach among the four.

## 2. A plausible definition of euthanasia

"Euthanasia" comes from two Greek words: "eu" and "thanatos." In the ancient Greek language, "eu" means "good" or "well," and "thanatos" means "death."

Etymologically, euthanasia is the good death, a sweet death, a death without pain. But in a deeper sense, not every kind of good death is euthanasia. We cannot call euthanasia every kind of sweet death.

If my grandfather dies while he is sleeping, his death is sweet, good, and without pain, but it is unusual to say that he died of euthanasia. In ethical contexts, when we talk about euthanasia, we refer to an *action* or an *omission* that causes a good death. On the ethical level, we think of euthanasia in terms of an intervention from the outside (to an induced death at the hands of others). For example, in an act that makes someone die painlessly.

Moreover, it is not sufficient that an action brings about a good death to define such an action as "euthanasia." Other factors are necessary. Particularly, a certain motivation (a good motivation) is required. Let us make an example. If tonight I pass by my aunt and kill her while she is sleeping, practicing on her a painless injection to get in advance the money she has left to me, is this a case of euthanasia? It is difficult to answer yes. Why is this kind of action not euthanasia? Because in this situation, I killed my aunt for *my* own interest. But the death that is involved in the concept of euthanasia should not be good for the subject who gives it, but for the subject who receives it. The specificity of euthanasia killing, compared to other forms of killing that can be classified as homicides, consists in the benevolent intention that inspires it.

The English expression "mercy killing," with which the Anglo-Saxons define euthanasia, captures this peculiar aspect of the so-called sweet death. Euthanasia is (identifiable with) death given by pity, by compassion. When the anticipation of the death of an individual is not aimed at his benefit but in favor of those who perform the action, we cannot speak sensibly of euthanasia.

If the killing of someone for his good adequately captures the general idea of euthanasia, further clarification is necessary to arrive at a plausible definition.

Firstly, it is necessary to specify that this mode of action does not only concern human beings but also extends to the animal world. It seems a peaceful fact, but in reality, it is overlooked by many definitions of euthanasia, in which we refer only to our species.

Secondly, the anticipation of death must be deliberate, that is, intentional, not something simply foreseen but not intended as an end or a means. Without this clarification, considered essential by the critics of euthanasia, the club of supporters of sweet death would increase excessively.

Taking into account these clarifications, we can therefore define euthanasia as *any type of external intervention with which we deliberately (intentionally) anticipate the death of a sentient being, aimed at his benefit.*

## 3. The forms of euthanasia

The general idea of mercy killing can unfold in various ways, and these ways give rise to six varieties of euthanasia. First of all, euthanasia can be:

- Voluntary
- Nonvoluntary
- Involuntary

Euthanasia is voluntary when it is the fruit of a choice, more precisely a free, informed, and conscious choice. Namely, euthanasia is considered voluntary when the subject to whom it is addressed expressly requires it or gives his or her consent. Euthanasia is judged as voluntary even when a person is no longer able to express his will to die, but he expressed it clearly previously when he was lucid in an early directive and confirmed this request at regular intervals.

Euthanasia is instead defined as nonvoluntary when there is no request for death or consent from a patient is not given because the subject who should eventually decide is not able to choose. This can happen in two cases: (i) when individuals are no longer self-conscious and they did not express consent or dissent when they could (this is the case, for example, of Alzheimer's patients at an advanced stage, or those suffering from senile dementia, or even those who have suffered severe brain damage due to an accident and maybe they are in a vegetative state); (ii) when individuals cannot be and will never be self-conscious (this is the case of infants who have very serious malformations or serious pathologies or all those who suffer from severe mental disability, i.e., major brain injuries).

Euthanasia is considered involuntary when the person killed is capable of consenting to her own death but does not do so, either because she is not asked or because she is asked and chooses to go on living. Obviously, killing someone who has not consented to being killed can properly be regarded as euthanasia only when the motive for killing is the desire to prevent unbearable suffering on the part of the person killed. In other words, we have involuntary euthanasia when, although there is the possibility of asking for consent, this is not asked for or given. But it is believed the same that the subject's death is better for him or her.

However, beyond being voluntary, nonvoluntary, and involuntary, euthanasia can be active or passive. Said in non-strict but simple terms, euthanasia is active when death is caused by an action and not by an omission or a series of omissions. Passive euthanasia means letting (someone) die more than killing (someone). Euthanasia is passive when the death is caused by an omission or a series of omissions and not by an action.

Putting together the previous features, we obtain six types of euthanasia:

- Voluntary active
- Voluntary passive
- Nonvoluntary active
- Nonvoluntary passive
- Involuntary active
- Involuntary passive

## 4. Four approaches to euthanasia

We can summarize the positions on the morality of euthanasia in the following four approaches:

- The sanctity of life approach

- The liberal approach
- The Utilitarian approach
- The Kantian approach

I will outline the salient features of these four approaches and finally evaluate which of them appears most plausible.

### 4.1 The sanctity of life approach to euthanasia

The "ethics of the sanctity of life" or "ethics of the unavailability of life" expresses an absolute prohibition against all forms of euthanasia, as well as against the kind of action that closely resembles euthanasia, which is suicide. According to the ethics of the sanctity of life, it is never permitted to anticipate our death. We ought to live our life until its natural end. "Absolute prohibition" means precisely that there is no circumstance whatsoever that justifies euthanasia and therefore the anticipation of someone's death aimed at her benefit. Absolute prohibitions are those prohibitions that do not admit exceptions. In the technical jargon of moral philosophy, prohibitions that admit exceptions are called "*prima facie* prohibitions." Those who move in a perspective of only *prima facie* and not absolute prohibitions do not seem to be able to exclude any class of action. Thus, the theoretical framework that seems to be behind such an extremist position on the issue of euthanasia is precisely a form of rigid deontology built with obligations and prohibitions that do not allow exceptions. The ethics of the sanctity of life are well expressed and well represented by the Catholic Church, which, in fact, has as its official position a clear closure toward euthanasia [1].

### 4.2 The liberal approach to euthanasia (the ethics of autonomy or self-determination)

The liberal approach to euthanasia appears to be diametrically opposed to the sanctity of life approach. Moving from the ethics of the sanctity of life to the liberal approach, one moves from an absolute unavailability of one's own life to an absolute availability. Roughly speaking, we can say that from the ethical point of view, what unites liberals (what the liberals have in common) is a special emphasis placed on the principle of autonomy or self-determination, which appears to be the principle hierarchically prioritized over all others (beneficence, non-maleficence, etc.). The principle of autonomy, or self-determination, expressed in terms of obligations or duties, prescribes respect for the free and informed choices of others. It maintains that actions or norms tend to be right to the extent that they respect the autonomous decisions of others. Therefore, recognizing the value of self-determination implies respecting the choices that express it. In particular, every person has the right to non-interference in the choices that concern the most intimate aspects of his or her life.

Attributing to the principle of autonomy (or self-determination) a preeminence (a primacy) over all other moral principles means that, from a liberal perspective, people's free and informed choices (i.e., rational and self-conscious beings) about themselves must always be respected. This also applies to choices regarding the last part of their life. If an individual, at the end of his or her life (but not only in this view, even earlier), chooses to anticipate his or her own death, according to liberals, it is right to allow him or her to achieve that goal. From these premises, it follows that the liberal approach is in favor of (considers permissible) suicide as an expression of free choice. But, since there is nothing wrong with suicide, it cannot be wrong to collaborate with it either; in fact, in this view that emphasizes self-determination, the essential moral evil of murder does not consist in taking the life of an individual, but in taking his life without his permission. It is not in itself wrong to kill a person. It is wrong to kill him without his consent. And so the liberal position is also in favor of voluntary euthanasia, that is, euthanasia that is expressly chosen by an individual. And it is in favor of voluntary euthanasia in both passive and active forms. The right to choose one's own death implies the lawfulness of assisted suicide, both in the form of withdrawal of therapies and in that of active interruption of life.

But this approach is contrary to forms of euthanasia that go beyond the free choices of individuals, namely nonvoluntary and involuntary euthanasia. In particular, liberals are opposed to involuntary euthanasia, in which one even goes *against* the will of the individual receiving the euthanasia (albeit for his alleged good). His consent is not requested, even though there is the possibility of asking for it. Or the consent is not received (a dissent is obtained), and despite this, the act of euthanasia is carried out.

Examples of liberal authors who move in a liberal ethical vision are Engelhardt and Dworkin. Engelhardt's conception must be seen in the context of a metaethical perspective in which there are no longer shared objective values, and therefore, rules must be built on the basis of agreements: we agree on which principles to mutually assume. If you do not want to be killed, I will not kill you, but if you want to be killed, I will accept your request. In Engelhardt's view, there is no objective good or evil to conform to; values (and moral norms) are constructed. I cannot do to you what you do not want me to do to you. But if there is no such opposition from you, then the prohibition ceases [2, 3].

### 4.3 The utilitarian approach to euthanasia (the ethics of quality of life)

This approach expresses the point of view of utilitarian theories about euthanasia. Utilitarianism considers an action right or wrong on the basis of its consequences in terms of good and evil and benefits and harms for individuals. This criterion is also applied to the moral evaluation of euthanasia. For utilitarians, when an act or omission that anticipates death produces better consequences for an individual, it is right to do so. Particularly for utilitarians, as the nature of an act does not matter because its consequences count, the distinction between passive euthanasia and active euthanasia is not relevant. If the first is right, the second is right too.

A good example of the utilitarian approach to euthanasia is given by Peter Singer, which we can take as a point of reference for the discussion. This Australian philosopher oscillates between (or lumps together) a form of hedonist utilitarianism, which declines the goods and evils, respectively, to be maximized and minimized in terms of pleasures and pains, and a form of preference utilitarianism, by which the goods and evils to be maximized and minimized are translated, respectively, into the satisfaction and frustration of the preferences or desires of the individuals involved in a certain context. A form of utilitarianism, this last one is connected to a subjectivist theory of value (good and evil consist solely of what an individual prefers or desires and what he opposes). Singer seems to favor the latter version of utilitarianism, but over the years, he has recognized the undoubted merits of hedonist utilitarianism as well.

In one of his most famous texts, *Practical Ethics* (1979 first edition; 2011 third edition), taking the utilitarianism of preference as his starting point, he arrives at the following conclusions on the topic of euthanasia.

From the basic premises of preference utilitarianism derives the moral permissibility of voluntary euthanasia: just as a person's preference to live counts as a relevant reason for not killing him or her, similarly the fact that this preference no longer exists, and there is even a contrary preference, that is, an explicit request not to be left alive, counts as a reason to indulge this desire. Preference utilitarianism, with the space it gives to autonomy, comes very close to the liberal approach.

Faced with legitimate misgivings about the procedures to be adopted to adequately identify an individual's preferences, Singer proposes a whole series of safeguards so that no mistakes can occur.

Regarding nonvoluntary euthanasia of those who were once self-conscious but are no longer so (due to an accident that has rendered them in a permanent vegetative state or due to a severely disabling brain disease) and who, when they could, did not provide indications of their wishes in the event of an irreversible loss of self-consciousness, Singer's position is as follows. He argues that if they are irreversibly deprived of psychological states, then their lives have no intrinsic value, and it is morally justified to no longer keep them alive. If, although they are irreversibly deprived of self-awareness, they are conscious (not in a vegetative state), then their life has value only if it contains more pleasure than pain. If this does not happen, there is no point in keeping them alive.

Regarding involuntary euthanasia, Singer expresses his opposition, but he seems to be mistaken because he exemplifies it with the so-called "suppression of useless mouths" by the Nazis ([4], p. 157). In reality, such a policy of extermination toward the weak and marginalized subjects of society cannot be framed within the framework of euthanasia because it does not fit the definition. The benevolent motivation that should be at the basis of all forms of euthanasia is missing. There was no benevolent intent on the part of the Nazis in anticipating the death of those people! On the contrary! It was certainly not practiced for the good of the individuals in question.

But one of the peculiar points of Singer's treatment, qualifying the way in which utilitarianism, and more generally consequentialism, looks at euthanasia, consists in canceling (nullifying) the distinction on the ethical level between active euthanasia and passive euthanasia. In a perspective in which it is not the nature of an act that matters, but the effects that flow from it, it makes no sense to accept the passive version of euthanasia and reject the active one. For those who move in a deontological perspective, there is an important moral difference between the execution of an act that has certain consequences—for example, the death of a malformed child—and the omission of something with the same consequences. If this doctrine is correct, the doctor who gives a child a lethal injection is doing something morally wrong, while the one who omits to give the child antibiotics, with full knowledge that without antibiotics the child will die, is not doing something morally wrong. But Singer is convinced that from a moral point of view, there is no difference ([4], p. 151).

## 4.4 The Kantian approach to euthanasia (the ethics of respect for persons)

The Kantian approach to the end of life is an approach developed in bioethics by some philosophers who are followers of the German thinker Immanuel Kant. They refer to the second formula of his famous categorical imperative to outline a solution that they believe is balanced to the issue of euthanasia. This formula, which aims to indicate a general criterion for choosing the right actions to take, states: "act in such a way as to treat humanity, whether in your own person or in that of any other, always also as an end and never simply as a means." On the basis of this principle, today's

Kantians have developed an ethics of respect for persons, which, in their view, must replace the ethics of the sanctity of life but also stand as an alternative to entirely consequentialist approaches, such as utilitarianism, and entirely liberal approaches. Respect for the dignity (for value in itself) of persons must be the guiding principle from which to derive moral norms, what is right and what is wrong. Today's Kantian approach does not coincide in its entirety with the theses advanced by the historical Kant (who, on the issues of the end of life, should be framed in the perspective of the ethics of the sanctity of life). It embraces his theoretical ethics while diverging from the outcomes in practical ethics.

A good example of today's Kantian approach to the end of life can be found in the pages of Massimo Reichlin's *Ethics and a Good Death*, which is worth following closely. For Reichlin, contrary to the advocates of the ethics of the sanctity of life, it is not life that should be sacralized, but the human person. Sacralizing life leads to an exasperated and *overzealous treatment*: the continuation of life at any cost. Instead:

> *the Kantian approach is completely alien from attaching value to the mere continuation of the biological process of life: life is worth living insofar as it is the life of a personal being. Dignity is not properly predicated of life, but of the person: what is expressed in respect for physical life is therefore not a respect for life as such, but rather a respect for the person who lives it ([5], p. 185).*

Respect for humanity as an end in itself, in fact, is not only valid in reference to others but also in reference to oneself. Just as the second formula of Kant's categorical imperative states. For Reichlin,

> *the traditional expression "duties towards oneself" (...) indicates those duties that the human being has towards his own rational nature, the duties that he has by virtue of being such a creature. (...) If there were no duties of this type, one could not speak of self-respect and say that, in certain cases, it is possible to lose it. The expression "self-respect" is precisely to indicate that there is a certain standard of behavior below which a human being cannot go without making himself an object of contempt on the part of himself, even before that of others». (...) certain behaviors, in which for example the human being surrenders his freedom to others, or treats his body as an available and commodifiable object, or nullifies his rational capacity through the use of narcotic substances, are detrimental to the respect that each one should have for the rational nature, as it is found in his own person ([5], pp. 186–187).*

Since we must respect ourselves, our dignity as persons, says Reichlin,

> *self-determination (...) does not constitute a sufficient reason for the legitimacy of actions. That is, it is not enough that a certain action is freely chosen by an adequately informed individual and does not cause harm to other people for it to be defined as morally licit or approvable. (...) therefore, an action can be morally wrong not only because it violates the preferences or rights of others, or causes harm to other people, but also because it is incompatible with self-respect as a rational creature, even if it is not at all harmful to other people ([5], p. 187).*

But according to Reichlin, not even the consent of the other individuals involved constitutes a sufficient criterion of lawfulness for action. "Much of contemporary bioethics tends to consider morally acceptable everything that is done between consenting adults." According to a postmodern liberal like Engelhardt, for example, "what is wrong with murder is not ending another person's life, but doing it without permission." For Reichlin,

> *The Kantian thesis is radically opposed to these approaches, admitting further constraints than that of the consent of the interested parties or of harm to third parties: even if they do not violate anyone's freedom of choice, nor constitute harm to other people, it is possible that certain forms of interpersonal agreement are nevertheless morally problematic because they are contrary to respect for the rational creature ([5], p. 188).*

The Kantian approach, therefore,

> *leads to denying the existence of a generalized right to die, in the sense of a claim, always possessed by the human individual and justified by his autonomy, to choose whether to continue living or not: respect for one's own rational nature morally constrains individual decisions in this regard, limiting the freedom to commit suicide even regardless of the harm or suffering inflicted on other individuals ([5], p. 190).*

This leads

> *to consider suicide morally unjustified in many cases, although not in all (as Kant seemed to conclude). Certainly it is unjustified when it is motivated by fleeting and inadequately considered feelings or desires, or by a momentary lack of interest or pleasure in life, or by contempt for oneself and one's own moral unworthiness, or finally by the prediction of an unfavorable balance of pleasures and pains; and it is certainly so in many cases of even serious illnesses in which the possibility of controlling the painful symptoms allows a sufficient exercise of one's moral personality, or of writing significant chapters of one's history. The Kantian argument does not seem to be able to absolutely exclude suicide when it is the only possibility to not radically compromise one's personal dignity ([5], pp. 191–192).*

In more general and rigorous terms, according to Reichlin, the Kantian approach is based on the second formula of the categorical imperative

> *justifies the intention to end one's life only in two particular cases: on the one hand, in the case of so-called altruistic suicides, in which the main intention is aimed at safeguarding other individuals and therefore one's death is intended only as a necessary means to that end; on the other, in the case in which physical pain radically precludes the exercise of moral personality. (...) The conditions posed by the second case seem (...) such as to almost necessarily require the intervention of another person to end the life of the sufferer (...) and it therefore seems necessary to hypothesize some form of assistance in suicide ([5], pp. 101–102).*

Consequently,

> *it seems clear that the principle of respect for the person justifies the use of analgesics in the terminal phase as it aims to protect the residual rational capacities of the dying person». (...) In these cases, the only effective remedy consists in using analgesic drugs in quantities that induce, with reliable predictability, death within a short time. In*

*DOI: http://dx.doi.org/10.5772/intechopen.1010897*

> *these extreme situations (...) the choice to die cannot be considered disrespectful of his rational nature, but rather intended not to degrade his dignity ([5], p. 194).*

Similarly, "choosing, or possibly arranging in advance, a deep sedation that induces coma and death by respiratory failure does not imply a disrespectful attitude towards one's humanity" ([5], p. 195). Finally, "even when the renunciation of life-sustaining treatments involves leaving room for death within a very short time, this choice does not seem to be in conflict with the principle of respect for the person" ([5], p. 198).

## 5. Critical evaluations of the debate

The Kantian approach appears to be the most balanced from the moral point of view because it rejects the excesses of the other three positions (traditional, utilitarian, and liberal).

Against the sanctity of life approach: it is difficult to live with an ethics of absolute duties and prohibitions. And it is hard to believe that throughout history, there have never been cases in which euthanasia would have been morally legitimate. Especially if one considers that until recently, there were no adequate analgesic therapies.

Against the utilitarian approach: a deontological theory, for which consequences are not the only relevant factor in determining whether an action is right or wrong, seems more appropriate. And, with regard to euthanasia, this also means not putting passive euthanasia and active euthanasia on the same level, as the utilitarians do. The former seems preferable.

Against the liberal approach: this position gives an absolute relevance to autonomy. But in ethics, there are other important moral principles. For liberals, it is sufficient that an action concerning ourselves is freely chosen and in full awareness to be morally justified. But such action could damage us or not respect our value as persons. Like when a person prostitutes himself or harms his body with alcohol and drugs.

Instead, the Kantian approach prescribes that an individual ought to respect the value of his person and therefore not irreparably harm his body or mind. But respecting the value of person does not mean that we are never justified to anticipate our death. There are anticipations of death that does not violate the respect for the value of our person. For example, in cases of altruistic suicide or when the level of suffering is unbearable. And we are at the end of our life (we have no more important chapters of our life to write).

Although I have expressed my preference for the Kantian approach, I nevertheless believe that something more can be granted to liberals. I think that we can reconcile the reasons of the liberals with the reasons of the Kantians by distinguishing two levels of evaluation, a legal level, that of the intervention of the public force, and a moral level.

From a legal point of view, the liberals are right. You cannot force a person (suffering from a certain disease) who has chosen in full consciousness (and with full information) not to continue a certain therapy to continue it against his or her will, even if the suspension would have a fatal outcome. And this seems to me to apply in more general terms as well. If I decide, even without a justifiable reason, to cut off a finger (I do not like it because it is crooked), law enforcement cannot—*must* not—intervene because I am—*must* be—the absolute sovereign of my body. However, from a moral point of view, the situation is different. It is completely unjustified to cut off a finger (i.e., to perform a mutilation of one's body) because one feels like doing it. But, even if it is wrong, no one should forcefully prevent me from doing it. You can beg me (by kneeling down) or try to convince me with all the possible reasons, but not with physical coercion. If, in the end, in my strange mind (of which I have full possession, however), I want to proceed in this direction, you cannot prevent me.

Emblematic in this regard was the case of a woman who, a few years ago, was diagnosed with gangrene in one of her feet. The doctors explained to her in every possible way that if the foot had not been amputated, she would have died, but they were unable to convince her. The lady, who in addition to being informed appeared lucid, tenaciously and obstinately opposed, denying her consent to the surgical operation. The inevitable outcome was her death. Although her action appeared unreasonable—losing a foot is an enormous trauma, but not enough to justify losing one's life—and highly questionable from a moral point of view, they certainly did not proceed to remove her by force and take her to the operating room, cutting off her foot against her will. It is in this sense that J. S. Mill is right when he asserts that everyone is absolutely sovereign over his own body.

In other words, the liberal option appears to be the most appropriate in the sphere of *public* ethics, that part of moral doctrine that deals with duties and rights publicly established by the community toward individuals. An area that does not ask what is the morally best choice for the subject, but rather: "what can the community impose on individuals, and what space should it not infringe?" In this perspective, behaviors that are assumed as rights on which others do not have the right to interfere do not necessarily also represent praiseworthy behaviors, and there is no claim to indicate what is morally recommendable for the individual regardless of whether others have a duty not to prevent him from doing so.

On ourselves, we have the right to make morally wrong choices. On the most intimate things in *one's* life, the self-conscious, rational individual must be free from external constraints, even if his or her choices are ethically questionable. And this freedom should not *only* apply to therapeutic choices. It also applies to choices that are not therapies.

By distinguishing the ethical from the legal level, one can thus recognize the reasons of both parties. The liberal proposal appears more plausible on the legal level; the Kantian option is more convincing on the ethical level.

Taking a liberal position also on the ethical level (and not only on the legal one), we have no argument to exercise even a moral suasion toward the lady who does not want her gangrenous foot to be amputated. While faced with a case like this, it is not only permissible but *obligatory* to do everything possible to persuade the woman to give her consent to the cutting of her foot. If we adopt an *ethically* liberal position, such persuasion makes no sense. The liberal on the ethical level would say: everyone is the master of his own life. Period.

*DOI: http://dx.doi.org/10.5772/intechopen.1010897*

## Author details

Francesco Allegri
Pegaso University of Naples, Italy

*Address all correspondence to: francesco.allegri@unipegaso.it

## References

[1] Sacred Congregation for the Doctrine of the Faith, Declaration on Euthanasia. 1980. Available from: https://www.vatican.va/roman_curia/congregations/cfaith/documents/rc_con_cfaith_doc_19800505_euthanasia_en.html [Accessed: May 4, 2025]

[2] Engelhardt HT Jr. Death by free choice. Modern variations on an antique theme. In: Brody BA, editor. Suicide and Euthanasia. Historical and Contemporary Themes. Dordrecht: Kluwer; 1989. pp. 251-280

[3] Engelhardt HT Jr. The Foundations of Bioethics. New York: Oxford University Press; 1996

[4] Singer P. Practical Ethics. Cambridge: Cambridge University Press; 1979

[5] Reichlin M. L'etica e la buona morte. Torino: Edizioni di Comunità; 2002

Section 4

# Patient Critical Care

Chapter 13

# Global Bioethics and Nursing

*María Del Pilar Sosa Rosas, Laura Jiménez Trujano and David Fernando Espinosa Esqueda*


## Abstract

Globalisation is a historical process that allows the development of countries from different aspects that include education, economy, health, ecology, politics, culture, production of products and services, technology, social networks, artificial intelligence, and care. The nursing profession has a fundamental role in the latter, as it has a training based on ethics and bioethics, which allows it to apply values in the direct care of the healthy and sick person. From the origin of the nursing profession proposed by Florence Nightingale, the influence of globalisation is observed, which in the nineteenth century is consolidated to the point that it influences the being and doing of different professions that to persist have adapted the concepts of the same to their environment. Especially during the twentieth century and so far in the twenty-first century, nursing is a profession that is immersed and participates in globalisation. In this sense, we must not lose sight that this profession is characterized by individual human treatment. The purpose of this article is to give an overview of the relationship between the bioethical principles of nursing and the development of globalisation. It contains an introduction to globalisation, ethical and bioethical aspects related to nursing, and conclusions.


**Keywords:** globalisation, nursing, bioethics, ethics, migration

## 1. Introduction

The nursing profession is dedicated to the care of healthy or sick human beings specifically since the nineteenth century and is a profession that is present in all countries that are part of the Earth. The way to provide care in their role as a professional is diverse according to the economic, social, cultural, political, environmental, ethical, and legal conditions of each of the nations that make up the six continents (Asia, Africa, America, Europe, Oceania, and Antarctica).

It is necessary to clarify that before the nineteenth century, nursing care was already provided. In some countries, there were nurses who provided it, some of them were part of religious orders or were religious. However, it should be noted that the word profession is used from a non-religious aspect during the nineteenth century, when capitalism as an economic current has a great influence in the different fields of human beings.

In the aforementioned century, the profession acquires a meaning from the social, when Max Weber exposes a whole systematization of the notion of profession that is related to work and capital (purchasing power, money), where he also gives it an ethical connotation and the sense of duty of the individual with society. Since then, different concepts of profession have been elaborated. We can say that regardless of the concept, during the twentieth century, the fact that professions exist has given rise to various meanings related to the word profession, a professional, professional identity, professionalisation, professional training, liberal professions, new professions, and professional crisis, which will not be developed in this chapter.

The profession is something that provides the human being with the theoretical and practical knowledge, skills, abilities, attitudes, and specific competencies to have a livelihood within society. It gives the opportunity to be part of a particular social group that requires ethical and bioethical values to relate to the concert of society in which it is found. Given that we are living in an era of globalisation, we can say that the profession is "an occupation that monopolizes a series of private activities on the basis of a large body of abstract knowledge, which allows the practitioner considerable freedom of action and has important social consequences" [1].

At the same time, Max Weber analyzes "some beliefs of primitive Protestantism, the idea of the duty that every man has in his profession" [2], an economic movement that was imperceptible to the members of the society at that time. We refer to globalisation, a term that is used by a few theorists, especially those who were related to market, trade, economic, and political concepts.

Göran Therborn "speaks of six waves of globalisation; the first from 400 BC to 800 AD, although he states that this period is not properly global; the second from 1500 to 1700, coinciding with the discovery of America and the first colonialism; the third from 1750 to 1815, with the Napoleonic wars; the fourth from 1830 to 1918, with the second European colonialism; the fifth from 1945 to 1989, which would cover the Cold War; and the sixth from 1990 onwards, which he calls self-assumed globalisation" [3]. The nursing profession is located in the fourth wave, having been initiated by Nightingale in 1859.

The origin of the concept of profession in the nineteenth century gives rise to the creation of a specific activity, which later is nurtured by theoretical concepts and practice in society, and fits with the term globalisation. Therefore, it is mentioned in the previous paragraphs, to understand that, in globalisation, we talk about work, economy, and public policies that determine the axis in which the human being will develop. In the historical moment of the mentioned century, the care of the healthy people, but especially the sick ones, is part of the daily life of the human being, of the family life, of the compassion for the other, which does not require a payment. It requires a willingness to care for the sick or healthy person without expecting anything in return.

The fourth wave of globalisation and the industrialisation of work occurred in the nineteenth century, when men had to spend more time away from home and were paid for working and women stayed at home doing various domestic activities, one of which was caregiving. The task of care during the beginning of industrialisation cannot be performed by the members of a family or by the religious orders that have been transforming their relationship with society. Care at that time becomes a necessity that has to be performed by someone, and it is then that Florence Nightingale appears.

When Florencia wrote her book of Notes on Nursing, what is and what is not?, she initiated and consummated her proposal of professional nursing, where care is going to be provided by a woman who is not in the family, nor in a religious order, she is a civilian woman, who may have to comply with the requirement of liking to care, she is a woman of society who will eventually receive payment for caring and with this the way was opened to consider care as a job, which requires training and continuous updating to exercise it.

The title "Notes on nursing, what is it and what is it not?", shows that the expression what is it philosophically interrogates the thing, the matter, in this case this knowledge, that is described. In other words, nursing comes into existence as a theoretical concept, thus allowing the possibility of developing and constructing itself "[4] as a profession and a science.

Nursing, which began as a science and art of care, began to be built as a profession, consolidating, and refining, recreating, transforming, and establishing communication with the people who live in the society. Over time, nursing takes a special place in the population and empathy begins as an intrinsic aspect of the nurse that persists during these first 166 years from 1859, the year it was created. Nursing will coexist with artificial intelligence and robotics, because this profession is distinguished by being a human act, the human is irreplaceable. The time that this profession has existed has allowed it to be built as a science of the human and to have a body of disciplinary knowledge that considers social, biological, psychological, spiritual, and scientific aspects and thus be able to contribute to other disciplines.

"Nightingale defined nursing as an ethical profession, as well as the ethical practices embedded in this discipline. She presented guidelines for the professional relationship with patients, such as the principle of confidentiality and the taking of decisions that could potentially affect them; ideas that are still valid today in the professional practice of contemporary nursing [5]," speech by Ms Sofía Rodríguez Jiménez. This speech allows reflection on the specific characteristics that the nursing professional must have for the treatment of the human being, to provide humane care, to understand the person in their state of disease, and to clarify the doubts of the sick subject. Nursing is a discipline that needs to be continually updated, which is why the purpose of this chapter is to reflect on the nursing profession as part of the globalised world in which we live. This profession applies ethics and bioethics when providing care to the human being, in each of the stages of growth and development during life or during accompaniment at the end of life.

The chapter is structured by three subtopics, the first one is the introduction to the topic where the terms profession, globalisation, and nursing are discussed, and then we move on to the development of the topic where the relationship between globalisation and nursing, ethics, and bioethics is discussed in depth, ending with the conclusions.

## 2. Nursing: From the profession to globalisation and its ethical and bioethical aspects

Health as a theme, action, function, right, gift, need, being well, has always been present in humanity regardless of the time we mention, whether before Christ or after Christ in the East and in the original cultures of America. During the centuries that the person has been alive in the world has been interpreted in different ways, the knowledge around it is diverse and even unimaginable, the actors to achieve it have been different within the different societies that coexist and have coexisted.

In its beginnings, health was conceived as feeling well to get ahead; therefore, the construction of knowledge and its application in practice with respect to the health of the human being is a construct that has tried to be tangible; the disease is more tangible than health. The concepts of health and disease are many and diverse for each era that the human being lives, in the society, and the culture of each country is different; the truth is that health as well as disease is something that the human being needs to live, so it is an indissoluble binomial, the person is neither completely healthy nor completely sick, and many human beings live with their illness; they get used to it and nursing is a fundamental pillar.

Due to the importance of the subject, in the past, present, and future of society, it is generally discussed in a particular way from public health, having social, cultural, and diverse structures. We have to recognize that, in most of the occasions, we fail to conceive that health and disease is a process that develops next to the economic and political aspect; it is somewhat paradoxical the fact that people do not take care of themselves to have health in a constant way, and at the moment they get sick, they lose all acquisition they have to recover it, which represents a great expense and difficult to carry by the families. From a political point of view, it is easier to talk about health promotion than to offer help in case of illness, because it is more expensive.

The point we are making is that since centuries ago, health has been related to the economic power of people, individuals, citizens, what changes is whether they will pay or whether the state will cover the expenses for the process of health and disease, only for health or only for the disease, or both will cover the cost. Thus, we say that globalisation, health, and disease have always had the same path in humanity, and the difference is made by economic resources, social and cultural barriers that are intrinsic in human beings, as well as technological advances, the willingness to help and solidarity that occurs between the members that make up society.

Globalisation is a very complex term, which is not easy to define, nor can its beginning be located in a single historical moment: Pieters Jan Nederveen "places its beginnings in 2000 to 3000 BC, highlighting the ability to exchange goods and information that has always accompanied human beings" [6], almost gives us to understand that possibly from the beginning of mankind, globalisation was already being thought of.

Others place it with the beginning of the colonial empires and the European community as Robertson Roland, who "cited five phases of the globalisation process; the first or germinal between the XV and XVII centuries; the second, called incipient globalisation, between the XVII century and the decade of 1870 A.D.; the third or take-off phase between the decades of 1870 and 1920; the fourth in which there was a struggle for hegemony, between 1920 and 1960; and the fifth and last, called uncertainty, between 1960 and 1990" [7].

Robertson Robbie, locates the beginning of globalisation in the nineteenth century with the progress that was made in communication and transport of people and "proposed the existence of three waves of globalisation; the first appeared with the commercial empires of the 16th and 17th centuries; the second with the industrial revolution from the 19th century; and the third after the Second World War [8]." In this sense, we can say that, from this author's analysis, globalisation is seen as modernity, and modernity influences all spheres of human beings.

It is in the nineteenth century, where the natural commercial activities that had been given in the human being begin to be monopolised by the nascent state in Europe with their respective institutions; there is a special interest in the purchase of goods through money, a situation that marks important differences in people, to appear the power of consumption through money and the creation of modern markets where Max Weber argues that

"Modern markets do not arise from the natural propensity to barter, payment in kind and exchange discovered by Adam Smith, nor do they arise from the rational choices of individuals. For their emergence several substantive conditions must first be developed, rational modes of accounting and administration, the enactment of formal law rationally interpreted and applied by jurists, the concept of citizenship, a science, advanced technology, a modern economic ethic, the separation of home and business economics, and the absence of absolute monopolies in the marketplace" [9].

Finally, there are authors who mention that the origin of globalisation is to be found in the decade of the fifties of the twentieth century, where there was a growth of the capitalist system throughout the globe after the Second World War. Castells and Conversi estimate that this movement was consolidated between 1980 and 1990 "coinciding with the appearance of ICTs, the intensification of physical communications and the worldwide expansion of goods, and, above all, capital markets, favoured by a new political climate" [10, 11].

With this historical tour, we reaffirm that it is not easy to have a single concept of globalisation, from the points of view of the social sciences, where the capitalist society has created different constructs, from the point of view of pure science, the ideal would be to have a single concept of globalisation, because through it we could be mentioning that this concept persists without any change, which would give it the strength to be considered universally, so that a concept that comes from the economy can demonstrate that it can influence science and thus avoid speaking of globalisation in health and care as something new in the future.

Another point that deserves a deeper analysis on globalisation is that since the revolutions that humanity has had, at the beginning it was by means of hand-to-hand wars, where the creativity of the human being himself is used to create weapons capable of destroying the human being himself in a matter of seconds. Later, we also talk about the industrial revolution that gave an important advance in the production of capital and creation of work, after the second decade of the twentieth century. We must consider the knowledge society, and now, during this second decade of the twenty-first century, we must analyze the relationship of human beings with robotics, technologies applied to communication, and artificial intelligence.

With this, the underdeveloped countries, which have always sought better economic performance in order to have less poverty, are being left at an apparent disadvantage. It would seem that this is something that is difficult for each of them to achieve individually, where the ideas of health, well-being, and happiness, which persist to this day, are very much in vogue.

In the twentieth century and so far in the twenty-first century, globalisation, which seems to be new to nursing, is in the hands of the different nation-states that make up the world, the developed countries have a greater economic progress, as they have more economic power than the underdeveloped countries. Taking into account the colonization of the American continent since the fifteenth century, and seen by European countries as countries without the strength to advance, currently some underdeveloped countries have been seen as emerging in the global economy and have provided economic goods worldwide, which will allow them to make the leap, not only economically, but also in knowledge, contributions to health and of course in nursing.

Little by little, a world order is created, between brackets, which at the end of the twentieth century is absorbed by "transnational companies – having negotiated with the government of the destination country the administrative, legal, and fiscal conditions – to establish businesses that create jobs and generate wages for nationals while, if it is the production of goods for export, it will result in foreign exchange earnings, improving the country's balance of trade, making it an attractive place for permanent foreign investment by companies that, in a globalized world, seek opportunities for expansion" [12]. This has led to a greater influence of institutions at both the national and international levels.

According to the International Monetary Fund (IMF) "globalisation represents a political choice in favor of international economic integration, wich for the most part has a gone hand-in- hand with the consolidation of democracy. Precisely because it is a choice, it may be challenged, and even reversed-but only at great cost to humanity" [13].

The World Bank (WB) says that "globalisation is best understood as an extension beyond national borders of the same market forces that operate at all levels of economic activity" [14], the Organization for Economic Cooperation and Development (OECD). "The globalisation is a process of intensification of the interconnections between the different sectors inside the world scene, which has affected in the state legal authorities, and in the traditional visión of the democracy and of the paper of the national Constitutions" [15].

The International Labor Organization (ILO), as the international organization that it is, understands that it has to have a specific position on this event that is present in developed and underdeveloped countries, its "basic argument is that global governance is a whole that goes from the local to the international level and requires strengthening from one end to the other. Adopting decent work as a global objective would help guide this process towards more equitable opportunities and outcomes for all" [16].

The International Council of Nurses (ICN), founded in 1899, is the world's largest and oldest health professional organization, "is a federation of more than 130 national nurses' associations (NNAs) representing the 28 million nurses worldwide" [17], and is responsible for making proposals for nursing professionals at the World Health Assembly organized annually by the WHO. It is the one who directs the nursing pathways at the international level, and we can say that this federation was born during the globalisation that took place during the nineteenth century; its birth is prior to the World Health Organization (WHO), to the ILO.

This federation has no concept of globalisation for nursing, what it recognizes in alliance with the Commission on Graduates of Foreign Nursing Schools is that "we can anticipate the arrival of a migration tsunami as, more than ever in the past, countries around the world look to the international supply of nurses to meet their staffing needs. The pre-existing inequality in the distribution of nurses around the world will be exacerbated by large-scale international recruitment by high-income countries looking for a "quick fix" to address their nursing shortages, which will increase inequalities in access to health care globally" [18]. Nursing professionals have sought better working conditions to adapt to today's globalisation.

With the concepts of globalisation of these three institutions and the position of the other two international institutions, we consider that in the globalisation movement, in addition to the participation of a number of authors, different social facts have also been related, the economy, financing, real estate, technology, the internet with its different platforms, telemedicine, social networks, information technology (which is having more and more power and influence in people's daily lives) and health. Intrinsically, humans seek to satisfy their political, environmental, ecological and cultural concerns, which in different ways contribute and have contributed to the creation of goods and services, which are necessary for the survival of human beings.

The five international institutions mentioned, over the years have become a pillar in the movement of globalisation that occurs in all areas of human beings worldwide, in this sense we have to consider that the nursing professional plays a triple role in this movement; the first related to the care they have to provide to the population in health and disease, the second when they become migrants in search of better opportunities and the third in that it makes an economic contribution to the interior of the regions where they work outside their place of origin.

It is necessary to analyze in greater depth the concept of globalisation that is used by the federations belonging to nursing, one aspect is to say that as nursing professionals we participate in globalisation, and a very different one is to explain how, perhaps this is because nurses have always thought about the needs of people related to health and disease, situations that have become political, and the federations although they do not say it openly have a political responsibility and the nurses at the base of the guild have to know the direction of the policy that decides the fate of nursing.

It is important to highlight that in 2025 and in the immediate future, it is necessary to train a greater number of nursing professionals to deal with the health-disease problems that arise in the world. The COVID-19 pandemic, which was in almost every country in the world and which is a biological example of globalisation. One of the challenges that we have to favor is the growth of the new generations in many of the countries of the world to have young people who want to study nursing, to encourage older adults who want to do so, the other crisis that is faced with the risk of increasing even more, is that there will be a larger aging world population that will be forced by social circumstances to take care of people who are in the same conditions.

In this sense we can say that on the one hand it is good to have a longer survival time, however, it is necessary to see how many human resources we have in health to contend with it, especially because it seems that the new generations are more interested in other types of professions, because they have realized that the health professions have a heavy workload, a greater risk of exposure to infectious diseases, require greater dedication to continuous updating and a greater risk to the demands.

If we start from all the concepts mentioned above, we realize that for the first time health-illness is considered as part of the economy since the nineteenth century, although it is not specified how it affects it. In this chapter, for the purposes that concern us, we locate the birth of nursing as a profession in globalisation, in the nineteenth century, with industrialization, where, although it is not named, we begin to talk about curing the disease in a more concrete way, especially because it begins an era where local, national, country or continent production becomes a necessity for the manufacture of goods that human beings require to live and health is one of those goods that requires investment either by the individual, the community, the nation or the state.

It is necessary to express that the creation of nursing as a profession by Florence Nightingale is not an isolated event, rather it is the result of several social aspects that are intertwined, one of them is the fact of the process of industrialisation shown in the battlefield, where politics is inserted as it is considered as part and advance of globalisation. Another fact is to speak of need, a word that has been in use throughout time and will surely remain for much longer. This word in nursing would give rise to the creation, during the first half of the 20th century, of the philosophy, theory or nursing model of the needs of the American nurse Virginia Henderson, which is still in use today.

Just as the term need appears, it is said of the concept of well-being that "it alluded to physical needs, to the protection of the development process, which requires a permanent surplus of organic energy beyond that necessary for mere survival" [19], this term clarifies that the deficiencies of the population must be solved, one of them, the lack of health, said deficiency is represented by the disease in its different manifestations that the human being can acquire.

It is at this historical moment when medicine, which has existed for more than a thousand years, is seen as a profession, and with it certain roles related to the occupation arise and a division of labour begins, in which the nursing professional will be dedicated to care as an occupation and the doctor to activities related to diagnosing disease and health.

Considering medicine as a profession, "Medical practice has to be part of the special institutionalization of scientific research and the application of science to practical problems, which is a characteristic feature of modern Western society. In general, it can be said that in the instrumental division of labor the institutionalization of all roles is a functional requirement for its effective realization [20]", when talking about the division of labor, it is clear that medicine could not, and cannot, resolve everything that humans need to cure disease.

Medicine is responsible for making diagnoses of diseases that for many years have been called medical diagnoses and creates a whole series of treatments that can be implemented in human beings, said treatments require another professional prepared to carry out and monitor the therapy: the nascent nursing professional is an actor who, from a social point of view, is seen as part of medical care, willing to attend to the needs of the patient, spending long hours with the patient, the nurse must be aware of their ethical values and economic provisions for their work.

Curiously, since its origin, regardless of the country in which it is located, nursing has created various categories for the provision of care to people, a situation that makes the employment relationship between health institutions and nursing complex, creating economic differences within the same guild. It must be recognized that nursing positions are sometimes created based on the needs of doctors, this is something that nursing will have to change in the future, in the sense that social needs are considered in terms of the health-disease process, the needs of the nursing profession.

Well-being is linked to the "gestation of a new conception of the State as an entity that collaborated to promote individual and national health. The State is even associated metaphorically with the function of promoting vigor and vitality. This anticipated the importance that health would play in the well-being ideologies of the twentieth century; an importance that is reflected in all British legislation passed between 1911 and 1946" [21], and with the happiness that a human being can feel when living with others, giving rise to social happiness, then it is said that if a human being, regardless of the country he is in, if he has health, money, work, he can be happy.

Without anyone noticing, by not considering the importance of daily life, within well-being, care is installed alongside the search for health when one has an illness, giving rise to a leading role for the person who provides care from a professional perspective; the nurse, however, since caring is part of daily life and is provided by women, it is not considered as valuable as medical work. Given this fact, it seems that the nursing profession was born outside of globalisation, which is the image that has been given for many years.

This vision is demystified by pointing out that globalisation gives rise to its appearance, not only in the economic field, but also in the political, ethical and communication fields. Apart from having studied nursing with nuns, Nightingale also knew about politics, being part of a family immersed in the English bourgeoisie, this fact propitious that she had a great influence and with it she started the current of globalisation in nursing care.

Apart from what has been described here, another aspect that links the nursing profession with globalisation is migration, which is as old as man himself. The Royal Spanish Academy defines migration as the geographical displacement of individuals or groups. This displacement is for different reasons economic, lack of work, environmental, political, wars, terrorism, at the beginning of the twenty-first century, in addition to those mentioned above, drug trafficking, religious, violation of human rights and even natural disasters that reduce the chances of survival of the groups that inhabit these geographic areas.

The United Nations (UN) reports through the Population Division of the Department of Economic and Social Affairs (DESA) "that the number of international migrants worldwide was nearly 281 million. International migrants represent approximately 3.5 per cent of the world's population, up from 2.8 per cent in 2000 and 2.3 per cent in 1980" [22].

Migration, speaking in terms of globalisation, has favored the exchange and creation of knowledge, in addition to bringing economic benefits to various countries. For this reason, in 1951 the International Organization for Migration (IOM) was created, which works with national and international government organizations to find solutions to the challenges that migration entails, due to the fact that "almost three out of four international migrants were between 20 and 64 years old, and 41 million were under the age of 20. Most international migrants reside in Asia and Europe (31%), followed by North America (21%), Africa (9%), Latin America and the Caribbean (5%) and Oceania (3%)" [23].

Migration as a social movement, placing it within globalisation, causes people who move to be identified as migrants, adopting an ethical model of each region, thus an international migrant is defined as "a person who moves away from their usual place of residence, either within a country or across an international, temporarily or permanently, for various reasons..." [24].

Migrants, regardless of the time in which they are located, require goods and services, one of which is to provide health care in the event of illness, which they can acquire in the countries they pass through, because traveling means changing eating habits, as well as hygiene and cleanliness habits. A migrant requires being cared for by medical and nursing professionals, as well as other members of the health team. In some countries, for example in the United States of America, the first point of contact in the case of disease is the nursing professionals.

As described in the previous paragraph, nursing professionals require observation, communication and cultural skills to be able to care for a migrant during the twentieth century. When nursing provides care to migrants on the six continents of the world, at the end of the twentieth century and beginning of the twenty-first century, they also became part of migration groups. "At the international level, the migratory flow of nurses has responded to the need to remedy the shortage of this personnel in industrialized countries. Among the main factors of attraction, as occurs with other population groups, the current salaries in the receiving countries stand out" [25].

The migrant nursing professional hopes to improve their living conditions by migrating to countries that offer them better salaries and high-quality continuing education, however this is not always the case. In some industrialized countries, nursing professionals who have been trained in their country for a period of 4 to 5 years are treated in these countries as cheap labor. Migrant nurses do not have access to the benefits of uniform allowances, the possibility of accessing continuing education and they are discriminated against. Inequity in the treatment of people violates human rights, which is why the validity of obligations and responsibilities is supported to establish a formal process to eliminate marginalizing practices" [26].

The fact that industrialized countries, faced with the need for trained nursing professionals to care for their population, issue calls for the migration of professional nurses from underdeveloped countries and do not receive the salary they are entitled to, as they have cheap labor, is just a small example of the disadvantage of globalisation in the sense that by not paying what is due, the industrialized country is making economic gains. This is where nursing makes an economic contribution to globalisation, a contribution that also accompanies its country of origin by sending remittances; this contribution goes to the gross domestic product of both countries.

Another point to consider within globalisation, is the fact that one of the possibilities that are seen for a greater development in the profession, is the advanced practice nurse, the concept is given by the CIE, and each of the countries that are within globalisation are adapting it according to their needs and the legal aspects that they consider of the profession, the advanced practice nurse would have and has the possibility of having an independent practice, which would give rise to nursing increasing its value in the economic market; until now the professional nurse is hired more by health institutions, companies than by the civilian population.

Possibly one of the topics that has the greatest impact on globalisation from the nursing perspective is the one related to ethics and bioethics. Ethics is a science that has existed since the time of the Greeks, and over time it has undergone changes during the more than 21 centuries that humanity has lived on earth. The word ethics comes from the Greek ethos, which means "character" or way of being of a person. In this chapter, it is conceptualized as "a conscious activity of the human being, according to its macro and microcosmic reality, whose action influences and is reflected, for better or worse, in the micro and macro society that we inhabit" [27].

Ethics has always been present in the nursing profession since its creation with Nightingale and has formed and is part of the study plans of this profession. It is considered a fundamental knowledge that must be applied during practice as a student, as a professional with human beings, because human beings have corporeality and character; their behavior is different when they feel vulnerable due to illness. During this process, they have greater verbal and non-verbal communication with the nursing professional, regardless of their stage of life.

The nursing professional is aware that human beings have dignity and must therefore be treated with respect. They also know that when faced with an illness, people suffer, so "the ethics of care is based on respecting the suffering of the person and being sensitive to their pain, providing protection to both the person and their companions to avoid isolation and the feeling of abandonment; if it is the patient, making them feel less of their disability" [28].

Knowledge of ethics in nursing is supported by "the first International Code of Ethics for Nurses was approved by the Council of National Representatives (CNR) of the Council of Nurses on July 10, 1953" [29]. This code is distributed in each of the member countries of this organization, the countries introduce it into the study plans of the profession, and a whole series of continuing education courses are held for nursing professionals.

It is emphasised that, in the preamble of the code, the four fundamental duties of nursing are mentioned: to promote health, prevent illness, restore health, and alleviate the suffering of the individual, the family, and the community, including respect for human rights, cultural rights, and the right to life and free choice, dignity, and be treated with respect.

Since the beginning of nursing, the nurse has been dedicated to the care of life and death, caring for the person during the course of life, from birth, growth, and development. The nurse provides care at the death of the person, in each of the stages that the human being goes through, according to the nature of the illness. When the person dies, the nurse accompanies him/her, and, if necessary, also accompanies the loved ones.

Following on from the previous paragraph, it must be added that, in nursing care, technology is also present through different electromedical devices, mobile phones, computers, at this time technology in its maximum expression, are part of the daily life of a sick person, including social networks, computers, and artificial intelligence, everything mentioned requires that the nursing professional continues to have the ability to continue communicating with people, as one of the pillars of the profession because it has always had the ability to establish the nurse-patient relationship based on empathy.

Nursing care "also includes respect for autonomy, privacy, confidentiality, reliability and fidelity. To provide this care, the nurse must make use of a fundamental element, the nurse-patient relationship, which is built on the ethics of respect for the other as a valid interlocutor, and intersubjectivity and effective communication, respecting the cultural aspects, values and beliefs of the person being cared for" [30].

Nursing has applied the code of ethics for several years, and it has been flexible in the face of the change that has occurred in global society. The said change is directly related to the life and death of the human being and therefore allows the introduction of bioethics in its being, doing and professional practice. The term bioethics is registered in 1927 by Fritz Jahr, German philosopher and educator, and Van Rensselaer Potter, uses it for the first time in his article "Bioethics the science of survival" [31].

The inclusion of bioethics in human life, as part of the social interrelation that occurs between the groups that make up both national and international society, implies an even greater commitment of professional responsibility to human dignity, which is why the CIE saw the need to update the code of ethics during the year 2021, in accordance with the times of globalisation that we are experiencing in 2025, where it seems that national and international institutions are a ray of hope for the large number of people who inhabit the earth.

"The ICN Code of Ethics for Nurses is a statement of the values, professional responsibilities, and areas of professional accountability for nurses and nursing students that defines and guides ethical nursing practice in their various roles and areas of practice. It is not a code of conduct but can act as a framework for nursing practice and ethical decision-making, in order to meet the professional standards set by regulatory bodies" [32].

In this chapter, "bioethics is understood as a discursive, deliberative and transdisciplinary discipline, which aims to integrate biomedical, ecological, economic, anthropological, historical and philosophical knowledge in the systematic study of the moral dimensions and behaviors of human beings around life to discuss the ethical challenges that they face today and in the future" [33].

The aforementioned code of ethics and the times of globalization that are being experienced in the nursing profession allow nurses to apply the principles of beneficence, autonomy, justice, fidelity, truthfulness, and confidentiality, to fulfill the fundamental responsibilities of the nurse: by promoting health, preventing illness, restoring health, alleviating suffering, and promoting a dignified death for the human being because nursing care is a universal need for the globalisation movement in which we live.

Globalisation requires us to know the values, beliefs, customs, needs, tastes, and languages of different peoples, which makes it essential to have highly qualified and prepared human talents in the various areas of life. "With creative and innovative capacities, flexible, but also rigorous" [34]. "Universities must be open to this type of higher education by offering options that generate and increase higher knowledge, as well as the understanding of these phenomena in order to contribute to their own well-being and that of their community" [35].

In this sense, we have to say that nursing professionals should have the knowledge of transcultural nursing; realistically, this cannot be the case, because one of the greatest challenges is to train nursing professionals. The response of nursing is to raise awareness and train professionals about the fact that human beings are cultural and diverse, and care should be provided regardless of race, religion, sex, socioeconomic level and culture, applying in a committed way observation, communication, ethics and bioethics, being here and being there when caring for human beings regardless of their age and stage of life.

This implies that bioethical knowledge be included in the training curricula of professional nurses so that during their professional practice, they apply the right of universal access to health care and attention, defend the dignity, freedom and worth of human beings, contribute to the development of health policies, collaborate and protect the natural environment, and understand and comprehend their role of care in the cultures that are present in the different countries of the globe.

Bioethics training is not only for students but also for nurses who practice their profession. In this case, it must be through continuing education, whether in person, remotely, hybrid, or through international exchange. Understanding that communication is also globalized, face-to-face communication is still important, although currently communication can also be face-to-face through platforms. This fact allows for interaction, but not immediate face-to-face empathy.

The commitment of nursing to the application of bioethics in this era of globalisation is being forested more rapidly, through the technology that favours reflection and reflection, on how nursing can conduct research with these tools without ceasing to do so as it has done up to now, requires further research on how globalisation influences the bioethics applied by nursing, in the education of professional and scientific care that is given through social networks, blogs, chats, without forgetting what the application of ethics and bioethics implies; within artificial intelligence, it must be seen more as a collaborator than as an enemy.

## 3. Conclusions

This chapter allows us to reflect on how globalisation has influenced the nursing profession over time, since its consolidation in 1859. This influence has been gradual and constant, which is why nursing has a hard time realizing that it is part of globalisation. This is possibly due to the fact that, for many years, it has been said that care has nothing to do with politics and economics.

In recent years, precisely with globalisation, weight and importance have been given from an economic point of view to activities that since the nineteenth century have been considered domestic; in this case, this is the care that is provided by the nursing professional. We hope that, in the near future, economic importance will continue to continue to be given to this, because it represents an advance for the nursing profession.

The term globalisation is very complex; however, it has been present in human life at different times, acquiring a greater presence from the nineteenth century with industrialisation; at the end of the twentieth century and beginning of the twenty-first century, it has strengthened even more in developed countries than in underdeveloped ones, impacting even more with the evolution of artificial intelligence, computing, telemedicine, and the promptness of communication through social networks, but the words of well-being, need, happiness, health continue to resonate in the population, concepts that are not so easily changed.

Globalisation has been present in the nursing profession since its creation, which has influenced it to acquire a greater commitment and responsibility in providing care to healthy and sick human beings during life and death.

The challenge for nurses is to apply the bioethical principles that emanate from their profession while respecting the culture of human beings who live in different ways in this era of globalisation that is more influenced by economic power than by human values, where this globalizing movement will gain greater influence with artificial intelligence and social networks.

Nursing professionals in these times of globalisation have to understand that one of the demands of globalisation is immediacy, a difficult situation to meet because curing an illness does not happen immediately, but rather according to the care provided; each person's response to the evolution of the health-illness process is different.

The nurse is characterized by knowing how to establish communication with the person she cares for. The said communication is more fluid in person, but in this moment that we live in and those to come, the capacity to manage communication through the different platforms and social networks that exist must be increased, being more responsible with the information provided because currently sick people can find out what they want with just one click; hence, society demands greater preparation from nursing professionals.

Welcoming the challenge of globalisation for nursing professionals, which in the not too distant future, will require that nurses be better prepared and more confident in the application of the principles of ethics and bioethics in the world population, which over time has more ethical dilemmas both in person, on platforms, in hybrid, where surely the code of ethics and bioethics that is transformed must consider all these aspects that the world is experiencing.

## Author details

María Del Pilar Sosa Rosas*, Laura Jiménez Trujano
and David Fernando Espinosa Esqueda
National Autonomous University of Mexico, Mexico City, Mexico

*Address all correspondence to: sosapilar932@gmail.com

## References

[1] Fernández PJ. Elements that consolidate the concept of profesión. Notes for reflexión; electronic. Journal of Educational Research. 2001;**3**(1):24

[2] Ballesteros LA. Handbook of Max Weber and the Sociology of Professions. Vol. 25. México D.F: National Pedagogical University; 2007. 254 p. Collection of more texts

[3] Therborn G. The World, a Guide for Beginners. Madrid: Alianza Publishing; 2012. 356 p. ISBN 8420673846, 9788420673844

[4] Núñez Carrasco ER. Understanding the nursing historical perspective of Florence nightingale. Nursing and Science. 2011;**XVI**(1):12

[5] Santillán ML. Florence Nightingale: Nursing and Care Theorist. Mexico: General Directorate of Cultural Diffusion, National Autonomous University of Mexico; 2020. Availabe from: https://ciencia.unam.mx/leer/1027/florence-nightingale-teorica-del-cuidado-y-la-enfermeria [Accessed: December 3, 2024]

[6] Pieters J, N. Periodizing globalization: Histories of globalization. New Global Studies. 2012;**6**(2):1-25

[7] Robertson R. Mapping the global condition: Globalization as the central concept. Theory, Culture and Society. 1990;7(15):15-30

[8] Robertson R. The Three Waves of Globalization. A History of a Developing Glonal Consciousness. Spain: Alianza Publishing; 2005. p. 390. ISBN 84-206-4591-5

[9] Max KS, Weber. Main Dimensions of his Work. Buenos Aires Argentina: Prometeo Books Publishing House; 2007. p. 138. ISBN 978-987-574-196-6

[10] Castells M. The Information Age. Economy, Society and Culture. 4th ed. Madrid Spain: Alianza Publishing; 2006. p. 488

[11] Conversi D. The limits of cultural globalization. Journal of Critical Globalization Studies. 2010;**3**:36-59

[12] de Méler Ugarte JL. History of Globalization. Vol. 282. Madrid, Spain: Ministry of Defense, Center for National Defense Studies; 2004. ISSN 0213-6864. Available from: https://dialnet.unirioja.es/servlet/articulo?codigo=4580078 [Accessed: December 7, 2024]

[13] International Monetary Fund. Globalization; a Framework for IMF Involvement [Internet]. N.W. Washington D.C.: International Monetary Fund; 2011. Available from: https://www.imf.org/external/np/exr/ib/2002/031502.htm [Accessed: December 13, 2024]

[14] World Bank. Is Globalization in Retreat? This Is What a New Study Reveals [Internet]. N.W., Washington D.C., United States of America: World Bank; 2023. Available from: https://blogs.worldbank.org/es/voices/la-globalizacion-esta-en-retirada-esto-es-lo-que-revela-un-nuevo-estudio [Accessed: December 4, 2024]

[15] Goig Martínez JM. The OECD in the age of the globalization: Development and influence. Law Journal UNED. 2016;**19**:111-150

[16] World Commission on the Social Dimension of Globalization Labour Organization. For a Fair Globalization.

The Role of the ILO; Report of the Director-General on the World Commission on the Social Dimension of Globalization. 1st ed. Ginebra, Suiza: The International Labour Office; 2004. p. 69. ISBN 92-2315787-0

[17] International Council Nursing. Who we are [Internet]. 2004. Available from: https://www.icn.ch/es/quienes-somos [Accessed: December 10, 2024]

[18] Shaffer FA, International Council Nursing. Comission on Graduates of Foreing Nursing School, International Centre of Nurse Migration. New Report Calls for Global Action Plan to Address Nursing Workforce Crisis and Prevent Avoidable Health Disaster [Internet]. Geneva, Switzerland: International Council Nursing; 2022. Available from: https://www.icn.ch/es/noticias/un-nuevo-informe-insta-un-plan-de-accion-mundial-para-abordar-la-crisis-de-fuerza-laboral [Accessed: December 13, 2024]

[19] Hobson JA. Imperialism: A Study, Mercantile Library. New York: New York James Pott Company; 2006, 1988, 1902. 412 p

[20] Ballesteros LA. Max Weber and the Sociology of Professions. Vol. 25. México D.F: Universidad Pedagógica Nacional Publishing; 2007. 249 p. Collection of more texts, ISBN 978-970-702-230-10

[21] Freeden M. History of 20th Century Political Thought; the Advent of the Welfare State. España: Akal Publishing S.A; 2013. 787 p. for the spanish languaje

[22] United Nations. Population Division of the United Nations Department of Economic and Social Affairs. Data on Migration [Internet]. 2020. Available from: https://www.un.org/es/global-issues/migration [Accessed: December 8, 2024]

[23] United Nations. United Nations Peace, Dignity and Equakity on a Healthy Planet [Internet]. United Nations; 2020. Available from: https://www.un.org/es/global-issues/migration [Accessed: December 7, 2024]

[24] International Organization for Migration. International Migration Law No. 34. Geneva, Switzerland: International Organization for Migration; 2019. 248 p. ISSN 1813-2278

[25] World Health Organization. The World Health Report. Working Together for Health. National Health Workforce Development Strategies. Geneva, Switzerland: WHO Press, World Health Organization; 2006. 211 p

[26] Pan American Health Organization. Series. Human Resources for Health. 61 Migration of Nurses from Latin America, Central America Area, Mexico and the Latin Caribbean. Washington, D.C.: Pan American Health Organization; 2011. 154 p. ISBN: 978-92-75-33260-3

[27] Tanur TB. For a humanistic medicine. CONAMED. July-September 1999;**12** ISSN-e 1405-6704

[28] Nava Galán MG. Conceptual model of nursing, its relationship of ethics and bioethics of care with the person and their dignity. Neurological Nursing (México). 2012:91-97

[29] Oguisso T, Hiromi TM, Fernandez de Freitas G, Barrionuevo Bonini B, Araújo da Silva T. First international code of ethics for nurses. Tex & Contex Nursing. 2019;**28**:e20180140. DOI: 10.1590/1980-265X-TCE-2018-0140

[30] Garzón N. Professional ethics and nursing theories. Aquichan. 2005;**5**(1):64-71

[31] Potter VR. Bioethics Bridge to the Future. Exlibrary ed. New York: Prentis Hall Publisher; 1971. p. 205

[32] Internacional Council of Nurses. The ICN Code of Ethics for Nurses Revised 2021. Geneva, Switzerland Ginebra: Internacional Council of Nurses; 2021. p. 32. ISBN: 978-92-95099-94-4

[33] BJK A, Sandoval-Ramirez M. Ethical competencies for the development of nursing care. Revista Brasileira de Enfermagem. 2018;**71**(suppl 4):1915-1920. DOI: 10.1590/0034-7167-0539

[34] Rodríguez C, Vío CP. Need for postgraduates in Chile. Quality in Education. 2003;**18**:21-39

[35] Muñoz J. Chile and the challenges of its new economic scenarios. University and Society. 2002;**4**(24):3-4

Chapter 14

# Redefining Medical Ethics in Esthetic Practice: Balancing Patient Empowerment and Professional Responsibility

*Sylvia Ramirez and Gunther Scherz*


## Abstract

This chapter examines the ethical challenges in esthetic medicine arising from the shift to "user-driven medicine," where patients influenced by social media seek specific procedures. Practitioners must navigate expectations amid misinformation and unattainable beauty ideals. Key issues include appearance and aging anxiety, subjective beauty measures, limited treatment evidence, social media's impact, commercialization, conflicts of interest, and non-medical practitioners performing procedures. Applying Beauchamp and Childress's ethical principles — autonomy, beneficence, non-maleficence, and justice—the authors stress the need for frameworks prioritizing patient safety and well-being. Proposed strategies include shared decision-making, comprehensive consultations, setting ethical boundaries, promoting transparency and education, integrating psychological support, and strengthening ethical and regulatory frameworks. The chapter concludes that balancing patient empowerment with professional responsibility is crucial for the future of the ethical esthetic practice. By aligning medical expertise with ethical principles, practitioners can ensure that esthetic medicine transcends mere physical enhancement, upholding individuality and the moral responsibilities of the medical profession.


**Keywords:** medical ethics in esthetic medicine, patient empowerment vs. professional responsibility, ethical challenges in user-driven medicine, social media influence on beauty standards, Beauchamp and Childress's four ethical principles

## 1. Introduction

Traditionally, the doctor-patient relationship adhered to a straightforward model: Patients consulted physicians for specific health concerns, received diagnoses, and followed prescribed treatment plans [1]. This dynamic was built on trust in the physician's expertise, with financial considerations playing a minimal role. However, this paradigm has evolved dramatically. In esthetic medicine, patients frequently arrive with predetermined treatment goals or aspirations for achieving a particular appearance, reflecting the emergence of "user-driven medicine" [2]. This transformation brings a host of ethical challenges to the forefront. The intersection of beauty's medicalization, rapid advancements in science and technology, increased accessibility to esthetic procedures, and the influential role of social media in shaping beauty standards demands a corresponding shift in ethical frameworks. For esthetic practitioners, addressing these ethical complexities has become a critical and urgent priority.

The title of this chapter, "Redefining Medical Ethics in Esthetic Practice: Balancing Patient Empowerment and Professional Responsibility," reflects the evolving tension between patient autonomy and professional judgment in modern esthetic medicine. Unlike traditional specialties, where physicians diagnose and prescribe treatments, esthetic medicine stands out for its consumer-driven nature. Patients often arrive with specific goals heavily influenced by social media, celebrity culture, and the growing accessibility of esthetic procedures. While this shift empowers patients to actively shape their esthetic journeys, it also presents distinct challenges, as practitioners must navigate pre-existing expectations in a landscape saturated with digital misinformation and unattainable beauty ideals [3].

This phenomenon, often termed esthetic fluency, represents a cultural shift in which conversations about cosmetic enhancements have transitioned from taboo to mainstream. Social platforms like Instagram, TikTok, and YouTube have normalized esthetic procedures, embedding them in the broader discourse of self-care and personal grooming. However, this newfound acceptance, while liberating, risks blurring the line between genuine self-expression and societal pressures, compelling practitioners to critically assess whether a patient's requests align with their overall well-being [3].

Ethical practitioners acknowledge patient autonomy as a cornerstone of medical ethics, affirming individuals' rights to make decisions about their bodies [1]. Yet, autonomy in esthetic medicine transcends mere consumer choice. Physicians are not transactional service providers; they are custodians of patient health. Unlike the purchase of material goods, esthetic procedures involve medical risks and ethical considerations that extend beyond financial capacity. To protect patients, decisions about procedures must rest on professional responsibility, clinical evidence, and a steadfast commitment to minimizing harm.

The phrase "just because we can do a treatment does not mean we should" succinctly captures the ethical essence of the physician's role in esthetic medicine. Practicing ethically requires discernment—the ability to refuse a procedure when it conflicts with a patient's best interests or when psychological vulnerabilities, such as body dysmorphic disorder, suggest that the intervention could cause more harm than benefit [3].

This chapter discusses these crucial tensions, examining how practitioners can navigate the balance between empowering patients to achieve their esthetic aspirations and upholding rigorous ethical and professional standards. By redefining the parameters of medical ethics within this consumer-driven domain, we propose a model of practice centered on patient safety, dignity, and holistic well-being. Viewed through this ethical framework, esthetic medicine transcends mere physical enhancement, emerging as a profound acknowledgment of individuality and the moral responsibility inherent in the medical profession's art and science.

In the field of medical esthetics, where care is elective and non-urgent, the importance of ethical practice is amplified within the broader framework of medicine.

Healthcare professionals are tasked with prioritizing patient welfare over self-interest, as neglecting this responsibility can result in significant harm [4]. Despite this imperative, the ethical discourse surrounding medical esthetics remains contentious. Often referred to as the "golden goose" of medicine due to its lucrative fee-for-service model, esthetic medicine has faced scrutiny for its perceived deviation from core medical values, particularly its focus on youthfulness within a market-driven paradigm [2].

The rise of social media as a platform for professional visibility, a practice termed "medutainment," further complicates this ethical landscape [5]. Sensationalized and promotional content frequently dominates, raising concerns about the balance between scientific rigor and self-promotion [6]. Patients, who expect high standards of professionalism, may mistakenly equate social media prominence with clinical expertise, highlighting the ethical challenges posed by this trend. As a result, esthetic medicine must undergo critical ethical evaluation to align its practices with foundational principles, ensuring that patient care retains its integrity amidst these evolving dynamics [7].

## 2. Rise of esthetic medicine: Global statistics

Medical esthetics encompasses non-invasive cosmetic interventions for the face and body, including procedures such as injectables (e.g., botulinum toxin and dermal fillers), energy-based treatments, chemical peels, and body sculpting. These treatments are administered by a range of practitioners, from specialized physicians to general practitioners and non-physician technicians, distinguishing them from invasive plastic surgery, which requires the expertise of specialized plastic surgeons.

The shifting consumer landscape, emphasizing wellness, beauty, and healthy aging, has elevated the visibility and acceptance of esthetic treatments, positioning them as essential components of self-care. A comprehensive McKinsey survey from October 2021, involving 10,000 consumers and 500 healthcare professionals across key markets, projects annual revenue growth for the industry of 12 to 14% over the next 5 years [8]. Supporting this trajectory, the American Society of Plastic Surgeons reported striking increases in non-invasive procedures from pre-pandemic levels, with botulinum toxin treatments up 73%, hyaluronic acid fillers rising by 70%, and non-invasive fat reduction surging by 77% [8].

This growing demand reflects a heightened societal focus on physical appearance, particularly in a digitally driven era. While esthetic procedures can empower individuals, they also expose patients to societal pressures to conform to prevailing beauty standards. The rapid evolution of the industry, driven by innovations and trends, raises concerns about safety, professionalism, and equitable access. Anchoring these practices in safety, authenticity, and holistic well-being is essential. Ultimately, esthetic procedures should not merely enhance appearance but foster confidence and self-worth. This chapter examines the ethical complexities of the field, addressing potential concerns and proposing strategies to uphold ethical standards amidst the dynamic growth of medical esthetics [9].

## 3. Heightened ethical obligations in medical esthetics

Practicing medical esthetics entails a unique set of ethical responsibilities distinct from those tied to life-saving medical interventions. Unlike critical procedures aimed at addressing life-threatening conditions, esthetic treatments focus on enhancing physical appearance, which introduces nuanced ethical considerations [10–12]. The absence of well-defined guidelines, the pervasive influence of societal beauty ideals, and the active role of healthcare professionals in potentially reinforcing and perpetuating these standards amplify the ethical challenges inherent in this field.

The decision-making process behind pursuing esthetic treatments is intricate, often shaped by external influences such as societal and interpersonal pressures, alongside the pervasive impact of social media. These factors frequently drive individuals to seek cosmetic procedures as a means of "fitting in" or aligning with shifting norms of "normalcy" [13]. However, it is essential to recognize that societal definitions of "normal" are fluid and continuously reshaped by external forces [14]. This susceptibility to psychosocial pressures becomes particularly pronounced during pivotal life events, such as divorce, which can significantly influence choices related to esthetic interventions.

Ethical considerations in medical esthetics extend far beyond the procedures themselves, encompassing the broader context of patient motivations, societal dynamics, and the ever-changing nature of esthetic ideals. For practitioners, addressing these challenges demands a nuanced understanding of the psychological and social factors that underpin patients' decisions, ensuring an ethical approach that prioritizes well-being and informed care.

The heightened ethical obligations in medical esthetics are further underscored by the field's rapid global growth juxtaposed with a lack of well-defined ethical guidelines. Unlike traditional medicine, which centers on saving lives and promoting health, esthetic medicine involves treatments—ranging from minimally to more invasive—that aim to enhance the appearance of otherwise healthy individuals. This contrast raises fundamental ethical questions. The Nuffield Council on Bioethics has highlighted the urgent need for greater ethical scrutiny given the increasing demand, aggressive marketing, and performance of invasive procedures. While cosmetic treatments can positively influence self-esteem and confidence, they also risk reinforcing societal appearance ideals tied to gender, age, and race, necessitating a careful and multifaceted ethical approach [10].

Compounding this concern is the limited discourse on ethics within esthetic medicine, particularly in non-invasive facial esthetics. Even in plastic and reconstructive surgery, a field more established in the medical hierarchy, ethical discussions are scarce; an extensive review found that only 0.01% of over 100,000 articles in the field addressed ethical principles [15]. This "ethics gap" has been attributed to factors such as differing priorities within subspecialties, discomfort with non-quantitative disciplines, and limited training in ethical concepts. Yet, medical esthetics, arguably facing even more nuanced ethical challenges, suffers from an even more pronounced absence of literature on ethical considerations. This gap underscores the critical need for comprehensive ethical exploration to address the implications of cosmetic and reconstructive procedures for both individual well-being and broader societal norms. Collectively, these challenges reinforce the necessity of heightened ethical vigilance in the practice of medical esthetics [14].

## 4. Ethical challenges in esthetic medicine

Esthetic medicine presents a distinctive set of ethical challenges, particularly as it emphasizes refining facial appearance. This section explores the ethical complexities inherent in the daily practice of this field (**Figure 1**).

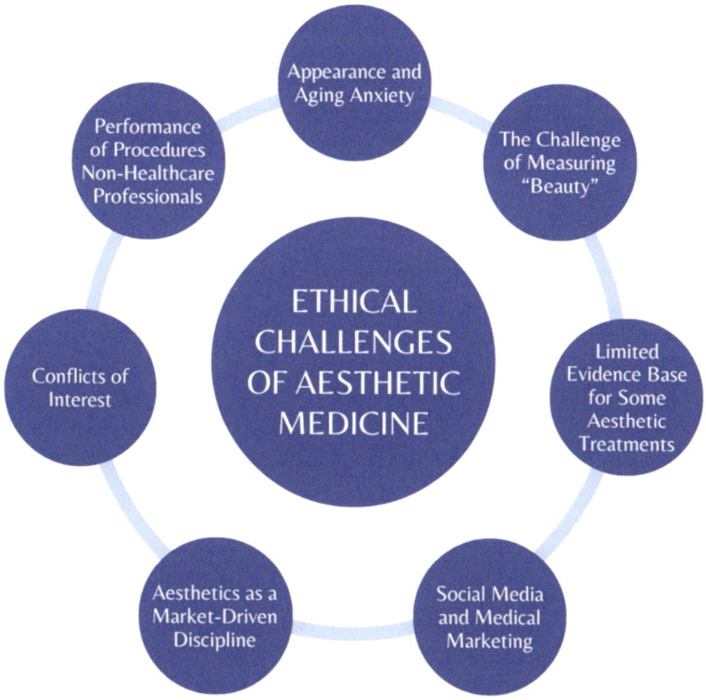
Appearance and Aging Anxiety
The Challenge of Measuring "Beauty"
Limited Evidence Base for Some Aesthetic Treatments
Social Media and Medical Marketing
Aesthetics as a Market-Driven Discipline
Conflicts of Interest
Performance of Procedures Non-Healthcare Professionals
ETHICAL CHALLENGES OF AESTHETIC MEDICINE

**Figure 1.**
*This figure gives a brief overview of the unique and complex ethical challenges that professionals in esthetic medicine face. It outlines these various challenges and helps explain the specific ethical issues in the field.*

### 4.1 Appearance and aging anxiety

The pervasive cultural belief that beauty equates to success, happiness, and societal acceptance is perpetuated by media that champions a narrow and restrictive ideal of beauty, emphasizing youth, symmetry, and thinness [14]. As a result, individuals often feel compelled to conform to these ideals, sometimes against their personal values. Women disproportionately bear this burden, while non-Caucasian individuals face additional pressures to align with Eurocentric beauty standards [16]. Furthermore, beauty norms are ever-changing, shaped consciously and subconsciously by societal influences. This cultural fixation on appearance and youth has led to heightened anxiety about one's looks and the natural aging process, driving many to pursue procedures aimed at meeting these unattainable standards [15].

Perceptions of what is "normal" are constantly evolving, influenced by exposure to idealized imagery that reshapes notions of attractiveness [17]. Studies show that repeated exposure to images of slim figures can shift individuals' body ideals and perceptions of attractiveness toward thinner standards, distorting their understanding of normalcy. These societal pressures can prompt individuals to alter their appearance, fueling demand for esthetic treatments [18]. While practitioners are not directly responsible for these dynamics, their approach during consultations can either mitigate or exacerbate appearance-related anxieties. Discussions of esthetic concerns must be handled delicately to avoid introducing new insecurities to patients.

Beyond appearance anxiety, aging anxiety represents another significant societal concern. Youthfulness remains a central criterion for attractiveness, fostering apprehensions not only about self-esteem but also about the social and professional consequences of visible aging [19]. Ageism, or prejudice based on age, exacerbates these fears, contributing to mental health challenges like depression among older adults. In promoting "anti-aging" treatments, practitioners risk perpetuating age-related stigma and reinforcing negative stereotypes about aging [20].

As esthetic professionals, it is essential to critically evaluate how language, practices, and treatments impact societal attitudes toward aging. Shifting the focus from youth-centered beauty ideals to an inclusive approach that values individuals at all life stages can help counteract the unintended consequences of ageism. By fostering a more compassionate, age-inclusive perspective, the field can contribute to a broader appreciation of beauty in all its forms.

### 4.2 The challenge of measuring "beauty"

Esthetic medicine faces a significant challenge in the subjective nature of measuring esthetic outcomes. Unlike other medical disciplines with objective benchmarks, beauty is inherently difficult to define, complicating the evaluation of cosmetic interventions. While esthetic scales or broad assessments of improvement are often used, these methods remain subjective and insufficiently standardized [21]. To address this gap, validated patient-reported outcomes like the Face-Q questionnaire have become invaluable. Specifically designed to assess patient satisfaction and quality-of-life changes following elective facial rejuvenation procedures, Face-Q has emerged as a critical tool in medical esthetics research. Despite its prominence in the academic literature, the consistent use of such measures in clinical practice is rare, highlighting the need for routine integration to better align patient and practitioner perceptions of success.

### 4.3 Limited evidence base for some esthetic treatments

Another ethical challenge lies in the limited evidence base supporting certain esthetic procedures, many of which are implemented in clinical settings without rigorous validation. Unlike medical therapies that undergo stringent safety and efficacy evaluations, emerging esthetic techniques often lack comprehensive clinical scrutiny. For example, polynucleotides derived from fish sources, such as salmon and trout, are widely used in Southeast Asia despite minimal clinical studies and an undefined mechanism of action [22]. Similarly, the injectable liquid polycaprolactone marketed as Gouri is frequently employed as a dermal filler despite no published clinical studies, with its website citing only early-phase trials involving 200 subjects [23].

This disparity in the level of scrutiny raises ethical concerns about patient safety, informed consent, and the financial implications of unproven treatments. While innovation is vital to the advancement of medical esthetics, the field's unique focus on elective procedures necessitates specific guidelines to ensure ethical practice and safeguard patient welfare. Establishing robust processes for evaluating new interventions is essential to uphold both scientific rigor and ethical responsibility.

### 4.4 Social media and medical marketing

The expansive reach of social media introduces a complex ethical landscape, as highlighted by Henrique M. and Patnaik D. in their exploration of its influence on beauty standards [24]. Unlike peer-reviewed medical literature, the digital domain lacks rigorous scrutiny, leaving it vulnerable to misinformation. Compounding this issue is the absence of institutional oversight in many regions, allowing social media to foster hype and exaggeration at odds with the integrity of medical practice. Despite these challenges, social media remains a vital tool for marketing, particularly in esthetic medicine and plastic surgery, amplifying its ethical significance.

Social media's influence on self-perception and psychological well-being is profound. While initially envisioned as a means of enhancing human connectivity, it has fueled a fixation on appearance, driven by filters, social influencers, and curated content. A study involving 763 individuals found significant links between social media use and markers of depression, social anxiety, appearance anxiety, and appearance rejection sensitivity [25]. Encouragingly, interventions such as limiting social media to 1 hour daily for 3 weeks have shown notable improvements in self-esteem among young women with body dysmorphic disorder, demonstrating the potential for small changes to counteract its negative effects [26].

The use of filters presents another ethical dilemma by promoting a narrow definition of beauty, epitomized by the so-called "Instagram face," characterized by elevated cheekbones, flawless skin, and full lips. This trend not only undermines individuality but fosters unhealthy comparisons with airbrushed versions of oneself, pushing individuals toward unattainable ideals. Similarly, the rise of influencers endorsing esthetic procedures complicates the landscape. Without formal credentials or oversight, influencers often present curated and sensationalized content that promotes unrealistic expectations while underemphasizing risks, complications, and maintenance requirements [27].

Social media also serves as a powerful channel for physicians to connect with patients, offering opportunities to build familiarity and trust. However, this accessibility raises ethical concerns. Pre-existing online connections can blur professional boundaries, potentially making it harder for physicians to deny inappropriate treatment requests. Navigating this dynamic requires practitioners to balance the advantages of engaging with patients online while upholding ethical standards [28].

As the digital era reshapes esthetic medicine, practitioners face the dual challenge of adapting to evolving cultural trends while maintaining ethical rigor. Thoughtful curation of social media content and a critical assessment of its impact on patient expectations are essential for fostering a responsible and trustworthy online presence. By striking this balance, esthetic physicians can harness the benefits of social media while mitigating its ethical pitfalls [29].

### 4.5 Esthetics as a market-driven discipline

The rise of social media and the internet has profoundly reshaped the marketing and advertising of cosmetic procedures, influencing how patients evaluate esthetic practitioners and understand treatments. Today, patients frequently enter consultations with a well-defined vision of their desired outcomes, reflecting a shift from the traditional "doctor-led" model to a more modern, "user-led" approach [30]. This evolution underscores the growing role of patient aspirations as the foundation for esthetic interventions.

Studies reveal that as many as 70% of patients depend on the internet to assess surgeons and explore procedures, highlighting the internet's critical influence on patient attitudes. However, this reliance on online information presents challenges for physicians, especially when patients arrive with fixed expectations that may not align with medical realities. Physicians are often placed in a delicate position, balancing the need to respect patient autonomy with their ethical duty to guide patients toward safe and appropriate choices [31].

The pervasive influence of social media in shaping perceptions of cosmetic procedures has prompted a call for clearer guidelines on its ethical use in esthetic medicine. The medical community must address the ethical complexities that arise as patients increasingly turn to social media for decision-making. Balancing patient autonomy with informed consent and professional responsibility is critical in ensuring ethical practice in this rapidly evolving, market-driven discipline.

As medical esthetics continues to thrive in this user-centric landscape, practitioners must navigate the fine line between honoring patient preferences and upholding their ethical obligations. By fostering transparent communication, providing evidence-based guidance, and adhering to ethical standards, the field can responsibly adapt to the changing dynamics of patient expectations in the digital era [32].

### 4.6 Conflicts of interest

The intricate relationship between physicians and the pharmaceutical industry casts a spotlight on financial conflicts of interest within medical esthetics, a concern magnified by the industry's proactive marketing and commercial focus. Esthetic medicine has become a significant business sector, with its growth fueled by this intersection of beauty and commerce [33]. A survey of American Society of Plastic Surgery members revealed the prevalence of these conflicts, with 75% of respondents acknowledging acceptance of gifts from industry representatives and 58% open to receiving them in the future. While such exchanges are often justified as tools for increasing awareness of new therapies, they are rarely discussed transparently, reflecting the nuanced and often uneasy stance physicians hold on the matter [34].

Collaboration between esthetic practitioners and the industry is widespread, with pharmaceutical companies supporting nearly 65% of all U.S. medical research, including clinical trials and consulting roles [35, 36]. However, these relationships can influence decision-making, consciously or subconsciously, creating ethical dilemmas. Society expects medical evaluations to prioritize patient welfare, yet evidence suggests that financial ties impact clinical outcomes. For example, a literature review found that studies with declared financial conflicts were seven times more likely to report favorable outcomes than those without such ties [37]. Similarly, physicians receiving compensation from pharmaceutical companies were 58% more likely to prescribe specific drugs, raising concerns about compromised objectivity. In plastic surgery, factors such as personal finances, surgical center ownership, and remuneration disparities further affect treatment recommendations [38, 39].

The American Medical Association (AMA) advises against industry funding for professional education to address these concerns. However, this guidance may be impractical in esthetic medicine, where pharmaceutical companies sponsor most conferences, training, and research for private practitioners. Navigating these challenges demands the development and enforcement of explicit guidelines to safeguard ethical decision-making and ensure patient-centric care in a field where financial interests and medical practice frequently intersect [40].

### 4.7 Performance of procedures by non-doctors and non-healthcare professionals

In several countries, non-physicians—including individuals without formal medical training—are permitted to perform non-surgical esthetic procedures. Regulations governing these practices vary widely, with no centralized database documenting the standards across regions. For instance, in the U.S., medical spas now outnumber physician-led cosmetic practices in 73% of major cities [41]. These facilities frequently employ non-physician operators with inconsistent training in dermatology and cosmetic techniques, leading to a lack of standardized oversight. Similarly, in the UK, a recent evaluation revealed that 23% of practitioners providing esthetic treatments are not doctors, nurses, dentists, or dental nurse professionals, highlighting significant variability in provider qualifications [42]. In contrast, countries like Singapore restrict injectable treatments to physicians and dentists, demonstrating a more cautious regulatory stance [42, 43].

The disparity in training and expertise among providers raises serious concerns about patient safety. While common complications such as bruising and swelling are generally mild and reversible, the surge in procedures has been accompanied by an increase in severe adverse events. Notably, vascular complications caused by dermal fillers, such as permanent blindness or stroke, though rare (estimated at 0.01–0.05% per treatment) [44], have become more frequent as the popularity of fillers grows. With over 4 million filler treatments conducted in the U.S. alone in 2022, the potential for harm underscores the need for stricter oversight [41, 44–46].

Theoretical and hands-on training deficiencies among beauty service providers pose a direct challenge to the ethical principle of non-maleficence. Ideally, only highly trained physicians should administer cosmetic procedures, with oversight and accreditation from recognized professional bodies. Recognizing these risks, licensing authorities in countries like the UK and Australia have begun tightening regulations for practitioner certifications. However, these efforts remain in the early stages, underscoring the urgent need for robust and enforceable standards to ensure patient safety and uphold ethical practice in esthetic medicine [47].

## 5. Beauchamp and Childress's four core ethical principles in esthetic medicine

Navigating the complex ethical landscape of esthetic medicine requires a systematic approach grounded in the established ethical frameworks. The Moral Theory of Principlism, introduced by Beauchamp and Childress in 1979, provides a foundational lens for this analysis [1]. Widely embraced across various domains of medical ethics, this framework is built on four key principles: respect for autonomy, beneficence, non-maleficence, and justice. These principles serve as a guiding compass for contemporary medical practice, ensuring that patient care aligns with ethical standards. The application of these principles within the evolving field of medical esthetics is discussed below, offering insights into their relevance and challenges in addressing the unique ethical dimensions of this discipline.

### 5.1 Autonomy

In medical esthetics, the principle of autonomy represents a cornerstone of ethical practice, obligating practitioners to uphold patients' rights to self-determination. Beyond fulfilling legal requirements, respecting autonomy emphasizes informed consent, patient-centered care, and a recognition of the subjective nature of beauty [17]. A patient's unique esthetic goals and expectations form the foundation of the consultation process, making transparent and empathetic communication essential.

However, autonomy does not equate to granting arbitrary requests based solely on personal preferences or financial means [10]. Physicians must act not as executors of demands but as ethical stewards, guiding patients toward treatment plans that align with professional standards and prioritize safety and well-being.

The informed consent process is central to respecting autonomy and requires more than securing a signature. It involves detailed discussions of risks, benefits, and alternatives tailored to individual patient needs [48]. Studies reveal that only 21–86% of patients retain information about risks post-operatively, underscoring the need for robust communication strategies [49]. Effective consent discussions should ideally last 15–30 minutes, though complex esthetic procedures may require even more time [50]. Combining oral and written communication enhances patient understanding, particularly for facial cosmetic treatments [51]. This highlights the necessity for personalized, well-structured consent processes in medical esthetics.

Informed consent is guided by three standards [52]: the professional standard, based on what physicians typically disclose; the reasonable patient standard, emphasizing information a prudent patient would need; and the specific patient standard, which accounts for individual patient values. Increasingly, the focus has shifted to the reasonable patient standard, fostering shared decision-making as a collaborative model. Shared decision-making integrates clinical expertise with patient values and preferences, creating a partnership where patients articulate their goals and practitioners provide evidence-based guidance [52, 53].

Despite its advantages, shared decision-making remains underutilized. A comprehensive review, focusing on complex choices related to breast reconstruction surgery, observed a notable absence of widespread adoption of shared decision-making in clinical practice, particularly among women considering postmastectomy breast reconstruction [54]. The U.S. Agency for Healthcare Research and Quality recommends the "SHARE" approach as a structured methodology for shared decision-making to better address these challenges [55]. However, shared decision-making remains a challenging and time-intensive approach. The medical esthetic community could benefit from targeted education and training initiatives aimed at improving proficiency in this consultation method. Embracing shared decision-making as the field progresses has the potential to facilitate a more harmonious collaboration between practitioners and patients, ultimately resulting in treatment choices that better align with the individual preferences and goals of esthetic medicine consumers [56].

## 5.2 Beneficence

The ethical principle of beneficence underscores the moral imperative for medical actions to prioritize the patient's welfare, fostering interventions designed to provide tangible benefits [7]. In medical esthetics, advancements in non-invasive procedures such as energy-based devices, botulinum toxin, and dermal fillers have shown effectiveness in addressing cosmetic concerns like wrinkles, skin laxity, and skin quality. However, the application of beneficence in this context is complicated by the inherently subjective nature of esthetic improvements, evolving societal beauty standards, and the lack of standardized endpoints for evaluating success [3]. This subjectivity often necessitates the use of patient-reported outcome measures (PROMs) to assess both appearance-related enhancements and health-related quality of life (HR-QOL). Tools like the FACE-Q Esthetic module, specifically validated for facial esthetic procedures, have proven valuable in capturing patients' satisfaction and perceived outcomes in clinical trials and studies [57]. Nonetheless, the routine adoption of these validated PROMs in everyday esthetic practice remains inconsistent, highlighting a gap between research findings and clinical implementation that warrants further exploration [58, 59].

Although debates about the integration of esthetic practices into the framework of core medical ethics persist, emerging evidence indicates that esthetic medicine transcends superficial beautification by addressing psychological and social dimensions of well-being. For instance, studies using the Beck Depression Questionnaire reveal that botulinum toxin treatments significantly reduce depression symptoms, demonstrating benefits beyond esthetic improvement [60]. Comprehensive reviews consistently underscore the psychological and quality-of-life benefits of multimodal approaches. The Harmony study, a multi-center, five-month prospective investigation employing validated patient-reported measures, serves as compelling evidence for the broader impact of esthetic procedures [61]. Combinations of fillers, botulinum toxin, skincare, and other serums led to significant improvements in patients' psychological well-being, social confidence, and perceptions of aging appearance. The Harmony study's results are striking, showing substantial improvements in various patient outcome measures. Beyond enhancing self-perception, these combination treatments positively influence how others perceive the treated individuals. In a related analysis, observers judged treated patients as more attractive, approachable, socially adept, friendlier, healthier, younger, and more successful at attracting others [62]. After treatment, people in the images were viewed as more educated, more financially successful, and having higher-level jobs compared to before treatment. These findings are consistent with the well-established "halo effect," where judgments of appearance influence perceptions unrelated to physical attributes [63]. Such evidence demonstrates that esthetic medicine aligns with the medical value of enhancing overall well-being, bridging physical and psychological health to deliver multidimensional benefits.

This underscores the genuine opportunity and responsibility borne by esthetic practitioners, as treatments can have far-reaching implications on a patient's quality of life, affecting how individuals are treated by others. The ethical principle of beneficence, in the context of medical esthetic procedures, highlights the potential positive impact on both individual well-being and social interactions, reinforcing the commitment to prioritize the patient's best interests.

### 5.3 Non-maleficence

The principle of non-maleficence, central to medical ethics, finds its origins in the ancient Hippocratic Oath, a timeless ethical guide attributed to Hippocrates that has profoundly influenced medical conduct across centuries [64]. Although the tradition of reciting the Oath during medical graduation ceremonies varies globally—some institutions maintain this practice while others do not—its foundational values remain deeply embedded in the ethos of the medical profession. A notable study reveals that 59% of physicians regard the Hippocratic Oath as highly significant, underscoring its continued relevance as a moral compass [65]. This enduring influence is reflected in the principles of non-maleficence, beneficence, confidentiality, and humility, which guides physicians to prioritize patient safety, uphold trust, and maintain ethical integrity in their practice. The enduring legacy of the Hippocratic Oath reinforces its role as a unifying ethical framework, transcending its ceremonial recitation to shape medical values in practice [66, 67].

The principle of non-maleficence, integral to medical ethics, is guided by three core tenets: avoiding intentional harm, exercising discretion in patient-driven treatment requests, and recognizing the boundaries of one's expertise [7]. In the context of medical esthetics, non-maleficence calls for practitioners to critically evaluate whether a procedure aligns with the patient's best interests rather than merely fulfilling their desires. This distinction between what "can" be done versus what "should" be done is pivotal, highlighting the ethical obligation to avoid unnecessary or potentially harmful esthetic interventions. While patient autonomy is a cornerstone of medical ethics, it must not override the clinician's professional judgment. Esthetic practitioners are thus ethically compelled to refuse procedures that fail to meet realistic expectations or align with the patient's holistic well-being. This requires not only technical competence but also a nuanced understanding of the patient's motivations, expectations, and psychological needs, reinforcing the commitment to ethical practice in esthetic medicine [68].

The persistent insistence of patients on undergoing esthetic treatments, especially with dermal fillers, combined with physicians complying with these requests, can result in a visually striking outcome referred to as the "overfilled face." This syndrome is characterized by excessively rounded apple cheeks, with an abnormal projection of facial fat pads, especially when smiling, rendering the patient in a perpetual squint. The multifaceted origins of this appearance include factors such as improper assessments, flawed techniques, unsuitable filler selection, and the cumulative impact of previous dermal filler treatments [62]. A behavioral factor contributing to this issue is known as "perception drift" [63]. In settings where an overfilled esthetic becomes widespread, the distorted look can become the norm and may even be considered an ideal of beauty. With each successive treatment, as patients and practitioners pursue wrinkle and line reduction, gradual alterations accumulate, obscuring the memory of their initial appearance. This augmented esthetic becomes the patient's new reality, drifting further from their natural baseline often without their awareness. As exposure to excessively manipulated facial features rises, there is a resulting perceptual shift in how attractiveness is defined and perceived.

The transverse facial septum, a structural element linked to the zygomaticus major muscle, plays a critical role in midface esthetics and the pathogenesis of the "overfilled face." This septum supports the deep medial and lateral cheek fat compartments, functioning as a "hammock" that maintains the facial structure at rest [69]. During smiling, the contraction of the zygomaticus major increases tension in the septum, resulting in an anterior and cranial shift of the midfacial fat compartments. This dynamic behavior can exacerbate the overfilled appearance, particularly in cases of excessive or improperly placed dermal fillers. These findings underscore the importance of incorporating dynamic facial assessments into esthetic procedures. Practitioners must evaluate patients not only in a static, resting state but also while the face is engaged in movement to ensure natural volumization outcomes. This approach minimizes the risk of creating unnatural projections and emphasizes the need for precise anatomical understanding and technique in midface augmentation.

The growing phenomenon of "filler fatigue," colloquially known as the "Big Dissolve," highlights increasing patient awareness and concerns regarding the risks of overfilled appearances, leading to a rise in requests for dermal filler reversals [69]. Although formal quantitative studies on this trend are scarce, clinical observations and patient consultations indicate heightened recognition of the esthetic and social pitfalls associated with overfilling. This paradox, where esthetic procedures intended to enhance well-being may result in distortion and negative perceptions, underscores

*DOI: http://dx.doi.org/10.5772/intechopen.1008821*

the need for cautious application. For instance, studies on women's motivations for lip fillers reveal that repeated exposure to augmented images intensifies the desire for such treatments, potentially driving anatomical distortion over time [70]. This reinforces the necessity for practitioners to balance the transformative potential of esthetic interventions with an acute awareness of their psychological and societal impacts. Judicious application, grounded in realistic patient education and discretion, is essential to mitigate the risks of the overfilled syndrome and uphold the ethical principle of non-maleficence.

### 5.4 Distributive justice

Distributive justice, a cornerstone of ethical medical practice, demands equitable access to care, ensuring that treatment opportunities are not unduly influenced by socioeconomic, demographic, or clinical disparities. In medical esthetics, this principle takes on added complexity due to the elective and non-essential nature of the treatments. While these procedures can significantly enhance psychological well-being and quality of life, their high costs often restrict access to affluent individuals, thereby perpetuating inequities in who can pursue these benefits [1].

The financial barrier inherent to esthetic treatments has led to a growing concern about a "two-tiered system of beauty," where access to youth-preserving and confidence-enhancing procedures is limited to those with greater financial means. This disparity underscores the challenge of achieving distributive justice in a domain so heavily influenced by market dynamics [4]. The ethical question arises: Should esthetic treatments that enhance well-being, although elective, be considered a form of healthcare that warrants broader accessibility?

#### *5.4.1 Financial and social barriers*

The cost of esthetic procedures creates a visible divide, fostering societal perceptions of beauty that are attainable primarily by the wealthy [13]. For instance, treatments such as injectables, energy-based devices, or advanced skin therapies often remain out of reach for individuals in lower income brackets. This issue mirrors the controversies surrounding access to semaglutide, a drug originally developed for diabetes but co-opted for off-label weight loss purposes. Dubbed the "Hollywood Drug," semaglutide has become a symbol of resource inequity, where market-driven demand for esthetic outcomes limits its availability for those with genuine medical needs [71].

Similarly, esthetic treatments risk being commodified to the extent that societal norms equate youth and beauty with success, compounding the pressures on individuals unable to afford such procedures. This commodification not only challenges the principles of equity but also highlights the moral responsibility of practitioners to address societal implications [22].

#### *5.4.2 Strategies for promoting equity*

Addressing these barriers requires innovative approaches to democratize access to esthetic care. Clinics and practitioners could consider implementing strategies such as:

1. Flexible payment plans: By introducing installment-based payment systems, clinics can make procedures more financially accessible, ensuring that economic constraints do not entirely exclude individuals from accessing care (Cantor).

2. Community outreach programs: Initiatives aimed at underserved communities, including pro bono treatments or subsidized care for individuals with specific needs (e.g., scar treatment after trauma), can enhance access.

3. Insurance collaboration: Encouraging the inclusion of certain medical esthetic procedures in insurance plans, particularly those with documented health benefits (e.g., treatments for conditions like rosacea or acne), could bridge the gap between esthetics and therapeutic care [72].

*5.4.3 Ethical considerations in practice*

The pursuit of distributive justice in esthetics must be balanced with the realities of market-driven dynamics and the elective nature of these procedures. Nevertheless, practitioners bear the ethical responsibility to acknowledge and address the societal implications of limited accessibility. Aligning individual patient care with broader social equity ensures that the benefits of medical esthetics do not remain the privilege of a select few but contribute to holistic well-being across diverse populations [22].

Practitioners also hold a unique position as advocates for systemic changes in policy and public perception. They can actively promote the integration of esthetic procedures with psychological and social well-being frameworks, emphasizing their potential contributions beyond physical enhancement [1]. Collaborative efforts with regulatory bodies to standardize pricing, transparency, and accessibility further underscore the ethical commitment to distributive justice [13].

## 6. Discussion/conclusion

This review provides a thorough and contemporary analysis of medical ethics as it pertains to non-invasive facial esthetics, addressing the complex interplay between societal trends and ethical practice. The growing demand for esthetic procedures reflects an intensified societal focus on physical appearance, often amplified by social media platforms that shape and perpetuate dynamic beauty standards. Social media not only drives patient aspirations but also introduces ethical dilemmas, including the normalization of unattainable ideals, the potential for overmedicalization of natural aging, and the prioritization of cosmetic enhancement over holistic well-being. These trends compel practitioners to navigate an evolving landscape where patient desires are influenced by external pressures, raising critical ethical questions about beneficence, non-maleficence, and justice. The practitioner's role in this context extends beyond technical expertise to include the responsibility to educate patients, manage expectations, and uphold ethical principles that prioritize realistic and safe outcomes in esthetic care.

In the patient-driven realm of medical esthetics, ethical practice necessitates a balanced application of the four fundamental principles: autonomy, beneficence, non-maleficence, and distributive justice. Social media's pervasive influence challenges autonomy by pressuring individuals to conform to unrealistic beauty ideals, while financial incentives and recognition-seeking behaviors within the esthetic community can undermine beneficence and non-maleficence. To uphold ethical integrity, practitioners must ensure patients make autonomous decisions through comprehensive, informed discussions about risks, benefits, and alternatives. Beneficence requires that interventions genuinely enhance the quality of life rather than merely fulfill fleeting esthetic desires, while non-maleficence demands vigilance against harm, including risks such as "overfilled syndrome." Distributive justice, though traditionally focused on equitable resource allocation, in esthetics involves addressing accessibility disparities arising from socioeconomic barriers. Adherence to these ethical principles becomes crucial as the field evolves amidst rising demand and societal pressures, enabling practitioners to navigate the complexities of balancing individual patient desires with the broader responsibility of ethical, equitable care in medical esthetics.

The practice of esthetic medicine exists within a unique ethical paradigm, shaped by the confluence of consumerism, social pressures, and professional medical standards. As explored throughout this chapter, the field is defined by the need to balance patient empowerment with the physician's responsibility to ensure safety, realism, and long-term well-being. This dual mandate requires more than just technical expertise; it demands a conscientious and holistic approach to patient care that is both ethical and empathetic.

To address the inherent tensions in esthetic practice, a multifaceted strategy is essential:

1. Strategic emphasis on shared decision-making

Shared decision-making (SDM) is a cornerstone of ethical esthetic practice [73]. SDM fosters an open, collaborative dialog, allowing practitioners to balance their medical judgment with the patient's esthetic goals. By leveraging tools like digital imaging, before-and-after comparisons, and decision aids, practitioners can offer patients a clear understanding of realistic possibilities, reducing dissatisfaction and mitigating the influence of unattainable beauty standards. This approach not only aligns treatment plans with the patient's values but also ensures decisions are evidence-based and grounded in ethical practice. By promoting patient ownership of choices while managing expectations, SDM enhances trust and satisfaction, creating a patient-centered framework for esthetic interventions.

2. Comprehensive consultation process

An extended and in-depth consultation process is critical to aligning patient expectations with realistic and achievable outcomes in esthetic medicine [74]. Beyond discussing procedural risks and benefits, these consultations should explore the underlying motivations behind a patient's desires, identifying potential psychological vulnerabilities such as body dysmorphic disorder (BDD) or the impact of social media ideals. Addressing these factors ensures that esthetic interventions contribute positively to patient well-being rather than exacerbating emotional challenges. For major or irreversible treatments, cooling-off periods provide patients, particularly younger individuals, the opportunity to reflect on their choices, reinforcing informed and thoughtful decision-making. For example, a young patient seeking rhinoplasty might benefit from a detailed consultation exploring motivations, emphasizing the permanence of surgery, and considering non-surgical alternatives such as filler rhinoplasty. If emotional vulnerability or external pressures appear to drive the request, recommending a cooling-off period combined with psychological counseling can help the patient approach the decision with greater clarity and confidence. This comprehensive approach enhances patient safety, satisfaction, and ethical care in esthetic practice.

3. Setting ethical boundaries

Practitioners must embrace the ability to say "no" when a requested procedure conflicts with medical best practices or ethical principles [3]. This approach requires cultivating professional courage and a clear understanding that autonomy is not an unbounded right. Just as a physician would not perform an unnecessary surgery, so too must esthetic practitioners prioritize non-maleficence by declining procedures that may harm the patient physically or psychologically. For instance, in a patient with a history of excessive filler use who then requests for more volume to their cheeks despite exhibiting signs of "overfilled face syndrome," risks of further treatments, including distorted facial proportions, should be discussed. Additional fillers may need to be discouraged and indeed, filler reversal combined with skin tightening treatments to restore a more natural look may be more appropriate, thus prioritizing the patient's long-term esthetic and health outcomes over their immediate desires.

4. Promoting transparency and education

Providing patients with accessible, evidence-based information—free from marketing bias—ensures that they can make informed decisions. Educational initiatives aimed at both patients and practitioners are equally important. For patients, these can include public health campaigns that address unrealistic beauty standards and emphasize holistic self-care. For practitioners, ethics training and professional development programs can strengthen their capacity to navigate complex moral dilemmas.

5. Integrating psychological support and holistic care

For esthetic medicine to holistically serve patient well-being, it must extend its focus beyond physical enhancements to address the psychological and emotional dimensions of care. Psychological screenings or partnerships with mental health professionals can help practitioners identify patients for whom esthetic treatments may not align with their emotional health, such as those with body dysmorphic disorder (BDD) or unrealistic expectations. By ensuring that treatments are suitable and supportive of the patient's overall well-being, this approach reduces the risk of emotional harm. Additionally, integrating skincare education, lifestyle counseling, and body positivity initiatives promotes a comprehensive understanding of beauty, emphasizing self-care and acceptance over reliance on procedural interventions. Such a holistic framework not only enhances patient satisfaction but also aligns esthetic practices with ethical principles, reinforcing the notion that true beauty encompasses physical, psychological, and emotional health.

6. Advancing ethical and regulatory frameworks

Global regulations reflect varying approaches to promoting justice and safety in esthetic practices. Unlike traditional medical specialties, esthetic medicine often lacks a formalized structure, such as residencies or fellowships, that ensures practitioners meet a baseline level of expertise before entering the field. This creates a situation where individuals with varying levels of training—from highly skilled dermatologists and plastic surgeons to non-physicians—can perform treatments. For example, in the UK, there is currently no legal requirement for practitioners administering injectable treatments such as botulinum toxin or dermal fillers to be licensed medical professionals [75]. This regulatory gap allows beauty therapists and other non-medical individuals to perform procedures, often with minimal or no formal training. The risks associated with this disparity include improper technique, insufficient knowledge of facial anatomy, and inability to manage complications such as vascular occlusion or allergic reactions, all of which directly compromise patient safety. For these reasons, the UK Health and Care Act 2022 was enacted to review licensing and qualification standards to ensure safe practice, emphasizing informed consent and robust documentation as both ethical and legal imperatives [76]. Discussions and consultations with experts in the UK are ongoing, and it is anticipated that revised regulations including a new licensing scheme will be introduced in the coming years.

In contrast, the Singapore's Ministry of Health enforces stringent guidelines to prevent unethical advertising and ensures that only licensed practitioners can perform approved procedures, prioritizing patient safety and transparency [77]. Laudatory terms and promotion of specific brands of cosmetic procedures are not permitted.

These legal frameworks underscore the broader responsibility of practitioners to align individual care with societal equity. Ethical advertising, for instance, prohibits sensational claims or endorsements that exploit patient vulnerabilities, while stringent data protection laws like GDPR (General Data Protection Regulation, enforced in various countries around the world) safeguard patient confidentiality [78].

## 7. Moving forward: Balancing ethical and legal commitments

The future of ethical esthetic practice depends on harmonizing the artistry of enhancement with the scientific and moral foundations of medicine. Navigating the delicate balance between patient autonomy and professional responsibility requires a collaborative and transparent approach, where shared decision-making, comprehensive consultations, and holistic care address both physical and emotional needs. Integrating ethical principles such as beneficence, non-maleficence, and distributive justice ensures that practitioners prioritize trust, respect, and patient well-being. By embracing these practices, esthetic medicine can transcend its cosmetic focus to become a discipline that combines the transformative potential of art with the rigor and compassion of healing. This evolution not only raises the standard of care but also reaffirms the profound moral responsibility practitioners bear in shaping perceptions of beauty and fostering patient confidence.

## Author details

Sylvia Ramirez* and Gunther Scherz
Cutis Medical Laser Clinics, Singapore, Singapore

*Address all correspondence to: dr.sylvia@cutislaserclinics.com

## References

[1] Holm S. Principles of biomedical ethics, 5th edn.: Beauchamp T L, Childress J F. Oxford University Press, 2001, £19.95, pp 454. ISBN 0-19-514332-9. Journal of Medical Ethics. 2002;**28**(5):332-332

[2] Maio G. Is aesthetic surgery still really medicine? An ethical critique. Handchirurgie, Mikrochirurgie, plastische Chirurgie: Organ der Deutschsprachigen Arbeitsgemeinschaft für Handchirurgie: Organ der Deutschsprachigen Arbeitsgemeinschaft für Mikrochirurgie der Peripheren Nerven und Gefässe: Organ der Vereinigung der Deutschen Plastischen Chirurgen. 2007;**39**(3):189-194; discussion 195-196. DOI: 10.1055/s-2007-965328

[3] Ramirez S et al. The primacy of ethics in aesthetic medicine: A review. Plastic and Reconstructive Surgery. Global Open. 2024;**12**(6):e5935. DOI: 10.1097/GOX.0000000000005935

[4] Cantor J. Cosmetic dermatology and physicians' ethical obligations: More than just hope in a jar. Seminars in Cutaneous Medicine and Surgery. 2005;**24**(3):155-160. DOI: 10.1016/j.sder.2005.04.005

[5] Bennett KG, Vercler CJ. When is posting about patients on social media unethical "Medutainment"? AMA Journal of Ethics. 2018;**20**(4):328-335. DOI: 10.1001/journalofethics.2018.20.4.ecas1-1804

[6] Buzzaccarini G, Degliuomini RS, Borin M. The impact of social media-driven fame in aesthetic medicine: When followers overshadow science. Aesthetic Surgery Journal. 2023;**43**(10):NP807-NP808. DOI: 10.1093/asj/sjad190

[7] Varkey B. Principles of clinical ethics and their application to practice. Medical Principles and Practice. 2021;**30**(1):17-28. DOI: 10.1159/000509119

[8] From Extreme to Mainstream: The Future of Aesthetics Injectables. McKinsey [Internet]; 2023). Available from: https://www.mckinsey.com/industries/life-sciences/our-insights/from-extreme-to-mainstream-the-future-of-aesthetics-injectables [Accessed: November 25, 2024]

[9] 2022 ASPS Procedural Statistics Release; plastic-surgery-statistics-report-2022.pdf

[10] Miller FG, Brody H, Chung KC. Cosmetic surgery and the internal morality of medicine. Cambridge Quarterly of Healthcare Ethics: CQ: the International Journal of Healthcare Ethics Committees. 2000;**9**(3):353-364. DOI: 10.1017/s0963180100903074

[11] Ramirez SPB, Scherz G, Smith H. Characteristics of patients seeking and proceeding with non-surgical facial aesthetic procedures. Clinical, Cosmetic and Investigational Dermatology. 2021;**14**:197-207. DOI: 10.2147/CCID.S296970

[12] Maisel A et al. Self-reported patient motivations for seeking cosmetic procedures. JAMA Dermatology. 2018;**154**(10):1167-1174. DOI: 10.1001/jamadermatol.2018.2357

[13] Archard D, Montgomery J, Caney S, Clancy T, Edwards J, Gallagher A, et al. Nuffield Council on Bioethics. Available from: www.nuffieldbioethics.org. (Cosmetic-procedures-full-report PDF)

[14] Furnham A, Levitas J. Factors that motivate people to undergo cosmetic surgery. The Canadian Journal of Plastic Surgery. 2012;**20**(4):e47-e50

[15] Chung KC, Pushman AG, Bellfi LT. A systematic review of ethical principles in the plastic surgery literature. Plastic and Reconstructive Surgery. 2009;**124**(5):1711-1718

[16] Bueller H. Ideal facial relationships and goals. Facial Plastic Surgery: FPS. 2018;**34**(5):458-465. DOI: 10.1055/s-0038-1669401

[17] Klassen AF et al. Measuring patient-reported outcomes in facial aesthetic patients: Development of the FACE-Q. Facial Plastic Surgery: FPS. 2010;**26**(4):303-309. DOI: 10.1055/s-0030-1262313

[18] Mele S, Cazzato V, Urgesi C. The importance of perceptual experience in the esthetic appreciation of the body. PLoS One. 2013;**8**(12):e81378. DOI: 10.1371/journal.pone.0081378

[19] Dimitrov D, Kroumpouzos G. Beauty perception: A historical and contemporary review. Clinics in Dermatology. 2023;**41**(1):33-40. DOI: 10.1016/j.clindermatol.2023.02.006

[20] Donizzetti AR. Ageism in an aging society: The role of knowledge, anxiety about aging, and stereotypes in young people and adults. International Journal of Environmental Research and Public Health. 2019;**16**(8):1329. DOI: 10.3390/ijerph16081329

[21] Liew S, Silberberg M, Chantrey J. Understanding and treating different patient archetypes in aesthetic medicine. Journal of Cosmetic Dermatology. 2020;**19**(2):296-302. DOI: 10.1111/jocd.13227

[22] Rahman E et al. A systematic review on the reinforcement loop in aesthetic medicine and surgery: The interplay of social media, self-perception, and repeat procedures. Aesthetic Plastic Surgery. 2024;**48**(17):3475-3487. DOI: 10.1007/s00266-024-04016-y

[23] Why Gouri [Internet]. Gouri Uk Training. Available from: https://gouritraining.co.uk/why-gouri/ [Accessed: November 25, 2024].

[24] Henriques, M. and Patnaik, D. (2020) Social Media and its Effects on Beauty, London, UK: IntechOpen. Available fromhttps://www.intechopen.com/chapters/73271 [Accessed: January 9, 2025]

[25] Hawes T, Zimmer-Gembeck MJ, Campbell SM. Unique associations of social media use and online appearance preoccupation with depression, anxiety, and appearance rejection sensitivity. Body Image. 2020;**33**:66-76. DOI: 10.1016/j.bodyim.2020.02.010

[26] Thai H, Davis C, Mahboob W, Perry S, Adams A, Goldfield G. Reducing social media use improves appearance and weight esteem in youth with emotional distress. Psychology of Popular Media. 2023;**13**:162-169. DOI: 10.1037/ppm0000460

[27] The Regulation of Social Media Influencers [Internet]. (Goanta C, Ranchordás S, editors. Elgar Law, Technology and Society series). Edward Elgar Publishing; 2020. Available from: https://www.e-elgar.com/shop/gbp/the-regulation-of-social-media-influencers-9781788978279.html [Accessed: November 26, 2024]

[28] Boen M, Jerdan K. Growing impact of social media in aesthetics: Review and debate. Clinics in Dermatology. 2022;**40**(1):45-48. DOI: 10.1016/j.clindermatol.2021.08.011

[29] Wismiarsi T, Pangaribuan C, Prayitno S, Ainin A. The influences of content interactivity on purchase intention: An engagement mediation. Multidisciplinary Science Journal. 2024;**6**:1-10. DOI: 10.31893/multiscience.2024094

[30] Hostiuc M, Hostiuc S, Rusu MC, Isailă OM. Physician-patient relationship in current cosmetic surgery demands more than mere respect for patient autonomy-is it time for the anti-paternalistic model? Medicina (Kaunas, Lithuania). 2022;**58**(9):1278. DOI: 10.3390/medicina58091278

[31] Wong WW, Gupta SC. Plastic surgery marketing in a generation of "tweeting". Aesthetic Surgery Journal. 2011;**31**(8):972-976

[32] Nisha Gupta. et al. (2020) The plastic surgery social media influencer: Ethical considerations and a literature review, Aesthetic Surgery Journal [Internet], 40(6). Available from: https://pubmed.ncbi.nlm.nih.gov/31738821/ [Accessed: 2024 November 26]

[33] Zarei E, Ghaffari A, Nikoobar A, Bastami S, Hamdghaddari H, et al. Interaction between physicians and the pharmaceutical industry: A scoping review for developing a policy brief. Frontiers in Public Health. 2022;**10**:1072708. DOI: 10.3389/fpubh.2022.1072708

[34] Steinman MA, Shlipak MG, McPhee SJ. Of principles and pens: Attitudes and practices of medicine housestaff toward pharmaceutical industry promotions. The American Journal of Medicine. 2001;**110**(7):551-557. DOI: 10.1016/s0002-9343(01)00660-x

[35] Purvis TE et al. Plastic surgeons' perceptions of financial conflicts of interest and the sunshine act. Plastic and Reconstructive Surgery – Global Open. 2018;**6**(4):e1733. DOI: 10.1097/GOX.0000000000001733

[36] Moses H, Martin JB. Biomedical research and health advances. New England Journal of Medicine. 2011;**364**(6):567-571. DOI: 10.1056/NEJMsb1007634

[37] Lopez J, Lopez S, Means J, Mohan R, Soni A, Milton J, et al. Financial conflicts of interest: An association between funding and findings in plastic surgery. Plastic and Reconstructive Surgery. 2015;**136**(5):690e

[38] Zbar RIS, Taylor LD, Canady JW. Ethical issues for the plastic surgeon in a tumultuous health care system: Dissecting the anatomy of a decision. Plastic and Reconstructive Surgery. 2008;**122**(4):1245-1252. DOI: 10.1097/PRS.0b013e318184597c

[39] Fresques H. ProPublica. Doctors prescribe more of a drug if they receive money from a pharma company tied to it. 2019. Available from: https://www.propublica.org/article/doctors-prescribe-more-of-a-drug-if-they-receive-money-from-a-pharma-company-tied-to-it [Accessed: January 9, 2025]

[40] Aesthetic surgery research funding: Where does it come from and to whom does it go? Aesthetic Surgery Journal|Oxford Academic [Internet]. . Available from: https://academic.oup.com/asj/article/41/12/1473/6012398. [Accessed: November 26, 2024]

[41] Valiga A, Albornoz CA, Chitsazzadeh V, Wang JV, Saedi N, Geronemus RG, et al. Medical spa facilities and nonphysician operators in aesthetics. Clinics in Dermatology. 2022;**40**(3):239-243. DOI: 10.1016/j.clindermatol.2021.11.007

[42] Zargaran D, Zargaran A, Terranova T, Khaledi H, Robinson A, Davies J, et al. Profiling UK injectable aesthetic practitioners: A national cohort analysis. Journal of Plastic, Reconstructive & Aesthetic Surgery: JPRAS. 2023;**86**:150-154. DOI: 10.1016/j.bjps.2023.06.057

[43] SMC | Guidelines on Aesthetic Practices for Doctors (2016 Edition) [Internet] [Internet]. SMC. Available from: https://www.healthprofessionals.gov.sg/smc/guidelines/guidelines-on-aesthetic-practices-for-doctors-(2016-edition; 2016 [Accessed: November 26, 2024]

[44] Schelke L, Decates T, Kadouch J, Velthuis P. Incidence of vascular obstruction after filler injections. Aesthetic Surgery Journal. 2020;**40**(8):NP457-NP460. DOI: 10.1093/asj/sjaa086

[45] Soares DJ, Hynes SD, Yi CH, Shah-Desai S, Irving SC. Cosmetic filler–induced vascular occlusion: A rising threat presenting to emergency departments. Annals of Emergency Medicine. 2024;**83**(1):59-67. DOI: 10.1016/j.annemergmed.2023.07.006

[46] Surgery AB of FC. American Board of Facial Cosmetic Surgery. How to Choose a Provider for your Injectable Treatments. American Board of Facial Cosmetic Surgery. Available from: https://ambrdfcs.org/blog/choosing-provider-for-injectable-treatments/; 2023 [Accessed: November 26, 2024]

[47] Medical Board of Australia - Codes, Guidelines and Policies [Internet]. Available from: https://www.medicalboard.gov.au/codes-guidelines-policies.aspx [Accessed: November 26, 2024].

[48] Autonomy and Consent. The Ethics of Consent: Theory and Practice|Oxford Academic [Internet]. Available from: https://academic.oup.com/book/32837/chapter-abstract/275317844?redirectedFrom=fulltext [Accessed: November 26, 2024]

[49] Sherlock A, Brownie S. Patients' recollection and understanding of informed consent: A literature review. ANZ Journal of Surgery. 2014;**84**(4):207-210. DOI: 10.1111/ans.12555

[50] Fink AS, Prochazka AV, Henderson WG, Bartenfeld D, Nyirenda C, Webb A, et al. Predictors of comprehension during surgical informed consent. Journal of the American College of Surgeons. 2010;**210**(6):919-926. DOI: 10.1016/j.jamcollsurg.2010.02.049

[51] Makdessian AS, Ellis DAF, Irish JC. Informed consent in facial plastic surgery: Effectiveness of a simple educational intervention. Archives of Facial Plastic Surgery. 2004;**6**(1):26-30. DOI: 10.1001/archfaci.6.1.26

[52] Spatz ES, Krumholz HM, Moulton BW. The new era of informed consent: Getting to a reasonable-patient standard through shared decision making. JAMA;**315**(19):2063-2064

[53] ACS [Internet]. Ethical Issues in Surgical Care. Available from: https://www.facs.org/for-medical-professionals/news-publications/books-and-manuals/ethical-issues-in-surgical-care/ [Accessed: November 26, 2024]

[54] Myckatyn TM, Parikh RP, Lee C, Politi MC. Challenges and solutions for the implementation of shared decision-making in breast reconstruction. Plastic and Reconstructive Surgery. Global Open. 2020;**8**(2):e2645. DOI: 10.1097/GOX.0000000000002645

[55] Bjønness S, Viksveen P, Johannessen JO, Storm M. User

participation and shared decision-making in adolescent mental healthcare: A qualitative study of healthcare professionals' perspectives. Child and Adolescent Psychiatry and Mental Health. 2020;**14**:2. DOI: 10.1186/s13034-020-0310-3

[56] The SHARE Approach [Internet]. Available from: https://www.ahrq.gov/sdm/share-approach/index.html [Accessed: November 26, 2024].

[57] Admqportfolio (2017) FACE-Q, Aesthetics - Q-Portfolio Measuring What Matters to Patients [Internet]. Available from: https://qportfolio.org/face-q/aesthetics/ [Accessed: December 16, 2024]

[58] Carruthers JDA, Glogau RG, Blitzer A, Facial Aesthetics Consensus Group Faculty. Advances in facial rejuvenation: Botulinum toxin type a, hyaluronic acid dermal fillers, and combination therapies--consensus recommendations. Plastic and Reconstructive Surgery. 2008;**121** (5 Suppl):5S-30S

[59] Stefura T, Kacprzyk A, Droś J, Krzysztofik M, Skomarovska O, Fijałkowska M, et al. Tissue fillers for the nasolabial fold area: A systematic review and meta-analysis of randomized clinical trials. Aesthetic Plastic Surgery. 2021;**45**(5):2300-2316. DOI: 10.1007/s00266-021-02439-5

[60] Wollmer MA, Magid M, THC K, Finzi E. Treatment of depression with botulinum toxin. Toxins. 2022;**14**(6):383. DOI: 10.3390/toxins14060383

[61] Cohen JL, Rivkin A, Dayan S, Shamban A, Werschler WP, Teller CF, et al. Multimodal facial aesthetic treatment on the appearance of aging, social confidence, and psychological well-being: HARMONY study. Aesthetic Surgery Journal. 2022;**42**(2):NP115-NP124. DOI: 10.1093/asj/sjab114

[62] Dayan S, Rivkin A, Sykes JM, Teller CF, Weinkle SH, Shumate GT, et al. Aesthetic treatment positively impacts social perception: Analysis of subjects from the harmony study. Aesthetic Surgery Journal. 2019;**39**(12):1380-1389. DOI: 10.1093/asj/sjy239

[63] The Decision Lab [Internet]. The Decision Lab - Behavioral Science, Applied. Available from: https://thedecisionlab.com/biases/halo-effect [Accessed: December 16, 2024].

[64] Hippocratic oath|Definition, Summary, & Facts|Britannica [Internet]. Available from: https://www.britannica.com/topic/Hippocratic-oath [Accessed: December 16, 2024]

[65] Indla V, Radhika MS. Hippocratic oath: Losing relevance in today's world? Indian Journal of Psychiatry. 2019;**61**(Suppl 4):S773. DOI: 10.4103/psychiatry.IndianJPsychiatry_140_19

[66] Oxtoby K. Is the Hippocratic oath still relevant to practising doctors today? BMJ. 2016;**355**:i6629. DOI: 10.1136/bmj.i6629

[67] Sioutis S, Reppas L, Bekos A, Limneos P, Saranteas T, Mavrogenis AF. The hippocratic oath: Analysis and contemporary meaning. Orthopedics. 2021;**44**(5):264-272

[68] Rethinking Autonomy and Consent in Healthcare Ethics | IntechOpen [Internet]. Available from: https://www.intechopen.com/chapters/53439 [Accessed: November 26, 2024]

[69] Cotofana S, Gotkin RH, Frank K, Lachman N, Schenck TL. Anatomy behind the facial overfilled syndrome:

The transverse facial septum, dermatologic surgery. Dermatologic Surgery: Official Publication for American Society for Dermatologic Surgery. 2020;**46**(8):e16-e22. DOI: 10.1097/DSS.0000000000002236

[70] Love M, Saunders C, Harris S, Moon Z, Veale D. Redefining beauty: A qualitative study exploring adult women's motivations for lip filler resulting in anatomical distortion. Aesthetic Surgery Journal. 2023;**43**(8):907-916. DOI: 10.1093/asj/sjad050

[71] Blum D. What Is Ozempic and Why Is it Getting So Much Attention? The New York Times [Internet]. Available from: https://www.nytimes.com/2022/11/22/well/ozempic-diabetes-weight-loss.html; 2022 [Accessed: November 26, 2024]

[72] Butt MD, Ong SC, Rafiq A, Kalam MN, Sajjad A, Abdullah M, et al. A systematic review of the economic burden of diabetes mellitus: Contrasting perspectives from high and low middle-income countries. Journal of Pharmaceutical Policy and Practice. 2024;**17**(1):2322107. DOI: 10.1080/20523211.2024.2322107

[73] Fan J, Li S, Qiang Y, Duan Z, Wu A, Wang R. Barriers and stimulus in shared decision making among aesthetic dermatologists in China: Findings from a cross-sectional study. Clinical, Cosmetic and Investigational Dermatology. 2024;**17**:1153-1164. DOI: 10.2147/CCID.S457802

[74] Essential Tips for Managing Patient Expectations in Aesthetic Treatments [Internet]. 2024. Available from: https://www.acquisitionaesthetics.co.uk/blog/essential-tips-for-managing-patient-expectations-in-aesthetic-treatments/ [Accessed: December 16, 2024]

[75] National Hair & Beauty Federation [Internet]. The Health & Care Act and the Future Licensing of Aesthetic Practitioners Q&As. Available from: https://www.nhbf.co.uk/documents/the-health-and-care-act-and-the-future-licensing-of-aesthetic/ [Accessed: December 18, 2024]

[76] Ministry of Health [Internet]. Phase 2 of Healthcare Services Act to Start on 26 June 2023. Ministry of Health. Available from: https://www.moh.gov.sg/newsroom/phase-2-of-healthcare-services-act-to-start-on-26-june-2023/; no date [Accessed: December 18, 2024]

[77] Medical Confidentiality in the Era of Digital Health [Internet]. Available from: https://www.sma.org.sg/news/2024/March/Medical-Confidentiality-in-the-Era-of-Digital-Health [Accessed: December 18, 2024]

[78] Nahai F. General data protection regulation (GDPR) and data breaches: What you should know. Aesthetic Surgery Journal. 2019;**39**(2):238-240. DOI: 10.1093/asj/sjy296

Chapter 15

# Expanding the Notion of 'Best Interests' in the UNCRC to Include Future Generations of Children

*Susan E. Zinner*


## Abstract

The United Nations Convention on the Rights of the Child (UNCRC), ratified in all nations except the United States, offers child plaintiffs a potent potential legal tool when challenging national and international policies which pose harm to the environment. While the litigation results have been mixed in recent years, the approach of the UNCRC and recent General Comments evidence a clear intention of respect for future generations and maintenance of a child-friendly approach for the future.


**Keywords:** climate change, UNCRC, children, intergenerational equity, international equity

## 1. Introduction

Anticipating an adulthood confronting existential challenges such as AI risks, bioterrorism, the collapse of important global infrastructure systems around the world and global warming and its impact, children today will inherit a future vastly different from our own. Young people will need new and flexible tools to respond to these crucial issues, many of which are being faced for the first time in human history. Grappling with the possibility of life-ending climate catastrophes caused by global warming, for instance, will call for innovative solutions and international cooperation.

One potential solution may be the United Nation's Convention on the Rights of Children (UNCRC), a [1] document created to affirm the rights of children everywhere and placing specific obligations on signatories. This article will explore the history of the UNCRC and its use as a tool to advocate for a safer world for both children today and for children not yet born. To illustrate its use, the author will focus primarily on climate change, but the UNCRC could potentially be used to address multiple future crises.

### 1.1 History of the UNCRC

The UNCRC was created in the era of another crisis; after the end of World War I, Englishwoman Eglantyne Jebb learned that the children of Germany and Austria were facing many challenges, including the deaths of their soldier fathers, meaning they were no longer able to financially support their families ([2], p. 19). In 1924, Jebb wrote the Declaration of the Rights of the Child, or the Geneva Declaration of the Rights of the Child [3], later adopted by the League of Nations ([2], p. 19–20). This document was historic in its approach. 'Children's vulnerability called for greater respect, not exploitation, because in other ways they were to be seen as being like adults, with developing and moral sensibilities and the capacity for work' ([2], p. 20). This concept of the vulnerability of children and the need to protect them was the societal framework embraced by many countries for the next few decades. In 1959, the U.N. adopted the Declaration on the Rights of the Child, which included specific rights of children to societal assets such as housing, medical care, and education although participation rights were not included ([4], p. 57). However, major social upheavals such as mass democracy, more women in the workforce, expanding ideas about equality and changing household roles led to the view in many developed countries that a more democratic model should also be adopted in parent-child relationships as well ([2], p. 21). Therefore, the ideal parent-child relationship became more focused on the developing autonomy of children and the role of parents in encouraging this growth.

The UNCRC, relying extensively on the Declaration of the Rights of the Child, evidenced this change in philosophy when it was drafted in 1989. The document reveals some of this tension between the obligation of parents and adults to protect children while, at the same time, granting them a great deal of autonomy and specific other rights. 'The Convention gives children their own rights, making them the subject of international law. The rights are in relation to their parents and to the state. The Convention gives parents obligations and certain rights' ([5], p. 31).

There was immediate international support for the UNCRC. The document, after obtaining the required 20 ratifications, became binding on September 2, 1990 ([6], p. 37). By mid-1993, 160 countries had signed the CRC or were States Parties via ratification or accession after ratification, making it the most supported international human rights document ever ([6], p. 37). The last two of 196 countries to ratify the UNCRC were Somalia and South Sudan in 2015, leaving the United States the sole country which has failed to do so [7]. Some child advocates believe that the UNCRC's prohibition of corporal punishment in schools and specific treatment of incarcerated juveniles, such as allowing solitary confinement in some cases, explains the U.S. reluctance to adopt the UNCRC.

## 2. Article 3 and best interests

Rights granted children under the UNCRC include subsistence, development, protection and participation rights ([8], p. 34). Both the State and parents have specific rights, 'but not above those of the child' ([5], p. 31). These rights are most clearly evident in Article 3, which mandates

1. In all actions concerning children, whether undertaken by public or private social welfare institutions, courts of law, administrative authorities or legislative bodies, the best interest of the child shall be the primary consideration.

2. States Parties undertake to ensure the child such protection and care as is necessary for his or her well-being, taking into account the rights and duties of his or her parents, legal guardians, or other individuals legally responsible for him

or her, and, to this end, shall take all appropriate legislative and administrative measures.

3. States Parties shall ensure that the institutions, services and facilities responsible for the care or protection of children shall confirm with the standards established by competent authorities, particularly in the areas of safety, health, in the number and suitability of their staff, as well as competent supervision (UNCRC, Art. 3).

Sutherland and McFarland note that the term "best interests," clarified in General Comment 14, ensures that, in the event that more than one interpretation is possible in a given situation, parents and other interested parties are to construe the UNCRC in favor of the child and that all decisions need to evaluate the impact on the child; the comment explains how this crucial analysis may be accomplished ([9], p. 5). The term "best interests" has typically been construed broadly even though it has also been criticized for 'enshrining a weak standard' ([10], p. 53). The elements of "best interests" include 'the child's views, the child's identity, maintaining family relations, the child's protection and care, education and health' ([10], p. 60). Although some critics have suggested that the "best interests" obligation refers to an interest possessed by the child as opposed to a defined right, there is a strong argument to be made that Article 3(1) intended the child to be a rights-holder despite specific language to that effect since this is the clear intent of the UNCRC ([10], p. 58–59). As Kilkelly notes, 'there is no Convention of the *Interests* of Children' ([10], p. 65).

An alleged violation of the UNCRC could impact children around the world except for those in the U.S. All actors are to consider the best interests of the child in making decisions impacting that child (Art. 3, UNCRC). Kilkelly notes that a 'plain reading of the text does not support the view that Article 3(1) contains a right', but the Vienna Convention's interpretive guidelines mandates a reading based on the intent of the UNCRC ([10], p. 57). Interpreting this term in the light of the entire document supports this view. Also, Doek notes that '[t]he most fundamental requirement for the implementation of the CRC is that the child is recognized and fully respected as a human being with rights' ([11], p. 55). Furthermore, 'rights imply duties' and 'if children have rights, then some adults have duties and responsibilities either to supply those things that children have a right to, or to refrain from interfering with those activities children have a right to engage in' ([12], 91). Should a narrow interpretation prevent this reading, Kilkelly argues that acknowledging that an interest (as opposed to a right) exists may still allow child advocates working together to achieve decisions that benefit children ([10], p. 64–66).

The obligation to accord great weight to this term has been justified for multiple reasons. The default position of the international community should be to act in children's "best interests" because children are more vulnerable than adults, this approach provides the best chance for them to achieve success as adults, because children did not ask to be born, ideal parental models espouse sacrifice for one's children and it creates a positive environment for future generations to thrive and develop ([13], 99–100).

Furthermore, assuming we acknowledge that all children possess certain rights, these rights belong to all the members of the group. 'They are universal. Once they depended on gender and race and on sexual orientation. Women were non-persons, black persons were kept in subservience by institutions such as slavery and apartheid' ([13], p. 43–4). The UNCRC, by granting specific rights to children, allows them to serve as agents. Once children possess the cognitive maturity to express their views, they may be considered to possess agency and therefore able to exert at least some control over decisions destined to impact their lives ([14], p. 439). Importantly, 'agents can negotiate with others. They are capable of altering relationships, of effecting changes in decisions. Agents can shift social assumptions and constraints... As agents, rights-bearers can participate' ([13], p. 46). Furthermore, there is evidence that many countries have failed to address the best interests of children in climate policy, including failing to gather statistics and the views of their child citizens ([15], p. 148), which indicates that a rights-based best interests approach could be effective. Those working to promote the best interests of the child will use this rights-based approach to advocate for children and define where the line between justice and injustice exists ([13], p. 47).

## 3. Article 12 and participation rights

The UNCRC also provides another tool to address injustices: that is Article 12 which provides for participation rights, although this right is limited to 'the child who is capable of forming his or her own views' (UNCRC, Art. 12(1)). Hart suggests that allowing for collaborative opportunities which engage children older adolescents and adults in joint decision-making is the best way to achieve this goal ([16], p. 84). However, he notes that, while this approach offers multiple benefits for all members of a society, it may be 'especially difficult for disadvantaged, low-income parents to understand, when they themselves have had no voice and see authoritarian child-rearing as the best approach for their child's success' ([1], p. 84–85). When exercised together, the right to seek and act in the best interests of the child (Article 3), after soliciting the views of the child-as-agent (Article 12), can become a potent tool in ensuring that children's views are heard and respected.

Freeman notes that the inherent vulnerability of children justifies prioritizing their interests since adults might tend to overlook them in an adult centric world ([13], p. 99). Furthermore, how each country responds to the needs of children will vary depending on the culture of that country. In this way, one can perhaps view the UNCRC 'not [as] a manual in the sense that it prescribes procedures. It does describe aims and ideals but so do other elements of a culture...which guides the behavior of its members' ([5], p. 31). Despite the vulnerability of children and the variability in how children are viewed in different nations, however, it is important to view children always as 'human beings rather than human becomings' ([17], p. 40). Society is not expected to wait until adulthood to acknowledge the centrality of the child in any decision affecting the life of the child.

Article 3 also references the well-being of the child. Well-being is 'what children feel and express' ([18], p. 181). Therefore, the role of Article 12 also becomes important as the vehicle to achieve child well-being and ensure that their interests are protected. Article 12 mandates the solicitation of the child's views in all matters affecting the child. One of these matters is surely the environmental future of our planet. Therefore, '[t]he principles of the UN Convention on the Rights of the Child (CRC) such as the principle of the best interests of the child have enormous potential for environmental litigation. It is important then to emphasize children as the link between the present generation and those yet to be born' ([15], p. 135).

This will no doubt strike the reader as inherently fair. An emphasis on fairness includes an obligation to future people, including future children, by those currently alive. This obligation manifests itself in several ways. First, intergenerational equity, a focus on our obligation to protect the earth and its resources, involves the fairness of passing on our planet in good condition to subsequent residents ([15], p. 136). In an interesting variation of John Rawl's thought experiment about allocation of societal resources, some philosophers have recently suggested that, if an individual does not know to which generation they will belong in this scenario, people will act rationally to protect and preserve vital resources and protect the environment from climate change ([19], p. 160). Brown Weiss has suggested that intergenerational equity is crucial since it supports the planet, sustains conditions and resources necessary to support human life and is needed to maintain a healthy human environment ([20], p. 37). While distinct from the UNCRC, the UNESCO Declaration on the Responsibilities of the Present Generation towards Future Generations acknowledges the importance of obligations to those not yet born [21].

Second, one should also consider international equity, which involves fairness between nations, and places greater obligations to mitigate damage, including future damage, by those who have contributed the most to the problem ([15], p. 134). Developed countries tend to be less vulnerable to climate changes and have more resources to both adapt and reduce their emissions ([22], p. 85). A future-sensitive response is needed given the 'greater sensitivity of children to environmental degradation and pollution', especially since they are likely to experience the consequences of unsustainable decisions ([23], p. 194).

## 4. Climate change and the UNCRC

One of the most significant of these challenges is climate change. The consequences of failing to act or not acting sufficiently to meet this threat are dire. They include 'extreme weather events, megadroughts lasting decades, severe coastal flooding, sea-level rise, melting glaciers and polar caps, desertification, deforestation, food supply disruptions, natural epidemics and pandemics, and a host of societal quandries like mass migrations, social upheaval, economic collapse and political instability' ([24], p. 80). Furthermore, scientists are aware that these climate changes impact human behavior. Hotter temperatures are expected to increase many crimes, including homicide, rape, burglary and car thefts ([24], p. 48). Finally, air pollution resulting from fossil fuels is already responsible for up to 10 million premature deaths annually; if we face hotter temperatures, then the threat of pollution impact increases since a hotter climate speeds up the chemical reactions which change tailpipe emissions into dangerous pollutants ([25], p. 51–2).

This potentially life-threatening scenario has impacted the measurements used by the Doomsday Clock, created to predict the likelihood of existential threats facing the world. The Bulletin of the Atomic Scientists did not include climate change as a risk immediately after World War II. However, the group expanded our understanding of the potential risk of climate change beginning in 2007, when the clock hands were moved from 7 minutes to 5 minutes before midnight and climate change was specifically cited as a primary reason ([24], p. 23). It has since moved forward in 2015 due, at least in part, to the risks posed by climate change. The current time is 90 seconds before midnight [26].

The theoretical Doomsday Clock has real-life implications at both the individual and societal level. There are major social investments and needed infrastructure required to prepare for the impact of climate change ([27], p. 59). One analysis found that at least 30 percent of the world's population is exposed to lethal heat conditions at least 20 days each year; assuming a "business-as-usual" model, this number will grow to 74 percent of the world's population if temperatures increase 4 degrees Celsius by 2100 ([28], p. 42). Such changes would be likely to lead to mass migration to cooler areas ([28], p. 43). The systems currently in place to address the needs of mass migration are currently unable to respond to a massive population shift where infrastructure needs might include transportation, road upkeep, adequate food supply and transportation of food and other goods, health care, care for vulnerable travelers, police and security issues, housing and other basic needs.

These interrelated issues arise because climate change has been deemed a "threat multiplier" by the Department of Defense ([28], p. 101) since it could exacerbate existing threats. Leigh notes that some of these threats might include a

> *totalitarian state might be more willing to develop a superintelligence that was focused on dominating humanity rather than on improving our well-being. A bioterrorism incident could be used as a pretext for an authoritarian crackdown. A brilliant and crafty artificial intelligence might deduce a way of delivering a knockout blow with atomic weapons—disturbing the fine balance between the nuclear powers. Like unknown risks, interacting threats raise the stakes and make it more vital still that we find ways of averting catastrophe ([28], p. 101).*

The realization over the past two decades that climate change is now characterized by systemic risk is one of the most significant changes in the field. These 'human-driven processes that interact with interconnected global socio-ecological processes… have complex, cross-scale relationships' ([29], p. 152). The move from a focus on external risks to more systemic threats is one of the more significant changes in existential studies ([30], p. xii). However, researchers have consistently shown that humans tend to discount future threats ([30], p. xii), especially if one happens to live in an unstable environment ([24], p. 86) and more immediate concerns predominate. Such a complex problem demands complex solutions. The study of such problems necessitates a new approach to climate change that includes a focus on justice and inequality as two of the primary drivers of climate change ([29], p. 152).

The sheer complexity of this challenge is also driven by the fact that 'policy deals largely in the world of immediate certainties, not distant hazards' ([28], p. 3). The blinders imposed by a tendency to focus on short-term threats, often at the expense of existential—and perhaps more likely—threats mean that many simply do not acknowledge climate change and its impact on the ways we will lead our lives. That is, 'we are lousy at judging the probability of rare but catastrophic events' ([28], p. 9). Furthermore, there is evidence that the more unstable a community or country, the less likely it is to consider existential future threats. As Leigh notes, 'highly unstable environments lead people to discount the future more, whereas stable environments lead to less steep discount rates…We should expect that climate change and biodiversity loss will decrease interest in existential risk studies in the coming decades, given that societies will likely be preoccupied with more immediate concerns' ([28], p. 86).

Just because it is human nature to ignore significant climactic changes, however, does not relieve humans of the responsibility to confront this risk. Justice mandates that individuals bear proportionate responsibility. All humans share some responsibility for climate change. The average American emits roughly 20 tons of carbon dioxide per year ([27], p. 23), for instance. However, an individual's ability to compensate for their part in this crisis varies considerably depending on geography.

The poorest countries consume the least material resources while generating limited greenhouse gases ([22], p. 85). Scientists have long acknowledged that wealthy households, especially those in the Global North, both use more resources which impact the environment negatively and used colonization and imperialism as tools to advance this agenda historically ([22], p. 85). Therefore, dynamic policies and laws are necessary to address climate change. After all, 'tackling existential risks is a political problem. Private citizens can achieve many things, but preventing nuclear war, averting bioterrorism, and curbing greenhouse emissions are fundamentally problems of government. Governments control the military, levy taxes, and provide public goods. So the values of those who run the country will determine how much priority the nation places on averting catastrophe' ([28], p. 14).

## 5. Intergenerational equity, climate change and the role of the UNCRC

In her ground-breaking work, *In Fairness to Future Generations*, Edith Weiss Brown proposed four principles for guidance in making intergenerational equity decisions. First, equitable allocations of natural resources should be made so that we recognize the needs of current and future generations. Second, since it may not be possible to predict the needs of future generations, the current generation does not have an obligation to make decisions which align with future values regarding natural resource use. Third, keep the guidelines simple and understandable. Finally, there should be wide acceptance of these guidelines [20]. Daly suggests that there are two schools of thought espoused by writers (generally not politicians): those who explain future equitable allocations without considering the role of future children and those who discuss the importance intergeneration equity and environmental preservation to protect future rights without addressing what this means for children ([15], p. 140). We lack a bridge linking current action and future generations with a concrete legal tool to achieve this purpose.

However, relying on crucial portions of the UNCRC, specifically Articles 3 and 12, noted above can help advance this theory. While other approaches, such as using language from the Constitutions of many countries, specifically the public trust doctrine [31] and selected human rights laws can also serve this purpose, this is beyond the scope of this article. Since intergenerational equity is "already an accepted frame for thinking about climate policy" ([32], p. 268), then [c]hildren in the present will possibly have legal standing, and can argue that they have already suffered harm, even if that harm is a failure in the present to consider their interests in the future" ([15], p. 144).

While laudable, the approach taken by the UNCRC has been criticized for several reasons. First, there is little emphasis on the collective rights of children, as opposed to an individual child ([17], p. 42–3). As Freeman writes (citing Smith [33]), '[t]he CRC is focused on the 'child,' not it should be noted 'children.' Its premise is the 'universal child" ([13], p. 89). 'Second, it is clear that the UNCRC is a Western centric document and addresses issues of concern primarily to those living in developed countries' ([34], p. 395), "best interests," a key term, may conflict with the child's views ([35], p. 34) and is also quite vague ([9], p. 12) and the UNCRC does not address the issue of cognitive development, referenced using the legal term "capacity" in the document, when soliciting the views of the child ([4], p. 66). Despite these flaws, when wielded effectively, it may offer the possibility of protection for current and future children facing multiple and complex future challenges.

## 6. Climate change litigation and child plaintiffs

Perhaps disappointed with the speed—or lack of it—with which nations are addressing the potential catastrophe of climate change, young people have initiated multiple lawsuits in the last decade or two. As of 2022, some 2180 climate lawsuits had been filed globally, including 34 cases brought forward by and on behalf of children and those under 25 years old [36]. Many of these claims are based on human rights arguments and the general failure of most countries to comply with the 2015 Paris agreement limiting global warming to less than 2 degrees Celsius ([15], p. 133). Also used as part of the legal reasoning in some of these cases is UNCRC General Comment 15 in 2021–2022, which explained that children's rights and health were linked to climate change (UNCRC). While some critics have suggested that there is not a strong enough link between climate change and child health ([34], p. 393) in the UNCRC, this link has been proven beyond a doubt in the world of medicine.

One of the earliest cases to tackle some of these issues was the *Oposa Minors* case where Philippine minors sued and won on behalf of children born and unborn in 1993 to stop logging by companies causing deforestation ([37], p. 182). However, the impact on logging in the Philippines remained unchanged and the reference in the court case to future generations is *obiter* ([37], p. 183), an incidental reference which is not legally binding. Both Sri Lanka and India have also acknowledged the need for intergenerational equity in similar cases ([37], p. 183–84). In Germany, a court in 2021 agreed with the young plaintiffs that the German government needed to do more to limit emissions, while Colombia's Supreme Court agreed with officials that the Amazon rainforest merited more protection ([38], Christian Science Monitor).

The American 2023 ruling in *Held v. Montana* resulted in a win for Montana children and adolescents when the court ruled in favor of the plaintiffs and said that the state is obligated to uphold its Constitution, which explicitly protects the rights of both current and future citizens to a healthy environment ([38], Christian Science Monitor). In Florida, a 2018 case resulted in the state setting renewable energy goals, while a case in Hawai'i brought by 14 young plaintiffs challenges the high greenhouse gas emissions produced by the state transportation system ([39], Progressive).

American children have been less successful than child plaintiffs in other countries since those countries are more likely to have adopted legally-binding human rights obligations or environmental rights are specifically protected in constitutions ([40], State of the Planet Report). The six major categories of lawsuits identified by Columbia University's Climate, Earth and Society organization include human and climate rights protected by international law or national constitutions, inadequate domestic enforcement of international climate change commitments such as the Paris Agreement, attempting to keep fossil fuels in the ground, corporate liability and responsibility by major industrial sources, climate disclosures and greenwashing involving misleading corporate assertions about their contributions to climate change and failure to adapt and its climate impact ([39], p. 31; [40], p. 3–4).

While the UNCRC does not reference intergenerational or international equity principals, it cites equality, health, education and non-discrimination ([37], p. 185) rendering it useful to child plaintiffs. General Comment 26, published in August 2023, however, directly addresses the issue of intergenerational equity and places requirements on member countries to consider the impact of potential environmental threats on current and future generations. Furthermore, children are given the right to pursue climate justice via litigation although this requirement is not legally enforceable.

*DOI: http://dx.doi.org/10.5772/intechopen.1009459*

Depending on the legal approach taken by signatory countries, these plaintiffs may nonetheless struggle to achieve the specific goals established by the UNCRC. For instance, countries incorporating the UNCRC principles evidencing respect for children's rights are often countries with a history of general respect for all human rights ([41], p. 442–63). Countries may incorporate the UNCRC principles in an informal way to promote internalization of the UNCRC values and norms or may be more formal and enact legislation or amend the Constitution ([42], p. 148). Of course, some signing countries failed to adopt any of these approaches, raising the question of how these rights are both known and enforced.

For countries which have signed the UNCRC and are actively working to achieve its goals, one legal challenge has been that '[c]laims for restitution are not usually made by individuals alleging that there will be harms in the future, but rather by those who are descendants of victims of injustice' ([15], p. 138). Most legal systems find it easier to remedy past injustices given that the harm is complete and it is possible to calculate damages in most cases. Even as some countries move towards incorporation of the idea of intergenerational justice into its laws and Constitutions ([15], p. 143–44), the law has been slower to embrace this concept. Anticipating a future harm and its future impact, even likely certain and irreparable harm, involves speculation. As noted earlier, reliance on Article 3 (best interests) and Article 12 (soliciting input from impacted children)—when combined with Article 24 of the UNCRC (ensuring that children reach the highest possible level of health, even when facing challenges such as environmental pollution) appears to provide a potent tool in protecting current and future children from damage associated with climate change.

## 7. Conclusion

The majority of children in the world today have a mostly-untested, but potent, tool available to protect their interests and right to a safer future by relying on these key provisions of the UNCRC, either directly or via reference to incorporated portions of the document into national or international law, policy or Constitution. The limited recognition from multiple courts acknowledging that right of child plaintiffs to pursue this legal strategy bodes well for future child plaintiffs. Leaders such as Greta Thunberg are likely to lead this legal charge in the future.

Reliance on terms such as "best interests," "well being" and the Article 12 expectation that a child's views will be solicited and listened to should be utilized and recognized as the formidable legal instruments that they are in protecting the future of children today and those yet to be born. Finally, the United States must consider ratification of the UNCRC to provide a safe future for our children.

## Author details

Susan E. Zinner
School of Public and Environmental Affairs, Indiana University Northwest, Indiana, USA

*Address all correspondence to: szinner@iu.edu

## References

[1] Convention on the Rights of the Child. Treaty no. 27531. United Nations Treaty Series, 1577. 1989. pp. 3-178

[2] Robinson S. Children's rights: Historic developments. In: Rutgers C, editor. Creating a World Fit for Children: Understanding the UN Convention on the Rights of the Child. New York: International Debate Education Association; 2011

[3] Available from: https://www.unicef.org/child-rights-convention/history-child-rights.

[4] Doel-Mackaway H. The right to participate in domestic law and policy development. In: Fenton-Glynn C, editor. Children's Rights and Sustainable Development: Interpreting the UNCRC for Future Generations. Cambridge: Cambridge University Press; 2019

[5] Flekkøy MG. Visions and voices: The UN convention on the rights of the child. In: Rutgers C, editor. Creating a World Fit for Children: Understanding the UN Convention on the Rights of the Child. New York: International Debate Education Association; 2011

[6] Himes JR. The UN convention on the rights of the child: More than a new utopia? In: Rutgers C, editor. Creating a World Fit for Children: Understanding the UN Convention on the Rights of the Child. New York: International Debate Education Association; 2011

[7] Oppier Y. Signatory States and Parties to the Convention on the Rights of the Child. Humanium; 2021. Available from: https://www.humanium.org/en/

[8] Amnesty International USA. Children's rights: The future starts here. In: Rutgers C, editor. Creating a World Fit for Children: Understanding the UN Convention on the Rights of the Child. New York: International Debate Education Association; 2011

[9] Sutherland E. Article 3 of the United Nations convention on the rights of the child: The challenges of vagueness and priorities. In: Sutherland EE, Macfarlane LB, editors. Implementing Article 3 of the United Convention on the Rights of the Child: Best Interests, Welfare and Well-Being. Cambridge: Cambridge University Press; 2016

[10] Kilkelly U. The best interests of the child: A gateway to children's rights? In: Sutherland EE, Macfarlane LB, editors. Implementing Article 3 of the United Convention on the Rights of the Child: Best Interests, Welfare and Well-Being. Cambridge: Cambridge University Press; 2016

[11] Doek J. What does the children's convention require? In: Rutgers C, editor. Creating a World Fit for Children: Understanding the UN Convention on the Rights of the Child. New York: International Debate Education Association; 2011

[12] Ladd RE. Rights of the child: A philosophical approach. In: Alaimo K, Klug B, editors. Children as Equals: Exploring the Rights of the Child. Lanham, Maryland: University Press of America; 2002

[13] Freeman M. A Magna Carta for Children: Rethinking Children's Rights. The Hamlyn Lectures. Cambridge: Cambridge University Press; 2020

[14] Jerome L, Starkey H. Developing children's agency within a children's

rights education framework: 10 propositions. International Journal of Primary, Elementary and Early Years Education. 2022;**50**(4):439-451. DOI: 10.1080/03004279.2022.2052233

[15] Daly A. Intergenerational rights are children's rights: Upholding the right to a healthy environment through the UN convention on the rights of the child. Netherlands Quarterly of Human Rights. 2023;**41**(3):132-154. DOI: 10.1177/09240519231195753

[16] Hart R. Introduction and meaning of children's participation. In: Rutgers C, editor. Creating a World Fit for Children: Understanding the UN Convention on the Rights of the Child. New York: International Debate Education Association; 2011

[17] Davis JM. Reimagining children's rights through the prism of sustainable development: Implications for educating children and young people. In: Fenton-Glynn C, editor. Children's Rights and Sustainable Development: Interpreting the UNCRC for Future Generations. Cambridge: Cambridge University Press; 2019

[18] Bradshaw J, Rees G, Keung A, Goswami H. The subjective well-being of children. In: McAuley C, Rose W, editors. Child Well-Being: Understanding Children's Lives. London: Jessica Kingsley Publisher; 2010

[19] Kim H. An extension of Rawl's theory of justice for climate change. International Theory. 2019;**11**(2):160-181. DOI: 10.1017/S1752971918000271

[20] Brown Weiss E. In Fairness to Future Generations: International Law, Common Patrimony, and Intergenerational Equity. Ardsley-on-Hudson, NY: Transnational; 1988

[21] UNESCO. Declaration on the Responsibilities of the Present Generations toward Future Generations. UNESCO; 1997. Available from: https://www.unesco.org

[22] Jones N. Beyond 'error and terror': Global justice and global catastrophic risk. In: Beard SJ, Rees M, Richards C, Rojas CR, editors. The Era of Global Risk: An Introduction to Existential Risk Studies. Cambridge: Open Book Publishers; 2023. DOI: 10.11647/OBP0336

[23] Desmet E. Children's rights and the environmental dimension of sustainable development. In: Fenton-Glynn C, editor. Children's Rights and Sustainable Development: Interpreting the UNCRC for Future Generations. Cambridge: Cambridge University Press; 2019

[24] Torres P. Morality, Foresight & Human Flourishing: An Introduction to Existential Risks. Durham, N.C: Pitchstone Publishing; 2017

[25] Hayhoe K. Heat. In: Thunberg G, editor. The Climate Book. New York: Penguin Press; 2023

[26] Available from: https://thebulletin.org/doomsday-clock/current-time/

[27] Wagner G, Weitzman M. Climate Shock: The Economic Consequences of a Hotter Planet. Princeton, N.J: Princeton University Press; 2015

[28] Leigh A. What's the Worst That Could Happen? Existential Risk and Extreme Politics. Cambridge, Massachusetts: MIT Press; 2021

[29] Kemp L. Ecological breakdown and human extinction. In: Beard SJ, Rees M, Richards C, Rojas CR, editors. The Era of Global Risk: An Introduction to Existential Risk Studies. Cambridge: Open Book Publishers; 2023. DOI: 10.11647/OBP0336

[30] Beard SJ, Rees M, Richards C, Rojas CR. Introduction. In: Beard SJ, Rees M, Richards C, Rojas CR, editors. The Era of Global Risk: An Introduction to Existential Risk Studies. Cambridge: Open Book Publishers; 2023. DOI: 10.11647/OBP.0336

[31] Treves A, Artelle KA, Darimont CT, Lynn WS, Paquet P, Santiago-Àvila FJ, et al. Intergenerational equity can help to prevent climate change and extinction. Nature, Ecology & Evolution. 2018;**2**:204-207

[32] Davies G. Climate change and reversed intergenerational equity: The problem of costs now, for benefits later. Climate Law. 2020;**10**:266-281. DOI: 10.1163/18786561-10030002

[33] Smith R. The third optional protocol to the UN convention of the rights of the child? Rights. 2013;**23**(2):305-322, cited in Freeman, Michael

[34] Fenton-Glynn C. The future research agenda: Where to from here? In: Fenton-Glynn C, editor. Children's Rights and Sustainable Development: Interpreting the UNCRC for Future Generations. Cambridge: Cambridge University Press; 2019

[35] Sutherland E, Barnes Macfarlane L. Introduction. In: Sutherland EE, Macfarlane LB, editors. Implementing Article 3 of the United Convention on the Rights of the Child: Best Interests, Welfare and Well-Being. Cambridge: Cambridge University Press; 2016

[36] Sabin Center Report 2023. Available from: https://climate.law.columbia.edu/sabin-center-unep-release-global-climate-litiation-report-2023-status-review.

[37] Atapattu S. Intergenerational equity and children's rights: The role of sustainable development and justice. In: Fenton-Glynn C, editor. Children's Rights and Sustainable Development: Interpreting the UNCRC for Future Generations. Cambridge: Cambridge University Press; 2019

[38] Hanes S. Suing the World to Save it. Children Pioneer a Right to a Secure Future. 2023. Available from: https://www.csmonitor.com.

[39] Gerhardt T. Youth Lead the Way on Addressing the Climate Crisis. 2023. Available from: https://www.progressive.org.

[40] Cho R. State of the Planet: Climate Lawsuits Are on the Rise. This Is What They're Based on. New York, NY: Columbia Climate School: State of the Planet; 2023. Available from: https://www.climate.columbia.edu

[41] Lundy L, Kilkelly U, Byrne B. Incorporation of the United Nations convention on the rights of the child in law: A comparative review. The International Journal of Children's Rights. 2013;**21(3**:442-463. DOI: 10.1163/15718182-55680028

[42] Hoffman S, Stern RT. Incorporation of the UN convention on the rights of the child in national law. The International Journal of Children's Rights. 2020;**28**:133-156. DOI: 10.1163/15718182-02801001

Chapter 16

# Rebuilding Lives: Areola and Nipple Complex Reconstruction

*Paola Gateño and Josefina Lattus*

## Abstract

This chapter will demonstrate the importance of the reconstruction of the nipple-areola complex in mastectomized women (breast cancer), the importance of free treatment, and the ethical bases treated from a psychological method of support to the patient, based on real cases and statistics. The importance of the protocol of this method is based on the patient's mental map and how, through reconstruction, the new connection of the body and mind of the patient to be treated can be achieved. Demonstrate the meaning and importance of this method created from the psychological and physical aspect, which has been based on the psychology of needs.

**Keywords:** mastectomy, reconnection, professional ethics, breast reconstruction, mental map

## 1. Introduction

Breast cancer is one of the most commonly diagnosed cancers in women. Likewise, it is the most feared disease among the female population since it provides psychological trauma due to the fear of mutilation and loss of femininity, which contributes to the distortion of self-image. The stages of depression, anxiety, and fear are frequent, causing behavioral and psychosocial problems [1]. For this reason, there have been many studies that have shown that the reconstruction of the nipple-areola complex has a value far from being only esthetic, but rather the experience of recovery, the return to a healthy state, the liberation from the treatment processes, and, in a way, a representation of the return to normality. It is a decisive step in the reconstruction of body image, which is affected by the disease [2]. It is for this reason that the professional must be very attentive to the needs of each patient as an individual, and therefore, professional ethics must be understood.

Aristotle associates the origin of the word "ethics" not only with êthos but also with éthos, "custom," and "habit" [3]. Therefore, ethics is not only linked to the things that build the man, such as the society, family, or place of origin, but also to the habit that this generates as these customs go on forming the character. So, ethics is a part of man that comes from an inner place; however, it is influenced by everything that has built that person, his life experiences, and that which is provided to him by nature.

Therefore, the profession cannot be separated from the individual himself. There will always be this human factor that will direct the person toward a final objective. Professionals have skills that come from themselves and others that they will have to acquire in order to achieve the best possible job.

 IntechOpen

Likewise, when a health professional commits himself to helping human beings who suffer from an illness, they ensure to provide care in accordance with the best that science and technology offer through a dialogic and dignified relationship, taking into account the family and community environment [4]. They are manifesting a bioethical facet.

The main objective of this study is based on interviews and testimonies from patients with breast cancer to recognize what characteristics are necessary in a health professional when caring for a woman with breast cancer, what changes between one professional and another, and what makes the real difference in how they go through the disease, as well as to demonstrate all of which surrounds the reconstruction process of the nipple-areola complex.

Considering the above, therefore, it is essential to take into account the patient's needs, which is why the heart of this research is directly linked to Maslow's pyramid of needs (1943) and the mental map of each patient.

## 2. Professional ethics in the reconstruction of the nipple-areola complex

Professional ethics in this field are difficult to define. As a first approach, it is important that there is a general understanding of the patient. A woman who has undergone a mastectomy is not only a mastectomized woman but also has her own inner world that is different from that of any other person. Part of getting that particular patient to experience the true feeling of healing is not by separating the woman's areola and nipple. It is important that the health professional take these parameters into account so that he or she understands the individuality of the patient within the environment presented. There are many points in common among these women. There may be words that are repeated within their stories, but just as there are similarities, there are many differences, and understanding this is what makes the difference in dealing with them from a professional point of view.

Additionally, ethics is linked to the sum of patterns that exist, thus the name of the Global Pattern, as a global pattern for the understanding of each case. The patients, after the reconstruction, will always be grateful, and that feeling of gratitude will be born within them. However, the warmth that the professional can show at the time of attending is very different from the warmth added to his technique and professionalism.

In **Table 1**, one can see a comparison of patient testimonies between two different professionals, one being only warm and the other using not only warmth but also professional ethics as a whole, which is added to morality, technique, protocols, experience, and ergonomics.

### 2.1 Global pattern (GP)

As previously mentioned, people are made up of their own internal world based on their life experiences. These give them the tools, or lack of them, to face up to situations that arise along the way. Coping is a type of response that is generated in the face of a stressful situation; that is, they are the tools and resources that the individual uses to handle external and/or internal situations that exceed the individual's resources [5].

So, with this in mind, we can understand that there are different ways to confront the experience of a mastectomy, which is why, as Perls, a Gestalt psychologist,

| Professional 1 | Professional 2 |
|---|---|
| Very affectionate | It changed my life |
| I felt welcomed | She is a wonderful, complete professional, she filled my soul |
| You can feel the warmth of the professional | She not only reconstructed my areola, but she also reconstructed my life |
| Very loving with me | She helped me feel complete again |
| You can tell the kindness of the professional | Being treated by her felt like the sun was rising again |
| An enjoyable experience, even though I thought it would be threatening | I never thought I could feel like a woman again, she made it happen |
| A very welcoming person | She is an angel who came to help me in every sense of the word |

**Table 1.**
*Comparison of patient testimonies based on professional approach: warmth alone vs. warmth combined with professional ethics.*

explains. He talks about the process of awareness, which allows the body to interact and contact its environment; to reach this, Gestalt puts emphasis on "becoming aware." Becoming aware of oneself, the environment, and the contact between them in the present, in the here and now, which according to the Gestalt point of view is called "Organismic Self-Regulation" [6]. In other words, this awareness is about giving the person the power to pay attention to what they feel at a given moment and hence also influence the perception they have of themselves as an individual and of the environment at a determined time. Therefore, in mastectomized women, there will always be words in common, subgroups in which they all feel identified regarding their mutilation process and illness. However, the experience of each one, the surrounding environment, and each thought were totally individual. Therefore, the ideal is that the professional takes the common aspects but does not take them as the absolute truth for all the patients, but rather as the starting point for the total comprehension of the person as a particular entity. This helps to enrich the reconstructive procedure, as the professional is a means; those who manage to go back are the same patients. It is up to them to find out what the procedure means to them and what it is going back to be. Therefore, it is necessary for the professional to know and adapt his mentality to this.

There are questions that should be asked before treating the patients, such as: What goes through the patient's mind when they tell her that she has breast cancer? What about the mutilation? Breasts have many extremely important meanings. They are the first source of connection we have with each other when our mother breastfeeds us for the first time. They represent femininity and sexuality, the ability to connect with a partner on a more intimate level. Be a mother. Be a woman.

When a woman loses her breasts, there is a total disconnection with all those areas as there is a loss in the way the person connects, and this connection is one of the ways in which one can heal. Bowlby is a psychologist who conceptualized what attachment can mean and how important it is for bonds, "which for convenience reasons I call attachment theory. It is a way of conceptualizing the tendency of human beings to create strong emotional bonds with certain people in particular and an attempt to explain the wide variety of forms of emotional pain and personality disorders, such as anxiety, anger, depression, and emotional withdrawal, that occur as a consequence of unwanted separation and emotional loss" [7].

What happens in the case of a mastectomy is that there is an unwanted loss of that which links them to others and themselves. So, effectively, this loss is going to have an emotional and psychological factor in the equation. On the other hand, there is a disconnection from another aspect, the physical one: when there is mutilation, sensitivity is disconnected or it is lost in the area of the scars where it was previously hypersensitive, either due to fibrosis or the emotional shock of what the procedure means. Therefore, when the complete reconstruction is achieved, including the nipple-areola complex, the women interviewed claim to have felt their breasts again. There is a reconnection on every level, whether with themselves, with others, and with touching that part of their body again and feeling the touch that it provokes.

Aristotle mentions that man is a social being, and it is true. When a connection of any kind is lost, in this case the person himself, he must connect with people; therefore, the professional must also take into consideration the importance of contact with others and for the patient to feel welcomed.

Taking everything into consideration, the professional must profess enough empathy to understand the difference between each patient. That is where the factor of change is found in how a patient does after reconstruction. In these cases, therefore, empathy means understanding what reconstruction of the nipple-areola complex means for each particular patient. See them as a whole. So it is by being able to interpret the patient's behavior and her needs individually from a global method.

### 2.2 The patient's needs

Abraham Maslow was an American psychologist who proposed the Theory of Human Motivation in 1943, where he developed the idea that people have five sets of needs and that these are presented in a specific order, so as they are satisfied, each set of needs will arise the requirement to satisfy the set that follows [8].

First of all, there are the basic physiological needs: eating, sleeping, drinking water, going to the bathroom, and the sexual needs of men.

When this first category is satisfied, the second category enters, which covers the need to feel safe and have the assurance that this need will be satisfied in the future. The need for love, friendship, and companionship continues.

The next category is the need for social recognition, status, and respect. The last category Maslow names is "self-fulfillment," since it has to do with feeling complete, doing what we want to do, and pursuing our desired dreams (**Figure 1**) [9].

By including Maslow's pyramid of needs, we can understand what reconstruction can mean for a woman. First of all, when given the diagnosis of breast cancer, the patient's first need will be to survive the disease. When this need is satisfied, the others begin to appear, such as feeling safe, loved, and accompanied.

In **Table 2**, you can see the words that are most repeated in the 123 testimonies and interviews of women who have been able to opt for reconstruction of the nipple-areola complex.

When a woman, after having lost her breasts, manages to reconstruct herself, for the most part, she feels complete. Just as Abraham Maslow said, this process is very similar to the pyramid, since she goes through a long process where something is missing that does not allow the person to move forward; however, the reconstruction procedure helps women feel "self-fulfilled" again by doing something they want to do in order to feel truly whole. A testimony from a patient mentions that "I did not

*DOI: http://dx.doi.org/10.5772/intechopen.1009746*

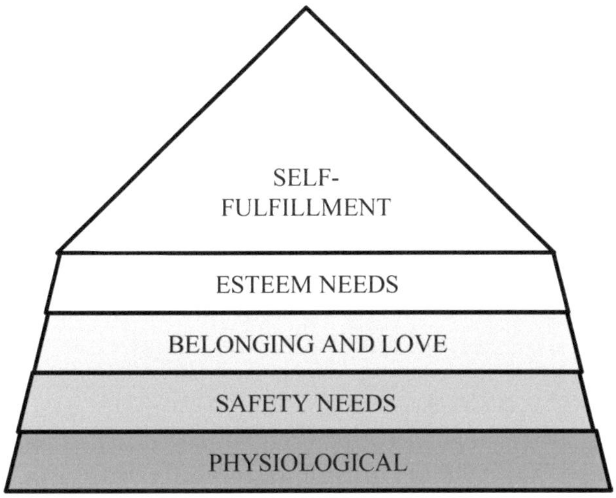


**Figure 1.**
*Adaptation of Maslow's pyramid illustrating the hierarchy of human needs.*

| Words | Percentage (%) |
|---|---|
| Feel again | 67.8 |
| Give back | 74 |
| Dignity | 84.6 |
| Femininity | 58.3 |
| Gratitude | 78.2 |
| Heal | 60.6 |
| Safety | 53 |

**Table 2.**
*Frequency analysis of terms in patient testimonials (n = 123).*

feel truly wholesome until I could see my breasts reconstructed, it is to feel that the disease has effectively disappeared." On the other hand, another patient confesses that "cancer was like sinking into a stormy sea, I swam and swam but the tide overwhelmed me, when I arrived at the foundation and managed to opt for the reconstruction of the nipple-areola complex, it was as if the sea was finally calm and I could get on that raft that was always in front of my eyes."

## 2.3 The gratitude

Gratitude in the reconstruction process of the nipple-areola complex is of utmost importance. Especially when it covers the issue of quality, since one thing has nothing to do with the other; however, it lends itself to misinterpretations.

Gratitude has a high impact on patients since this happiness manages to release a hormone, like when you win a prize; it is free; it is a gift. This itself causes that feeling of well-being in a patient, which is why it is the sum of each of these factors and protocols to achieve the total reconnection of a cancer patient.

### 2.4 Protocols

Professionals, thanks to the experience that this profession provides, create necessary protocols, whether general or personal, to achieve certain objectives. Linked to the need of the health personnel to the promise of preserving the patient's life, the protocols to follow in the caring of the patient must be juxtaposed; therefore, the know-how of the reconstruction procedure is closely connected to the understanding of the mental map and this method (GP). The main object is to adhere to the protocols, given that the protocols have been created based on ethics and the patient's improvement in order to help them in using all the tools available.

### 2.5 Reconstructing lives

What cancer causes in the lives of patients is that reality becomes like a fragmented photograph: how they see their body, their life, the past, the present, and the future. Everything becomes fragmented, and it is very difficult to put the pieces back together in order. A patient in an interview mentions, "it's like you have to put together a puzzle but you can't find where the pieces go." After they emerge from this whirlwind of cancer, from this wave, as one patient mentions, "it is like that respite when you can rebuild yourself again and feel that you have the right to do so."

Given the above, several social programs have been created around the world, for example, in South America and also in the Middle East regarding the insertion of the psychology program that must be implemented before being able to care for this type of patient. This is because there is a feeling that once the cancer is gone, the reconstruction could generate, in the thoughts of these patients, that the entity in which they believe, therefore, the faith they profess, could "punish" them. There are testimonies in many Islamic cultures and also in South America, so it is important to treat this issue delicately, not to take lightly the psychology of the woman who chooses this procedure since it entails a history behind it, not only personal but also cultural, that leads to making the decision of reconstruction. The Global Pattern of each patient will take the professional to the limit, and having this psychological program implemented, both to prepare for reconstruction and to understand the patient to be treated, is transcendental.

## 3. Conclusions

This study has addressed the importance of professional ethics in the process of the reconstruction of the nipple-areola complex in women who have undergone mastectomy due to breast cancer. Throughout this analysis, the importance of an integrated approach has been highlighted, which does not only consider techniques or professionalism but also integrates empathy, individual understanding of each patient, and the application of the Global Pattern (GP) model.

The discoveries reveal that the reconstruction of the nipple-areola complex goes beyond something merely esthetic: it is a healing process that will allow the patient to reconnect with herself, with her identity, and with her environment.

With regard to this, professional ethics must maintain the focus on respect for the individuality of each patient, avoiding generalizing and contemplating the diversity of emotional, psychological, and cultural experiences.

Likewise, the importance of protocols and free access to these procedures became evident. The promulgation of programs that allow free and quality reconstruction not only acts on the physical recovery of patients but also on their emotional well-being. The positive impact of free treatment in this process will achieve a feeling of relief and gratitude, which adds to the fact that it is important to guarantee this type of procedure as part of the right to well-being.

On the other hand, this work has highlighted that there is a willingness for patients to prepare themselves psychologically before and after reconstruction. Taking into consideration the importance that religion, culture, and previous experiences can have in the experience of this intervention. They must be accompanied professionally and, in that sense, be sensitive to these types of aspects to avoid generating internal conflicts in patients and strengthen a healthier adaptation to this new reality.

Finally, it is concluded that the success of breast reconstruction is not based purely on the precision of the procedure technique; in fact, it undermines the health professional's ability to integrate and respond to the emotional, social, and psychological needs of each patient. When a woman manages to see herself as a whole again, true healing occurs, and it is the professional's duty to make the process possible through the secret of excellence when reconstructing the nipple-areola complex, which is ethics added to professionalism, ergonomics, and human error. So, health personnel must understand the difference between each patient, which will generate the real difference at the time of attending.

## Acknowledgements

The translator, Francisca Conran, conducted a thorough review of the manuscript to ensure that the English in this research was as accurate as possible, making the necessary corrections.

## Author contributions

Paola Gateño is the director and founder of Fundación FEMPO. She has been the main manager of this project, which has been done under casuistry, and since the foundation, with the experiences of her patients and as she was observing and studying each case. Josefina Lattus is a psychologist at the foundation and a member of the board. She has had significant engagement with the patients through interviews and testimonies to gather the necessary data for the study conducted.

## Funding sources

The FEMPO Foundation is the entity supporting this research, offering oncological patients the opportunity to express themselves through testimonies and providing the necessary resources to make this research possible.

## Conflict of interest statement

The author has no conflict of interest to declare since she was the main manager and promoter of the manuscript, and also, the study was done based on her casuistry and personal experience in the field of oncological paramedical micropigmentation, supported by its own foundation (FEMPO).

## Statement of ethics

In this study, ethical approval was not required since it is a study carried out from their own experience and based on interviews with patients from the FEMPO Foundation, which consents that this ethical approval has not been required. These patients signed an informed consent that underlines their participation and shows their agreement to be part of this search.

## Data availability statement

All data from this study can be found in our references; therefore, they are available to the public and do not require any specific conditions to access this information.

## Author details

Paola Gateño*† and Josefina Lattus†
Fempo Foundation, Chesterton, Santiago, Chile

*Address all correspondence to: gateno.paola@gmail.com

† These author contributed equally.

## References

[1] Mendes IS, Souza GA da S, Neves MF das, Lima FPS, Freitas STT de, Andrade AO, Lima MO. The impact of mastectomy due to cancer on body image and self-esteem. Mundo Saúde. 2016;**41**(4):703-710. DOI: 10.15343/0104-7809.20174104703710

[2] Gateño, Caraccioli P. Essay on professional ethics aspects of cosmetic and medical tattoos. In: Current Problems in Dermatology, Cosmetics and Medical Tattoo. Vol. 56. Swtizerland: Karger Publisher; 2022

[3] Araos San Martín J. La ética de Aristóteles y su relación con la ciencia y la técnica. Diálogos Educativos. 2003;**6**: 13-38. Available from: http://revistas.umce.cl/index.php/dialogoseducativos/article/view/1281/1286

[4] Servín-Hernández D, Servín-Jiménez AS. Transformar la faceta bioética clínica por medio del pensamiento complejo y la compasión. Bioethics Update. 2023;**9**(1):23-36. DOI: 10.24875/BUP.22000016

[5] Acosta-Zapata E, López-Ramón C, Martínez-Cortés ME, Zapata-Vázquez R. Funcionalidad familiar y estrategias de afrontamiento en pacientes con cáncer de mama. Horizonte Sanitario. 2017;**16**(2):139-146. DOI: 10.19136/hs.v16i2.1629

[6] Burga R. Terapia gestáltica. Revista Latinoamericana de Psicología. 1981;**13**(1):85-96. Available from: https://www.redalyc.org/pdf/805/80513106.pdf

[7] Bowlby J. "El apego". Tomo 1 de la trilogía "El apego y la pérdida". Barcelona: Paidós; 1998

[8] Kremer W, Hammond C. Maslow's hierarchy of needs pyramid. BBC Magazine. 2013. Available from: https://247caregivingproducts.com/lifenow/Maslow_HierarchyOfNeeds_Pyramid_BBC.pdf

[9] Reid-Cunningham AR. Maslow's Theory of Motivation and Hierarchy of Human Needs: A Critical Analysis. PhD Qualifying Examination School of Social Welfare University of California, Berkeley. 2008. Available from: https://fouziyagm.wordpress.com/wp-content/uploads/2014/05/maslows-hierarchy-of-needs-a-critical-analysis.pdf